RESEARCH IN
COMMUNITY
AND
MENTAL HEALTH

Volume 2 · **1981**

RESEARCH IN COMMUNITY AND MENTAL HEALTH

A Research Annual

Editor: ROBERTA G. SIMMONS
Department of Sociology
University of Minnesota

VOLUME 2 · 1981

Ai JAI PRESS INC.
Greenwich, Connecticut

CONTENTS

LIST OF CONTRIBUTORS

Rebecca G. Adams

Department of Psychiatry, Social
Psychiatry Study Center, University
of Chicago

Dale A. Blyth

Schools and Adolescent Development
Project, Center for the Study of Youth
Development, Boys Town, Nebraska

Hendricks Brown

Chief Statistician, Department of
Psychiatry, Social Psychiatry Study
Center, University of Chicago

Richard Bulcroft

Department of Sociology, University
of Minnesota, Minneapolis

Diane Mitsch Bush

Department of Sociology, University
of Arizona, Tucson

Anita M. Cohen

Doctor of Jurisprudence,
1216 Robinson Blvd., Philadelphia

Rosalie Cohen

Department of Sociology, Temple
University, Philadelphia

Alfred Dean

Department of Psychiatry, The Albany
Medical College, Albany

Bruce P. Dohrenwend

Social Psychiatry Research Unit,
College of Physicians and Surgeons,
Columbia University, New York

Walter M. Ensel

Department of Psychiatry, Albany
Medical College, Albany

Debbie Felt

Department of Sociology, University
of Minnesota, Minneapolis

Lily Hechtman
Clinical Director, Department of Psychiatry, The Montreal Children's Hospital, McGill University, Montreal

Paul C. Holinger
Department of Psychiatry, Michael Reese Hospital and Medical Center, Chicago

Sheppard G. Kellam
Director of the Social Psychiatry Study Center, University of Chicago

Nan Lin
Department of Sociology, State University of New York at Albany

James N. Logue
Senior Environmental Epidemiologist, Geomet, Inc., 15 Firstfield Road, Gaithersburg, Maryland

Jon Lorence
Department of Sociology, University of Minnesota, Minneapolis

B. Claire McCullough
Department of Sociology, University of Maryland, College Park

Mary Evans Melick
Senior Research Scientist, Special Projects Research Unit, State of New York Office of Mental Health, 44 Holland Avenue, Albany

Jeylan T. Mortimer
Department of Sociology, University of Minnesota, Minneapolis

Daniel Offer
Chairman, Department of Psychiatry, Michael Reese Hospital and Medical Center and Professor of Psychiatry, Pritzker School of Medicine, University of Chicago, Chicago

Lenore Sawyer Radloff
Center for Epidemiologic Studies, National Institute of Mental Health, 5600 Fishers Lane, Rockville, Maryland

Donald S. Rae

Statistical and Mathematical Applications Branch, Alcohol, Drug Abuse and Mental Health Administration, National Institute of Mental Health, 5600 Fishers Lane, Rockville, Maryland

Morris Rosenberg

Department of Sociology, University of Maryland, College Park

Patrick E. Shrout

Social Psychiatry Research Unit, College of Physicians and Surgeons, Columbia University, New York

Roberta G. Simmons

Department of Sociology, University of Minnesota, Minneapolis

Elmer L. Struening

Director of Epidemiology of Mental Disorders Research Unit, New York State Psychiatric Institute, 722 West 168 Street, New York City

Edward F. Van Cleave

Department of Sociology, University of Minnesota, Minneapolis

INTRODUCTION

In accord with JAI policy, the articles for this volume are almost all based on analyses of research data. In this case, all authors were invited to submit articles concerning their research in community or mental health.

As it has turned out, most of the articles in this volume of *Research in Community and Mental Health* focus on some of the linkages depicted in the following diagram:

Independent Variables	Intervening Variables	Dependent Variable
Social position ↑↓ Social and Life Stressors	Mediating Mechanisms	Mental Health Indicators of Distress

The impact of social position and of potentially stressful life events upon mental health forms a major theme of the book.[1] The articles in the first section (IA) look at the self-image as a dimension of mental health; those in the second section (IB) focus on depressive affect and action; while those in the next segment (II) include a variety of mental health dimensions. Findings indicate that persons in the following categories and social positions are more likely to show mental health distress: *females* (Radloff and Rae, Logue *et al.*, Dohrenwend and Shrout, but also see Dean *et al.* and Holinger and Offer); *non-whites* (Radloff and Rae, Holinger and Offer); individuals of low *socio-economic status* (Radloff and Rae, Dean *et al.*, Logue *et al.*, but also see Dohrenwend and Shrout); the *physically ill* (Radloff and Rae, Dean *et al.*); those with recent *life-event losses* (Radloff and Rae, Dean *et al.*); and persons with *less social and family support* (e.g., the *unmarried*. See Radloff and Rae, Dean *et al.*, Mortimer and Lorence, Holinger and Offer). However, it should be noted that while in a great number of studies females score higher in measures of depression, it is males who apparently have a higher suicide rate. The verbal indications of depression are associated with being female, while males are more likely to take serious action.

Several articles examine the effects of major, potential life stressors upon mental health. Some authors use the life-events loss measures (Radloff and Rae, Dean *et al.*, Logue *et al.*) or the effects of poverty or illness (Radloff and Rae, Dean *et al.*); one chapter examines the long-term impact of a natural disaster (Logue *et al.*), while others look at the effect of being a teenage mother (Brown *et al.*), having a hyperactive child in the family (Hechtman), and reaching puberty (Blyth *et al.*). The authors generally perceive the relationship between a potential stressor and experienced distress as mediated by key variables. Results suggest that a stressor will be less harmful in cases where there is social and family support (see Mortimer and Lorence, Holinger and Offer, Logue *et al.*, Radloff and Rae, Dean *et al.*, Rosenberg and McCullough), in certain organizational environments rather than others (Blyth *et al.*), and in situations where there are better financial and physical health resources (Logue *et al.*, Dean *et al.*). Furthermore, Radloff and Rae hypothesize that certain categories of people—women, those of low socio-economic status—are socialized to respond less adquately to a stressor. As part of their sex-role learning or social status training, they are more likely to perceive themselves as helpless and powerless, and therefore are less apt to solve problems well. These problems then, unsolved, are more likely to cause distress.

The role of the family, both as a deflector of stress and as a unit of study, receives much attention in this volume (Hechtman, Brown *et al.*, Rosenberg and McCullough, Dean *et al.*, Mortimer and Lorence). Also, as in Volume 1 in this series (Elder and Rockwell, Fischer *et al.*, Langner *et al.*, Smith and Fogg, Clausen and Huffine, Pearlin and Lieberman, Greenley),[2] important long-term longitudinal data sets are analyzed here. Hechtman's study involves a five and ten year follow-up of families with hyperactive children; Brown *et al.* analyze the effect upon a woman ten years later of originally having been a teenage mother; Mortimer and Lorence restudy college freshmen when they are seniors and again 10 years later in order to ascertain degree of personality stability and factors impacting on the self-image at the three points in time.

The final two articles in this volume are somewhat different than the rest in tone. Dohrenwend and Shrout deal directly with the issue of measuring mental illness and suggest an approach for locating and classifying cases both within the general population and within labelled symptom groups. Cohen and Cohen examine societal definition and control over the mentally handicapped and mentally ill. Laws allowing or mandating sterilization for such individuals without their consent have survived into the present era in multiple states.

It is hoped that these studies as a whole present a valuable example of current research linking potential sources of stress to level of mental health, augmented by a very brief look at measurement issues and societal reaction.

Roberta G. Simmons
Series Editor

NOTES

1. These issues are also dealt with in Volume 1 of this series: e.g., See Pearlin and Lieberman, "Social Sources of Emotional Distress." Pp. 217–248 in Roberta G. Simmons (Ed.), *Research in Community and Mental Health*, Volume 1. Greenwich, CT: JAI Press, 1979.

2. See *Research in Community and Mental Health*, Volume 1. Greenwich, CT: JAI Press, 1979.

Part I

THE EFFECTS OF MULTIPLE DETERMINANTS ON ONE MENTAL HEALTH DIMENSION

Section A

EFFECTS UPON THE SELF-IMAGE

SELF-CONCEPT STABILITY AND CHANGE FROM LATE ADOLESCENCE TO EARLY ADULTHOOD

Jeylan T. Mortimer and Jon Lorence

Social scientists have long debated the degree of stability of personality as the individual moves through the life course. Psychoanalysts and some developmental psychologists believe that its main contours are set by the end of childhood (Lidz, 1968; Kagan and Moss, 1962; Luborsky and Schimek, 1964). In contrast, there are sociologists who argue that the personality is highly responsive throughout life to new social pressures and experiences, particularly at the time of important role transitions (Brim, 1970). Some have attempted to resolve this issue by taking an intermediate stance; according to this perspective, basic predispositions, constituting the "core" of personality, are formed rather early in life, while specific or more "peripheral" changes occur later in response to new environmental circumstances (Bloom, 1964; Yarrow and Yarrow, 1964: 500;

Research in Community and Mental Health, Volume 2, pages 5–42
Copyright © 1981 by JAI Press, Inc.
All rights of reproduction in any form reserved.
ISBN: 0-89232-152-0

Cottrell, 1969). Whereas this position is plausible, the extent to which personality attributes are stable or unstable can only be determined empirically, through systematic longitudinal research that assesses the same persons through different phases of the life cycle.

The present study examines the stability and change of the self-concept during the transition to adulthood, utilizing a panel of highly educated men. The self-concept is a central facet of personality and a widely recognized indicator of mental health. The objectives of the study are two-fold: first, to ascertain the stability of the self-concept over a 14-year period; and second, to identify those life experiences that contribute to its maintenance and to its change.

Unfortunately, the time and resources necessary to conduct longitudinal studies have limited the accumulation of findings that address the degree of personality consistency through time. There have been relatively few studies across broad phases of the life course, beginning in infancy, early childhood or adolescence, and continuing through the adult years. Highly notable instances of such long-term longitudinal research are the Berkeley and Oakland studies (Siegelman et al., 1970; Block and Haan, 1971; Jones et al., 1971; Peskin and Livson, 1972; Elder, 1974), the Fels study (Kagan and Moss, 1962; Moss and Kagan, 1972), the Terman study of the gifted (Oden, 1968), and the Grant study of Harvard men (Vaillant, 1977). Other research covers more limited time periods, such as the years in college (Katz, 1968; Heath, 1968; King, 1973; Feldman and Newcomb, 1969), or those spanning the teens to the twenties (Offer and Offer, 1975; Symonds, 1961; Golden et al., 1962; Bachman et al., 1978).

These studies, taken together, highlight the persistence of individual characteristics from childhood and adolescence to adulthood. This persistence is manifest whether personality is defined behaviorally, such as by dependency, spontaneity, or aggressiveness (Kagan and Moss, 1962; Tuddenham, 1971; Crandall, 1972); intellectually, by grades in school or by performance on intelligence and achievement tests (Kagan and Moss, 1962; Bloom, 1964; Oden, 1968); motivationally, by level of task involvement and perseverance (Kagan and Moss, 1962; Oden, 1968; Block and Haan, 1971; Vaillant, 1974); interpersonally, by strength of "object relations" (King, 1973); or in terms of subconscious processes, such as defense mechanisms (Vaillant, 1974) or fantasy projections (Buben, 1975; Symonds, 1961). Research on early and middle adulthood also indicates considerable stability in intelligence, vocational interests, self-confidence, and values (Kelly, 1955; Kuhlen, 1964).

Some investigators, instead of confining their attention to trait continuity, have focused on overall life adjustment, as gauged by clinical assessment of mental health, personality test performance, the acquisition of normal adult roles, or occupational achievement. Some have begun their research by purposely selecting a sample (or a sub-sample drawn from a larger study) on the basis of evidence of adequate functioning (see Cox, 1970; Golden et al., 1962; Vaillant, 1977; Vaillant and McArthur, 1972). These persons are then followed through life, and their adjustment monitored in succeeding periods. Other investigators have divided their samples at the last period of data collection into better and more poorly adjusted groups, and then have examined the attributes of each in earlier periods (Grinker, 1962; Oden, 1968; Siegelman et al., 1970). What is again most striking about this research is the substantial stability of adjustment and mental health, in spite of the diversity of operational definitions and the variations in methods employed (see also Offer and Offer, 1975; Block and Haan, 1971; Fischer et al., 1979).

Though not all persons follow the same path to adulthood, continuity appears to be considerably more prevalent than discontinuity. In fact, several investigators have commented that they began their studies of the transition to adulthood expecting to find high levels of disturbance, turmoil, and change, corresponding to the classic portrayal of conflict in late adolescence (Erikson, 1959), only to find stability over time (Offer and Offer, 1975; Grinker, 1962; Haan, 1972; Katz, 1968; King, 1972 and 1973; Bachman et al., 1978: 220–221). Thus, those who manifest high levels of adjustment during adolescence are generally found to have experienced relatively untroubled childhoods and good school adjustment. When followed into adulthood, these persons continue to show, sometimes decades later, an absence of neurotic traits, strong interpersonal relationships, and adequate adaptation to adult roles (Haan, 1964; Oden, 1968; Vaillant, 1977).

Stability of personality is generally measured by correlations of observer ratings of behavior or test scores between time periods. High stability implies that an individual's position, relative to others being studied, remains similar. Scores at one time thus predict subsequent score values. However, strong correlations do not necessarily mean that measures have remained constant over the period of observation (though this may occur), since there can be uniform change among members of a group. For example, mean self-esteem scores may fall as a group moves into early adolescence (Rosenberg, 1979: Chapter 9), while the members' positions vis-à-vis one another could persist. Using this correlational criterion, and drawing heavily on the Fels data (Kagan and Moss, 1962), Bloom (1964:177) has estimated that approximately half the variance in a number of important adolescent characteristics (e.g., intellectual interest, dependency, and aggression) can be predicted by the age of five.

While the stability of personality, whether defined by global measures of adjustment or by continuity in specific traits, has been frequently demonstrated, it is difficult to explain this phenomenon. Stability of a personality attribute or behavioral pattern, in the very simplest case, may be attributable to the fact that, once developed, it persists over time without being significantly influenced by the environment. Rosenberg calls this "static stability" (personal communication). Such persistence may mean constancy, such as a relatively unchanging characteristic like intelligence, or a persistence of advantage or disadvantage relative to others, like maintaing one's position at the top of the class. By early adolescence, the honors student may have developed sufficient achievement motivation and competitiveness to sustain continuously outstanding academic performance.

Alternatively, stability could be due to continuous external influence, as persistent social and environmental conditions support constancy, or the maintenance of one's position relative to others (see Bloom, 1964:223; Wheaton et al., 1977; 89–91). Rosenberg calls this situation one of "dynamic stability"— individual attributes remain stable over time as a result of supportive life experiences (personal communication). In this case, the personality attribute or behavioral pattern changes when environmental support is withdrawn. For example, stability in parental nurturing could support a child's feelings of confidence throughout the years of childhood and adolescence; stability of parental encouragement could engender continuously high grades. Removing supportive parental behaviors would cause a deterioration in the child's confidence and performance.

In this latter situation, the individual should not be viewed as a mere passive recipient of external influence, but is more likely an active selector and molder of the situational context. According to Cottrell (1969), "Much of our activity and striving, perhaps most of it, is directed toward establishing and maintaining social contexts supportive of desired identities, or toward changing contexts that impose unwanted identities" (see also Rosenberg, 1979:Chapter 11). For example, a sense of personal competence may promote values and skills which enable the individual to achieve high levels of work autonomy. This autonomy, in turn, will reinforce this positive self-attitude (Mortimer and Lorence, 1979b).

In our judgment, the understanding of personality stability, as well as change, requires considerable attention to these processes of individual-environmental interaction. But without systematic longitudinal study, it is difficult, if not impossible, to separate cause from effect, to ascertain the extent to which earlier personality attributes contribute to, and/or result from, surrounding environmental forces. Moreover, multivariate causal analysis is necessary to examine the effects of environmental forces on the personality, and to assess stability net of these influences.

In this research, we examine personality stability and change by studying the self-concept. Whereas prior longitudinal studies of personality development from childhood and adolescence indicate that important personality traits remain stable over long periods of time, these studies have not focused explicitly on the self-image. In the absence of empirical evidence covering broad phases of the life course, plausible arguments can be made both for and against self-concept stability.

On the one side, from Cooley's "looking glass self" (1902) to Rosenberg's "principle of reflected appraisals" (1979), there is a persistent theme in social psychological thought that the self-concept is responsive to the opinions of significant others. According to James (1892:197), the individual "... has as many different social selves as there are distinct groups of persons about whose opinion he cares." Moreover, according to Rosenberg's (1979) "principle of social comparison," individuals compare themselves with others in making self-judgments. Since the network of significant others changes over time, and because even when this network is constant, its members' opinions can change, the self might be expected to be correspondingly transitory. Taking a rather extreme position, Gergen (1972) has argued that the individual is so responsive to the pressures of immediate situations that the idea of a coherent sense of self is entirely illusory. Furthermore, the self-concept might be expected to be influenced by changing circumstances and achievements in different phases of life; e.g., by scholastic achievement during the school years (Purkey, 1970), and by occupational attainments in adulthood (Cohn, 1978; Bachman et al., 1978; Rosenberg, 1979:Chapter 5).

But there are also good reasons to believe that the self-image will be stable over time. This expectation conforms to the person's phenomenal experience as well as to the conceptualizations of social psychologists (Allport, 1955; Shaver, 1969:47). For Erikson (1959), the establishment of identity is the critical developmental task of adolescence, after which it remains quite stable. In fact, the preservation of a consistent and stable sense of self has been postulated as a major motivational goal (Lecky, 1945; Epstein, 1973; Rosenberg, 1979; and Korman, 1970). Finally, as indicated by our discussion of dynamic stability, stable environmental circumstances, of both a social and non-social character, may continuously support constancy in the self-image.

Whereas estimates of self-concept stability within phases of the life course do indicate a high degree of persistence, they leave substantial proportions of the variance unexplained, indicating the potential for change and responsiveness to external influence. For example, Engel (1959) has estimated that self-concept stability over two-year periods during high school is a rather high .78 (corrected for unreliability). Bachman and his colleagues (1978: 98) report a corrected stability coefficient of .40 over an eight-year interval from ninth grade to five years following high school graduation. Finally, Kelly's (1955:675) study of personality change in a sample of engaged couples, first contacted in early adulthood, indicates that self-rating stability is .56 over a 20-year period (again corrected).

In the present study, we first assess the stability of five dimensions of the self-image over two periods—from college entry to graduation, and from graduation to ten years after college. We then attempt to understand the processes of stability and change by estimating a complex causal model of self-image development. This causal analysis focuses on the individual's sense of personal well-being, an important component of self-attitudes and a critical indicator of mental health. The analysis enables examination of the implications of psychological well-being at earlier times for subsequent social, academic, and occupational attainments, as well as the effects of these experiences on well-being at later time periods.

DATA SOURCE

The data were obtained from 1966–67 male graduates of the University of Michigan. Upon entry to the University in 1962 and 1963, the men joined an extensive research project on the impacts of college life, which extended through their college careers. Since the initiators of that study, Theodore Newcomb and Gerald Gurin, were interested in the development of friendship patterns, three-quarters of the 650 freshmen chosen for the original study resided in the same dormitories; the others were chosen randomly. Four years later, 150 additional seniors were randomly chosen to compensate for freshman sample attrition (see Gurin, 1971, for a complete description of the study design). Thus, while the initial selection of students from the total student body was not entirely random, the college panel was not chosen in a manner that would be selective on the basis of differences in the self-concept. The data from the earlier study that are analyzed here were obtained during freshman orientation week, prior to the beginning of classes, and during the senior year, close to the time of college graduation.

In 1976, the authors successfully located 610 members of this panel, or 88 percent of the 694 men from whom data had been obtained in the senior year. Eighty-four percent of those who were found returned a mailed questionnaire that assessed the psychological attributes that were measured earlier, including measures of the self-concept, post-graduate educational and work histories, marital status, and occupational experiences.[1] Although data on 512 of the graduates were obtained in 1976, information at the time of entry to college was available for only 442 of these individuals. The analyses presented in this paper include only the men for whom questionnaire data are available at all three time periods.

This panel is highly advantaged, with respect to their social origins and their destinations. Ninety-three percent came from intact families, with both parents alive and living together. Only six percent had experienced a parental death, divorce, or separation. Fifty-three percent were first born or only children. The majority of their fathers were in professional or managerial occupations; less than 10 percent were blue collar workers. Fifty-two percent of the fathers, and 36 percent of the mothers, were college graduates. In 1962 and 1963, at the time of entry to college, only 29 percent of their families had incomes under $10,000; almost 20 percent were above $20,000.

By the time of the 1976 survey, more than half the panel (55 percent) had obtained the highest academic and professional degrees (including Ph.D., medical, law, dental, and divinity) and an additional 24 percent had received master's degrees. As shown in Table 1, the occupations of the graduates are concentrated

Table 1. Percent Distribution of Occupations

	Percent
Doctor	19.7
Dentist	3.6
Lawyer	18.8
Physical or Biological Scientist	6.8
Social Scientist	8.1
Elementary or Secondary Teacher	4.3
Artist, Writer	3.6
Managerial or Other Person-oriented Occupation	21.9
Other Technical Occupation	9.5
Blue Collar Worker	1.8
Other	.5
No Response or Inapplicable	1.4
Total	100.0
	n=442

at the higher professional and managerial levels. Thus, as indicated by their family backgrounds and their early adult educational, occupational and income attainments (see Table 2), the sample may be considered a rather elite group.

The present study therefore examines the development of the self-concept from late adolescence to early adulthood in a group of highly educated men.[2] This panel is probably not unlike persons of the same cohort who attended other highly selective colleges and universities. King's (1973:11) random sample of 600 entrants of Harvard College in 1961 and 1962 is quite similar in terms of

Table 2. Percent Distribution
of Income

	Percent
Under $3,000	.9
$3,000–4,999	1.8
$5,000–9,999	4.3
$10,000–14,999	14.0
$15,000–19,999	23.1
$20,000–24,999	18.3
$25,000–29,999	13.6
$30,000–34,999	6.6
$35,000–39,999	4.5
$40,000 +	10.2
No Response	2.7
Total	100.0
	n=442

fathers' occupations, parental education, family income, birth position, and in-
tactness of family of origin. Moreover, Korn (1968a:217) reports that of men
who entered Stanford in 1961 and subsequently graduated, 65 percent were in
graduate school by 1966, a figure quite similar to the 75 percent of our panel that
received advanced degrees.

The distinctive character of this group must be kept in mind in interpreting the
findings of the study. These persons have come from very advantaged family
environments, have graduated from a highly selective university, and have suc-
ceeded in entering the most prestigious occupational positions. They have, in the
aggregate, experienced a quite favorable life course. This pattern of life events
would be expected to engender and continually reinforce a positive self-image.
Though the characteristics of this sample probably restrict the variance in the
self-concept and the range of life experience that would be obtained in a more
representative group, the patterns indicated here will hopefully provide insight
into basic processes of self-concept development.

Table 3.   Observed Variables in the Self-Concept Constructs Based on the
Semantic Differential Scale[a]

Construct	1962–63 Freshman Year		1966–67 Senior Year		1976	
	$\bar{x}$	s.d.	$\bar{x}$	s.d.	$\bar{x}$	s.d.
Well-being						
Happy . . . . . . Unhappy	5.58	1.28	5.38	1.26	5.49	1.15
Relaxed . . . . . . Tense	4.59	1.66	4.15	1.65	4.19	1.51
Confident . . . . . . Anxious	4.38	1.63	4.53	1.57	4.88	1.39
Sociability						
Social . . . . . . Solitary	4.74	1.73	4.56	1.72	4.35	1.69
Interested in Others . . . . . . Interested in Self	4.75	1.57	4.57	1.54	4.37	1.50
Open . . . . . . Closed	4.65	1.69	4.65	1.64	4.48	1.69
Warm . . . . . . Cold	5.37	1.23	5.22	1.32	5.14	1.26
Competence						
Strong . . . . . . Weak	5.31	1.23	5.29	1.13	5.48	1.03
Active . . . . . . Quiet	5.40	1.52	5.29	1.43	5.15	1.57
Competent . . . . . . Not too Competent	5.80	1.01	5.81	.93	6.17	.68
Successful . . . . . . Not too Successful	5.77	.98	5.46	1.05	5.68	.92
Unconventionality						
Impulsive . . . . . . Deliberate	3.80	1.67	3.86	1.60	3.32	1.42
Unconventional . . . . . . Conventional	3.87	1.58	3.95	1.54	3.98	1.58
A Dreamer . . . . . . Practical	3.08	1.65	3.25	1.62	2.90	1.52

[a] The range for all variables is 1–7. (High scores indicate closer correspondence to the title.) Figure 1 and
Figures A-2 to A-4 in Appendix A give the measurement parameters describing the relationships between the
indicators and the constructs.

Table 4.   Observed Variables in the Self-doubts Construct[a]

	1962–63 Freshman Year		1966–67 Senior Year		1976	
	$\bar{x}$	s.d.	$\bar{x}$	s.d.	$\bar{x}$	s.d.
In the list below are some problems and issues which people often mention as sources of concern to them. For each statement, consider how much you have thought about or been concerned about the issue during the last year or two.						
Problems of concentrating—the fact that I am restless and bored, unable to concentrate for very long.	2.16	1.00	2.31	1.01	1.76	.88
A feeling that I am always acting, never being true to myself or being myself.	1.82	.94	1.66	.87	1.57	.79
Whether I am a normal person.	1.93	.93	1.65	.86	1.36	.61
Social sensitivity—a feeling that I get hurt too easily.	1.94	.94	1.88	.96	1.72	.76
4. Very concerned						
3. Somewhat concerned						
2. A little concerned						
1. Not at all concerned						

[a] Figure A-1 in Appendix A describes the relationships between these indicators and the self-doubts construct.

DATA ANALYSIS

Dimensions of the Self-Concept

We begin the analysis with an assessment of self-concept stability over the 14-year period of study. Current conceptualizations of the self-image feature its multidimensional character (Epstein, 1973; Shaver, 1969:47–48; Wells and Marwell, 1976; Brim, 1976). According to Rosenberg (1979:279), "the self-concept is the totality of the individual's thoughts and feelings with reference to himself as an object." To measure the self-concept, we used a semantic differential scale composed of 29 bi-polar characteristics, and five additional items in the same section of the questionnaire. On the basis of substantive considerations and an exploratory factor analysis, the following self-concept dimensions were identified: well-being, sociability, competence, unconventionality, and self-doubts (see Tables 3 and 4).

Though most research on the self-image focuses on self-esteem, Rosenberg (1979) clearly distinguishes self-esteem or the individual's *evaluation* of self—self-acceptance, self-liking, and a sense of personal worth—from other components. Because of the diversity in the use of the term, "self-esteem" (see Wells and Marwell, 1976:Chapter 5), and because none of the five dimensions considered here are patently evaluative, we prefer to think of them as components of self-attitude that are conceptually independent of, though perhaps empirically related to, self-esteem. It is probable that the degree of importance attached by the individual to the attributes signified by each of these dimensions would moderate their associations with self-esteem (see Rosenberg, 1979:18-19; Breytspraak and George, forthcoming).

There is substantial evidence that self-esteem is an indicator of mental health, as it has been found to have an inverse relationship to symptoms of anxiety, depression, and emotional disturbance (Rosenberg, 1965:22-25, 149-167, and 1979:54-55; Kaplan and Pokorny, 1969). The five self-concept dimensions under consideration in this study may also be broadly indicative of mental health and adjustment.

The first dimension is well-being (see Table 3), signifying the perception of self as happy, relaxed, and confident.[3] Because the sense of well-being is a widely-used criterion of psychological health (Gurin et al., 1960; Grinker, 1962; King, 1973; Erikson, 1959:118; Cox, 1970; Luborsky and Bachrach, 1974; Wessman and Ricks, 1966), and because the items in this construct appear to have the greatest intuitive appeal as indicators of positive affect and morale, we have chosen this dimension for an extensive causal analysis of self-concept change over time. In fact, given the high face validity of the well-being construct as an indicator of affective state, the reader may question its conceptualization as a dimension of the self-concept. But because it is clearly also within the domain of "the totality of thoughts and feelings" pertaining to oneself, we believe it is highly qualified for inclusion in an investigation of the self-image.

The second dimension taps the individual's evaluation of his interpersonal qualities. High scorers view themselves as social, interested in others, open, and warm. The ability to form close interpersonal relationships, which these attributes likely indicate, is a core feature of psychoanalytic and other definitions of mental health (Vaillant, 1977; King, 1973; Erikson, 1959; Grinker, 1962).

The third construct, competence, indicates the assessment of self as active, strong, competent, and successful, and thus seems to capture elements of Osgood's (Osgood et al., 1957) "activity" and "potency" dimensions. Franks and Marolla (1976) identified a very similar competence dimension in their factor analysis of a semantic differential scale (see also Monge, 1973). High scores on these items suggest a well-developed sense of personal efficacy, another widely-recognized criterion of mental health and maturity (French, 1968; Smith, 1968; White, 1973; Heath, 1976; Pearlin and Schooler, 1978).

The last construct in Table 3, unconventionality, is the most difficult to interpret as an indicator of mental health and adjustment. On the one hand, viewing the self as impulsive instead of deliberate, unconventional versus conventional, and a dreamer rather than practical, may reflect independence from social pressures and practical concerns and an ability to express impulses without rigid control. King (1973:213-215), using extensive interviews and projective tests, interprets increases in controlled impulse expression during the college years as evidence of growth toward healthy personality (see also Korn, 1968b). But this constellation of self-perceptions may also suggest withdrawal and a lack of responsiveness to social control.

Table 4 presents the items indicating the fifth dimension, self-doubts—that is, the perception of self as hypersensitive, unable to concentrate, as always acting, and as abnormal. These measures are reminiscent of Erikson's classic portrayal of the disturbed adolescent (1959), and also appear to correspond to Rosenberg's (1979:227–229) depiction of self-concept disturbance in adolescence—involving high levels of self-consciousness, "a seemingly false presenting self . . . lacking in spontaneity, artificial, or conspicuously intended for effect" (283). The fact that the means of each of these items show appreciable declines between the freshman year and ten years following graduation indicates a lessening of these problems in the group as a whole.

Some confirmation for the interpretation of these self-concept dimensions as indicators of morale derives from their correlations with three measures of satis-faction[4] obtained in the 1976 survey. The first column of Table 5 shows the correlations of factor-based scales (weighted sums of items) for each of the five self-concept dimensions, with overall job satisfaction. All correlations are in the predicted direction, and all but one—that involving sociability—are statistically significant. Clearly, those who have a strong sense of well-being and competence report higher satisfaction. In contrast, the self-concept dimensions of "unconventionality" and "self-doubts" are negatively related to job satisfaction. Turning to marriage, a second major sphere of life involvement, an identical pattern is apparent: those with more positive self-perceptions are more happily married (column 2). Once again, sociability is the only dimension that is unrelated to the criterion. Finally, the 1976 respondents were asked one question designed to assess their overall life satisfaction. There are significant relationships between this indicator and all five self-concept dimensions (see column 3).

These associations attest to the validity of the self-concept constructs (Wells

Table 5.   Correlations of Self-concept Constructs with Satisfactions in Work, Marriage and Life as a Whole

	Work Satisfaction	*Marital Satisfaction*	*Life Satisfaction*
1976 Self-Concept Construct			
Well-Being	.215	.256	.373
Self-doubts	−.232	−.307	−.415
Sociability	.064[a]	.038[a]	.118
Competence	.219	.144	.224
Unconventionality	−.099	−.233	−.206

[a] $p > .05$

Figure 1.   Measurement Model of the Well-being Construct.

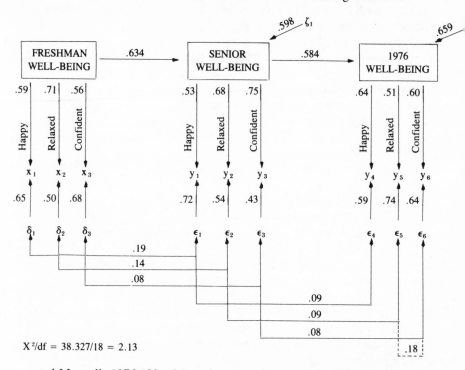

X²/df = 38.327/18 = 2.13

and Marwell, 1976:183–184) and support the contention that these five dimensions of the self-image, with the possible exception of "sociability," are plausible indicators of satisfaction with, and adjustment to, life. If mental health may be broadly defined in these terms (see Vaillant, 1974 and 1977), the self-concept constructs are also indicative of psychological well-being.

Self-Concept Stability through Time

The first major analytic task is to ascertain the level of stability of the self-concept over time. In order to do this accurately, it is necessary to separate "real change" in the five psychological dimensions underlying the observed items from change attributable to measurement error. In recent years, Jöreskog and his colleagues (Jöreskog, 1973; Jöreskog and van Thillo, 1972; Werts et al., 1973) have developed maximum likelihood confirmatory factor analysis, a highly useful statistical method to assess stability.

In confirmatory factor analysis, unobserved or "latent" constructs are defined in terms of the covariation of their measured indicators. The relationships among the latent constructs can then be estimated. In longitudinal research, this procedure has two important advantages over conventional regression techniques. First, both random and systematic measurement errors can be included in the causal model, and thereby more precise parameter estimates obtained. Second, this procedure incorporates a goodness-of-fit test (chi-square divided by the degrees of freedom) which allows one to determine whether the parameter estimates of the hypothesized model are reasonable. Chi-square values that approach the degrees of freedom represent a good fit to the data. Since recent research that applies confirmatory factor analysis to longitudinal data attests to the power and utility of this method (Jöreskog and Sörbom, 1977; Kohn and Schooler, 1978; and Wheaton et al., 1977), this technique was selected for the analysis. The parameters were estimated by the computer program LISREL (Jöreskog and van Thillo, 1972) which utilizes an iterative, maximum likelihood algorithm. The input to the program in each analysis was a variance-covariance matrix of the observed measures.[5]

Figure 1 presents the "measurement model" for the construct representing well-being, the perception of self as happy, relaxed, and confident. In this figure, the observed exogenous or independent variables are designated by x's; and the observed endogenous variables, by y's. The unobserved "latent constructs" are designated above these variables. Numbers to the left of the arrows from the constructs to the indicators represent the factor loadings (analogous, when squared, to the "true score" variance of each indicator).

The residual or error variances of the indicators are represented by deltas (for the exogenous variables) and epsilons (for the endogenous variables). Failure to take these random errors of measurement into account (as well as the correlations of errors within constructs) generally reduces stability estimates. Double-headed arrows connecting the error terms, between and within constructs, indicate the presence of correlated error, which may reflect influences such as test factors or memory effects.

The factor loadings, residuals, and correlated errors of the indicators are the measurement parameters. These are to be distinguished from the causal parameters; i.e., the estimates of relationships among the latent constructs. Since estimating all relevant measurement and causal parameters simultaneously would cause problems of model identification and exceed the limits of the LISREL program, it is first necessary to investigate the measurement parameters in a serial fashion, and to establish a criterion whereby those of small magnitude may be eliminated from further consideration.

Therefore, in developing these models, we followed the sequential procedure suggested by Sörbom (1975). Some parameters were fixed at zero initially, as when we hypothesized no significant paths between variables. The LISREL program gives first-order partial derivatives that indicate whether allowing parameters to be free rather than fixed at zero would significantly improve the model. Although the partials are not customarily followed too closely (theoretical considerations should dictate the placement of causal paths), they serve as a check to make certain that no important parameters have been left out. If we found large first-order partial derivatives indicating relationships that were theoretically justifiable,[6] they were then allowed to be freely estimated. If found to be statistically significant,[7] they were retained subsequently. Otherwise, they were fixed at zero. In the final stage, the entire model, including both measurement and causal parameters, was re-estimated (with all non-significant parameters fixed at zero).

In estimating this model, we assume that the freshman construct directly affects the same construct at the time of graduation. The latter dimension, in turn, influences well-being a decade later. Corresponding to the assumption of no direct effect from the earliest to the latest period, this path is fixed at zero.

The standardized solution is given in Figure 1 (and in subsequent figures). The estimated parameters (all of which are statistically significant) provide a rather good fit to the data, as indicated by the ratio of the chi-square value to the degrees of freedom, which is 2.13. Consonant with our assumption that freshman well-being has no direct effect on 1976 well-being, the corresponding partial derivative is quite small, suggesting that this path would not be significant if included in the model. (Moreover, by multiplying the paths from freshman to senior well-being and from senior to 1976 well-being, an estimated correlation of .370 is obtained, which is the same as the true score correlation between the freshman and 1976 constructs.)

What is most remarkable about this model is the high level of stability of the self-image that it suggests. The two stability paths should be considered quite precise since both random and systematic errors of measurement have been removed in estimating the coefficients. In fact, more than 40 percent of the variance in the sense of well-being in the senior year of college can be explained by the same construct four years earlier. (The unexplained variances in the endogenous constructs, not the residual paths, are given in the figure and noted by the Greek letter zeta. Thus, since 59.8 percent of the variance in "senior well-being" is unexplained, 40.2 percent is explained.) And while a much longer time period—ten years—has elapsed between the two later times, the stability coefficient of .584 is not much smaller than before. Thirty-four percent of the variance in 1976 well-being can be explained by the respondents' reports of well-being in the senior year of college.

To investigate the degree of stability in well-being from year to year across these two time periods, it is possible to estimate the average yearly stability by taking the xth root of observed stability, where x equals the number of years intervening. For the four-year stability coefficient, from the freshman to the senior year in college, to be .634, it would be necessary for the average stability to be .892 ($\sqrt[4]{.634} = .892$). This estimate is quite close to that reported by Bachman and his colleagues (1978:291) for self-esteem during the almost identical four-year period from one to five years following high school graduation. His stability estimate for this period is .69, corrected for unreliability, indicating .91 as the yearly stability coefficient.

For the ten-year period from college graduation to 1976, the stability in the sense of well-being is .584, indicating a yearly stability of .948 ($\sqrt[10]{.584}$ = .948). Kelly's (1955:675) stability estimate over a 20-year period of adulthood is likewise quite comparable, suggesting a yearly stability in self-ratings of .971.

Yearly equivalence in stability is not entirely plausible, since one might expect to find the most rapid change in the self-concept immediately following major role transitions (Bloom, 1964; Van Maanen, 1976). However, this exercise suggests the substantial consistency that is implied by these coefficients, and provides a measure of equivalence by which stabilities over different time periods can be compared. Moreover, the comparison of our self-concept stability estimates with those of other studies, made possible by this method, enhances the credibility of our findings.

The stability estimates across the five constructs appear in Table 6. (Measurement models for the other four constructs are given in Appendix A.) The competence dimension is the most stable, both during the earlier (.775) and the later (.792) periods. The sense of competence or personal efficacy is apparently rather well-formed by college entry, and remains quite persistent thereafter. Self-doubts is the least stable—.506 in the first period of data collection, but becomes more stable in the succeeding period.

Because of the longer duration of time between the second and third measurements, the similarity of the stability coefficients over the four-year and ten-year periods indicates that the self-concept probably becomes *more stable* as the individual moves into adulthood. For each of the five dimensions, the estimated annual stabilities increase over time. Thus, during the period from entry to college to graduation, the yearly stabilities range from .843 to .938; during the following ten-year period they range from .945 to .977. Even though the coefficients for the earlier period are quite large, these figures suggest even greater stability following college graduation and confirm the widespread assumption that personality becomes more stable with age (Bloom, 1964).

Taken altogether, these analyses support Erikson's (1959) thesis that the indi-

Table 6.   Stability of the Self-Concept Constructs over Time

	Freshman to Senior Year		Senior Year to 1976	
	4-Year Stability	Estimated Yearly Stability	10-Year Stability	Estimated Yearly Stability
Self-Concept Constructs				
Well-Being	.634	.892	.584	.948
Self-doubts	.506	.843	.647	.957
Sociability	.640	.894	.566	.945
Competence	.775	.938	.792	.977
Unconventionality	.649	.898	.730	.969

vidual's sense of identity is largely formed by the end of adolescence. If these five self-concept dimensions can be considered indicative of life satisfaction and mental health, as was argued earlier, the findings suggest that these phenomena may also become increasingly stable over time, in spite of the changes in life circumstances that occur during the transition to adulthood.

Causal Analysis of the Development of the Self-Concept over Time
While relatively high stability in five dimensions of the self-concept has been found, it has yet to be determined whether this stability is "static" or "dynamic" in character. The effects of external forces on the self-image remain to be investigated. As noted earlier, on the basis of both theoretical principles and empirical observations, one would expect to find that self-attitudes are responsive to the opinions of significant others and to other life experiences. In the present analysis, we examine a wide range of possible influences on the self-concept. Because of the extensiveness and complexity of this causal analysis, we restrict our attention to the sense of well-being. Earlier, it was found (see Table 5, row 1) that well-being is associated with more successful adjustment to work and family, and with life satisfaction. King (1973) considers a positive mood, which high scores on this construct would imply, as essential to an ability to adapt to life's problems:

> When a person is happy . . . he is more likely to be open to stimuli and to use exploratory activity, to become engaged with the environment. He is more likely to consider various alternatives for action. Under these circumstances, the possibilities for all kinds of learning are enhanced. (85)

If this is true, one might expect to find that earlier levels of well-being facilitate subsequent social, academic, and occupational achievements.

INTERPERSONAL SOURCES OF WELL-BEING

The literature on human development emphasizes the importance of social support during the highly formative years of childhood and early adolescence. The family is the central social context for the formation of personality (Yarrow and Yarrow, 1964). Previous longitudinal studies highlight the significance of close and supportive parent-child relationships for healthy personal outcomes in adulthood. Regardless of the specific conceptualization of the dependent variable— e.g., overall adjustment, absence of symptomatology, competence and adaptive capacity, strong interpersonal relationships, or level of functioning in social roles—the quality of earlier relationships in the family is outstanding in its predictive power (King, 1968; Peskin and Livson, 1972; Siegelman et al., 1970; Offer and Offer, 1975; Vaillant, 1974 and 1976). Cross-sectional research on self-esteem also points to the importance of parental interest, involvement (Rosenberg, 1965: Chapter 7), acceptance and understanding (Carlson, 1963) for the child's development of a positive sense of self.

The fact that early parent-child relationships have been singled out as crucial variables in the development of mental health and self-esteem suggests several questions regarding their continuing importance in later periods of life. To what extent does the parent-son relationship remain stable over time, providing a continuingly supportive context for post-adolescent development? Does consistency in the family environment contribute to the observed stability of well-being in subsequent life phases? Previous studies indicate that parent-child relationships are highly stable in childhood and adolescence, particularly for sons (Hunt and Eichorn, 1972; Crandall, 1972). It is plausible, therefore, to assume that the family of origin would remain a significant source of support in this transitional period, as the individual adapts to new adult roles in occupational, family, and other contexts.

Two questions, included at each of the three time periods, are the observed indicators of family relations. Because they were asked separately for each parent, there are four indicators of parent-son relations.

1. How well do you feel your parents understand you and what you want ouf of life? (Very well, fairly well, not too well, or not at all).
2. How close do you feel to your mother and to your father? (Extremely close, quite close, fairly close, not very close)[8].

Because social class has repeatedly been found to be positively related to the quality of family relationships (see, for example, Kohn and Carroll, 1960; Rosenberg, 1965) and because it is also associated with a positive self-image in adolescence (Rosenberg, 1965 and 1979:130), it is necessary to control socio-economic status in the investigation of family effects. We have included a socio-economic background construct in the causal model of self-concept development, consisting of the father's (x_8) and the mother's (x_9) educational level, family income (x_{10}), and occupational prestige (x_{11}).

However, this is also the period of life in which the individual establishes independence from the parents, and increasingly turns to peers for companionship, support, and intimacy (Erikson, 1959). We might expect, on this basis, that the association between the quality of family relationships and the sense of well-being would weaken in the late adolescent and early adult years. Alternative sources of interpersonal support during the college years are friendships and involvement with peers in extracurricular activities (Grinker, 1962). There are two indicators of college social activity in the senior year questionnaire: (y_8) "How active would you say you have been in extra-curricular activities on campus this year?" (Extremely active, quite active, moderately active, or not very active); and (y_9) "Could you please list on the following page all of the groups that you belong to now or have ever belonged to at Michigan?" (The number of groups listed is the second indicator of college social activity.)

Following graduation, one might expect that the family of origin and college friends would increasingly be displaced by the family of procreation (for those who marry) as the primary source of social support. Several studies indicate the advantage of married persons with respect to psychological well-being (Gurin et al., 1960; Bradburn, 1969; Glenn, 1975; Pearlin and Johnson, 1977). We therefore include the respondent's 1976 marital status in the causal model, coded 1 if married (72 percent) and 0 if single, divorced, or separated.

Academic and Occupational Experiences as Sources of Well-Being
In discussing the determinants of the self-concept, Rosenberg posits the "principle of self-attribution": "There can be little doubt that we draw conclusions about ourselves largely by observing our behavior and its outcomes" (1979:72). This principle is highly consonant with Kohn's "generalization" thesis (Kohn, 1977; Kohn and Schooler, 1973 and 1978), that occupational activities have wide-ranging effects on attitudes and psychological functioning. According to their formulations, persons who can attribute achievements to their own actions would have more positive self-images.

Research on college students highlights the importance of academic achievement for satisfactory adjustment and self-esteem (Katz, 1968; Becker et al., 1968; King, 1973; Vaillant, 1974; Grinker, 1962). According to Katz (1968:24), "Grades are, for many students, the central reality of academic life." In the causal model of self-concept change, there are three measures of academic performance: rank within the high school, grade point average over the four years of college, and post-graduate educational attainment (as indicated by highest degree).

Kohn and Schooler's 1964 survey (1973:103) showed that occupational conditions indicative of self-direction were significantly related to self-confidence and self-deprecation, even after education and other facets of work had been controlled. Other research has demonstrated a positive association between socioeconomic status and self-esteem (Luck and Heiss, 1970; Gurin and Gurin, 1976; Jacques and Chason, 1977; Rosenberg, 1979:Chapter 5). Accordingly, we also investigated the implications of occupational attainments during the transition to adulthood as sources of enhancement of well-being.

The measures of occupational achievement, beyond college, are income and work autonomy. The income measure is gross annual income in wages or salary earned from the respondent's main job (see Table 2). This measure was used, instead of total personal or family income, because it was considered an appropriate indicator of *individual* occupational achievement and success. The work autonomy construct is measured by three items:

(y_{11}) Overall, how much autonomy do you have in making important decisions about *what* you do at work and *how* you do it? (Complete autonomy; a great deal of autonomy; a fair amount of autonomy; some, but not much autonomy; almost none at all.)

(y_{12}) How much innovative thinking does your job require? Do you have to think of new ways of doing things, solving problems, presenting ideas, etc.? (a tremendous amount; a great deal; a fair amount; some, but not much; almost none at all.)

(y_{13}) Overall, how challenging would you consider your present job? (Very challenging; somewhat challenging; Only a little bit challenging; not at all challenging.)

These indicators, adapted from Kohn and Schooler (1974), assess the opportunity for self-directed thought and performance at work. Our previous analyses of the data indicate that occupational autonomy is the most salient work experience for psychological change (Mortimer and Lorence, 1979a and b). (A measure of occupational prestige was also included in a prior estimation of the well-being model, but was dropped because of its extremely weak relationship to the psychological dimension.)

HYPOTHETICAL CAUSAL MODEL OF THE DEVELOPMENT OF WELL-BEING

The hypothetical causal model is displayed in Figure 2. Well-being in the freshman year, relations with family in the freshman year, family socio-economic status, and high school class rank are the exogenous predetermined variables. Family relations at the end of the senior year, college social activity, and college grade point average (GPA) are "first layer" endogenous variables. The first two intervening variables represent social support during this four-year period, the last signifies academic achievement. All three are hypothesized to positively affect the sense of well-being at college graduation.

This model permits exploration of "selection effects"—the implications of freshman well-being for college social activity and academic achievement. We assume, however, that because the character of family relationships will have

Figure 2. Hypothetical Causal Model of the Development of Well-Being.

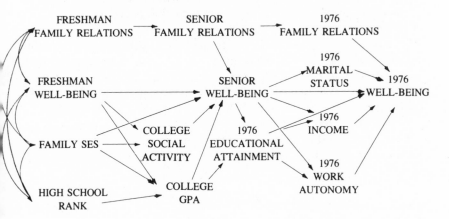

been stabilized long before the college years, they will be unaffected by freshman well-being and other variables in the model. (Still, the child could have played a major part in establishing the character of these relationships earlier; see Yarrow and Yarrow, 1964:522).

To control social class in estimating the independent effects of other variables, a direct path from family socio-economic status to well-being in the senior year of college is included. Since students of high social class background would likely be more comfortable and proficient in adapting to the social and academic aspects of college, it was also thought that this construct would have positive impacts on social activity and academic performance. Over time, the three academic achievement indicators were expected to be causally related, with high school rank predicting college grade point average, and college grades, in turn, related to 1976 post-graduate educational attainment.

It should be noted that we are assuming that well-being in the senior year is an effect, not a cause, of the intervening constructs (family relations, college social activity, and GPA). Therefore, we do not attempt to estimate reciprocal effects. Also, as in the earlier "stability" models, the three constructs representing well-being are assumed to be causally related at *contiguous* time periods, but the effect of well-being in the freshman year (time 1) on the same construct measured in 1976 (time 3) has been set to zero. The same assumption is made with respect to family relationships.

Turning to the period from the senior year to 1976, the quality of relations with the parents in 1976, marital status, post-graduate educational attainment, income, and work autonomy were expected to have positive direct effects on well-being. In addition, educational attainment was expected to have indirect effects on the psychological dimension through its impacts on income attainment and work autonomy. Consistent with the findings of previous research, we predicted that there would be significant selection effects from psychological well-being in college to marital status, educational attainment, income, and work autonomy ten years later. Thus, well-being at the time of graduation from college was expected to facilitate adult attainments.

Because of the limitations of the version of the LISREL program available to us, it was not possible to estimate this full causal model at once, including data from all three time periods. Therefore, the following strategy was adopted. We initially investigated the relationships between the predictors and the criterion up to the senior year, and then estimated the model, including only the constructs from the senior year to 1976. Deleting all those variables found to have no significant relationship to well-being in the two preliminary analyses made it possible in the final stage to re-estimate the entire model, including data from all three time periods.[9]

CAUSAL MODEL I: The Development of Well-Being from the Freshman to the Senior Year in College

The model shown in Figure 3 was estimated as specified. The measurement

Figure 3. Causal Model of Well-being: Freshman to Senior Year. $X^2/df = 255.202/179 = 1.43$ (Significant Correlations of the Residuals of the Observed Variables are Given Next to the Figure.)

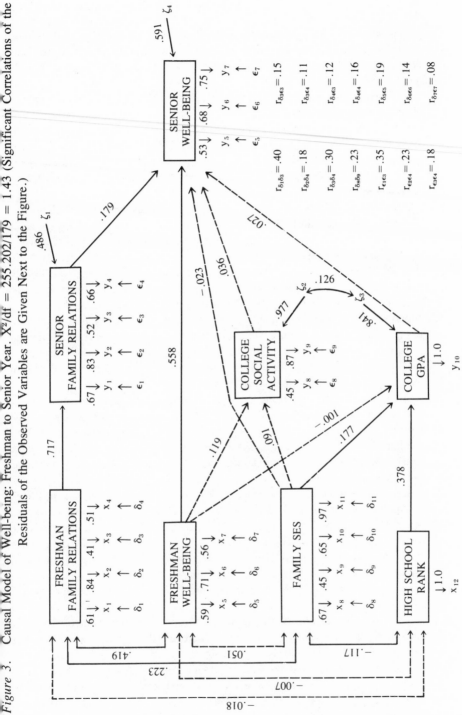

25

parameters of the well-being construct were fixed at the values shown in figure 1.[10] (Non-significant paths are indicated by dashed arrows.) The chi-square value divided by the degrees of freedom is 1.43 (n = 371) indicating a good fit to the input variance-covariance matrix.

The most striking feature of this first causal model is the high stability path from the freshman to the senior psychological construct. In comparison to the earlier "measurement" model of Figure 1, including no external variables, the stability coefficient has declined from .634 to .558. This rather small difference suggests that family relationships, college social activity, and academic achievement account for very little of the stability in well-being from the time of entry into college to graduation four years later.

A second important finding regards the effects of the parent-son relationship on well-being over the four-year period. The family construct is highly stable over time (.717); in fact, it is even more stable than the psychological dimension. In 1962–63, at the time of the students' entry into college, the true score correlation between the family and well-being constructs is a rather substantial .419. By 1966–67, at the end of the senior year, this correlation has declined somewhat to .354 (as shown in Figure 4). The path coefficient, indicating the effect of support from the family on the psychological dimension in the senior year, net of the effects of socio-economic status, earlier well-being, college social activity, and grade point average, is .179 (see figure 3). Consistent with the assumption that there are no direct effects from freshman family relations to senior well-being, the corresponding partial derivative is very close to zero.

A third notable feature of the model is the absence of significant paths relating the college social activity and academic performance constructs to the self-concept dimension. The sense of well-being in the freshman year was unrelated to high school rank; nor did this psychological construct have significant "selection" effects on the intervening measures of college social activity and grade point average.[11]

In accord with previous research, family socio-economic status was positively correlated with freshman family relationships (.223), but the social class construct had no significant relationship to either the freshman or to the senior well-being dimensions. The significant path (.177) from the socio-economic background measure to college grade point average may reflect the advantages of children of highly educated parents in coping with academic demands. As was anticipated, there is a rather substantial path (.378) from high school rank to college academic performance.

In summary, the only variables found to have significant direct effects on well-being in the senior year of college were the quality of relationships with parents and the same psychological dimension measured four years earlier. While it is somewhat unexpected to find that the college variables do not influence the perception of self as happy, relaxed, and confident, conceptualizing the self as a complex, multifaceted phenomenon makes these results quite plausible. Though investigators have reported that grades are of importance to students, it may be that well-being, for most students, is not a dimension of the self-image that is affected by academic performance. Given the multidimensionality of the self, it is reasonable to suppose that achievement will only affect those aspects of the self-concept that are directly implicated by that behavior. As a result, academic performance, as indicated by grade point average, would likely influence the individual's evaluation of his intellectual aptitudes, but would not affect his general sense of happiness or well-being, unless this kind of achievement were very highly valued.

College social activity was included in the model to represent the level of social involvement and support from others in college; the indicators assessed extracurricular involvements and organizational memberships. It has been argued, however, that the really important social experiences in college are the more informal ones, the close and sometimes intimate relationships formed with peers (King, 1973; Katz, 1968). But we have no measures of such relationships.

CAUSAL MODEL II: The Development of Well-being from the Senior Year in College to a Decade Following Graduation

The causal model in Figure 4 represents the development of a sense of well-being during the decade following college graduation.[12] Judging from the fact that the chi-square value, divided by the degrees of freedom, is a rather small 1.96, this model also represents a fairly good fit to the data (n = 346). In this figure, we again find very strong stability in the psychological dimension. Multivariate controls result in only a slight decline from the stability coefficient estimated previously (Figure 1)—.584 to .515. As before, the intervening experiences relating to family of origin, marriage, educational attainment, and occupational achievements cannot account for the stability of this construct over a ten-year period.

Consistent with the previous four-year period, Figure 4 shows that the family variables remain extremely stable (.598) in early adulthood.[13] Of greater interest is the continuing pattern of decline in the importance of family relations for a sense of happiness and well-being. As noted earlier, the true score correlation between these constructs in the freshman year was .419. By the senior year, this association dropped to .354, and by the end of the first decade following college graduation, it has fallen still further to .203 (not shown). When the effects of the senior self-concept dimension and the marriage and achievement variables are taken into account, the path from 1976 family relations to 1976 well-being is reduced to an insignificant .087.

This pattern suggests that the son's relations with his parents become less important for his sense of well-being as he moves into adulthood. The crucial formative influence of the family of origin occurs earlier, as indicated by the substantial correlation between the family and well-being constructs in the freshman year of college, after which both the psychological dimension and the character of relationships with the family remain quite stable. The correlations of the family variables with the three observed indicators of well-being provide

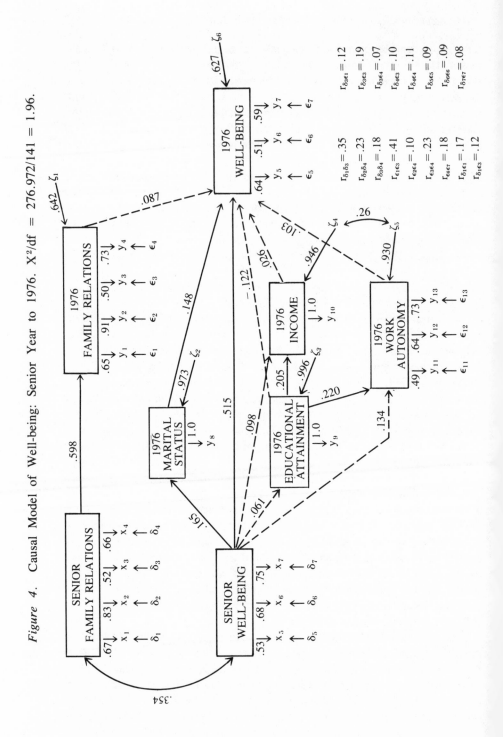

Figure 4. Causal Model of Well-being: Senior Year to 1976. $X^2/df = 276.972/141 = 1.96$.

further insight into the dynamics of these weakening family effects (see Table 7). It is noteworthy that in the freshman and senior year, perceptions of closeness and understanding in the relationship with the father are of greater consequence for a sense of well-being than the same indicators of relationship with the mother.

In our society, marriage is a widely recognized hallmark of the transition to adulthood. The significant path in Figure 4 (.165) from well-being in the senior year of college to marital status in 1976 suggests that those who were happier in 1966–67 have been more successful over the intervening period in establishing and maintaining their marriages. Furthermore, there is a significant path (.148) from marital status to well-being in 1976. This is a clear illustration of ''dynamic stability''—senior well-being increases the chances of getting married, and being married, in turn, strengthens 1976 well-being. The indirect effect of earlier well-being upon subsequent well-being, through marriage, is thus to enhance the stability of the self-image.

This overall pattern of results suggests that in early adulthood, relations with the spouse partially replace relations with parents in sustaining psychological well-being. It could be argued, however, that marital status is a rather inadequate measure of social support. Marriage should sustain a positive outlook only if the relationship with the spouse is gratifying and supportive. There were no measures in the 1976 survey, paralleling the parental relations indicators, of marital closeness and understanding.[14] But even though marital status is an imperfect proxy for social support, the result is quite consistent with prior research (Gurin et al., 1960; Bradburn, 1969; Glenn, 1975; Pearlin and Johnson, 1977).

To further investigate these relationships, this model was estimated as a ''full information model,'' allowing both measurement and causal parameters to be free. When this is done, the 1976 well-being construct changes so that the happiness item makes a much larger contribution to its definition. The factor loading for this item jumps from .641 to .873. In this analysis, the 1976 family relations construct has a significant effect on 1976 well-being (.171), and the path from marital status to this psychological dimension also increases (.214). The first result occurs because the happiness item is the only observed variable in the construct that has significant correlations with the family relations indicators (see Table 7). This suggests that ''happiness'' continues to be influenced by the family, whereas being relaxed versus tense, and confident versus anxious, are no longer affected by relations with parents. Taken together, the central finding is upheld; relationships with the family of origin have a declining effect on two of the three indicators of well-being.

Nevertheless, even in this second period, interpersonal relationships are of greater importance than achievements in enhancing well-being. None of the three attainment constructs—post-graduate education level, income from the main job, or work autonomy—had significant effects on this dimension of the self-image. Post-graduate educational achievement, an important form of human capital investment, increases 1976 income and work autonomy. However, there is a

Table 7. Correlations of the Family Relations Variables with the Well-Being Variables

	Freshman			Senior			1976		
	Happy	Relaxed	Confident	Happy	Relaxed	Confident	Happy	Relaxed	Confident
Family Relations Variables [a]									
Father Understands	.320	.152	.089	.355	.191	.239	.236	−.003 [b]	.054 [b]
Close to Father	.339	.160	.179	.310	.134	.137	.189	−.025 [b]	.054 [b]
Mother Understands	.225	.129	.053 [b]	.247	.097	.183	.169	.017 [b]	.066 [b]
Close to Mother	.278	.119	.063 [b]	.227	.075 [b]	.075 [b]	.145	−.021 [b]	.036 [b]

[a] These variables are paired with the well-being indicators by time, i.e., freshman family relations with freshman well-being, etc.
[b] $p > .05$

direct negative path from post-graduate educational attainment to the psychological construct, perhaps reflecting the high aspirations that education can instill, which almost reaches statistical significance (t = 1.84). The path from work autonomy to well-being is in the predicted direction, but is quite weak (t = 1.21). Nor were there significant "selection effects" from the earlier psychological dimension to these three attainments. Apparently, the sense of well-being in the senior year did not facilitate subsequent educational and occupational achievement.

These negative findings may once more be attributable to the specific dimension of the self-concept under consideration. The sense of competence, in contrast, was found to be significantly enhanced by experiences of work autonomy during the identical period and to promote both occupational attainments Mortimer and Lorence, 1979b).

CAUSAL MODEL III: *Development of the Sense of Well-being from Entry to College to Ten Years Following Graduation*

By deleting those constructs found to have no significant effects on the sense of well-being at the three time periods, we have reduced the number of variables sufficiently to re-estimate the entire model (see Figure 5). As in Figures 2 and 3, the relationships of the family and well-being constructs to their indicators have been fixed. The chi-square value divided by the degrees of freedom is 2.09, indicating a good fit to the input data (N = 386).

This final model highlights, in summary form, the results obtained earlier. It demonstrates the high level of stability of the self-image through college (.575) and over the ten years following graduation (.557), and the declining importance

Figure 5. Final Causal Model of Well-being: Freshman Year to 1976. X²/df = 234.003/112 = 2.09.

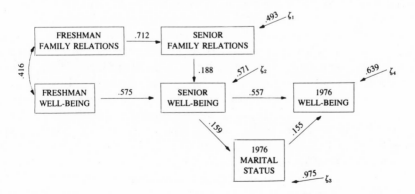

of relationships with parents in sustaining a positive outlook. It also shows that psychological well-being is a significant antecedent and consequent of marriage.

SUMMARY AND DISCUSSION

There are three central conclusions of this study. First, the research demonstrates a striking stability of five dimensions of the self-concept over a 14-year period spanning late adolescence to early adulthood. We have labelled these dimensions well-being, self-doubts, sociability, competence, and unconventionality. The four- and ten-year stability coefficients range from .51 to .79. When translated to yearly averages, these figures yield estimated stabilities from .84 to .98. In general, the findings suggest increasing stability of the self-image as the individual undergoes the transition to adulthood. They therefore support the widely-held view that the development of identity occurs prior to adulthood; i.e., in adolescence or childhood, and thereafter remains quite stable over time (Erikson, 1959; Bachman et al., 1978; Rosenberg, 1979). If these five dimensions of the self-image can be interpreted as indicators of adjustment and mental health, and there is good reason to do so, the results suggest that these pheonomena, too, remain highly persistent over time.

Secondly, the causal analysis of the development of a sense of well-being confirms the importance of social support from the family in sustaining a perception of self as happy, relaxed, and confident. At the time of entry into college, family relationships appear to play an important part in enhancing or detracting from psychological well-being. The impact of support from the parents steadily weakens over time, and becomes supplanted, in early adulthood, by support from the spouse.

The third major implication of the study is that the self-concept should be conceptualized as a multi-faceted phenomenon. As noted previously, our causal analysis of the development of competence in the ten years following college showed that this self-concept dimension, in spite of its high stability over time, is significantly affected by experiences of autonomy in the work environment— decision-making ability, innovative thinking, and challenge. The same occupational experiences, however, had no discernible effect on the perception of self as happy, relaxed, and confident. Academic achievement, as indicated by high school rank, grade point average, and post-graduate attainment, likewise had negligible associations with this dimension of the self-image. This divergent pattern of findings, in the two causal analyses, reaffirms Rosenberg's insistence on the multi-dimensional character of the self-image.

We have not performed similar causal analyses of the other three self-concept dimensions, and therefore lack the empirical evidence necessary to determine whether the causal antecedents of well-being are the same for them. Further research is necessary to assess whether well-being is like other self-perceptions—such as sociability, unconventionality, and self-doubts—in being significantly influenced by the family, and whether a sense of competence is unique in its sensitivity to work experiences.

The general lack of importance of non-family related variables, coupled with the fact that even the family constructs had rather weak net effects after the freshman year, suggest that the aspects of the environmental context studied here are of rather little importance in sustaining the sense of well-being during the transition to adulthood. External forces, at least within the range that can be observed in this sample, do not account for the remarkable pattern of stability in this dimension of the self-concept. Using Rosenberg's terminology, the weight of the evidence appears to be in favor of ''static,'' rather than ''dynamic'' stability. In interpreting this evidence, however, it must be remembered that the men who participated in this research project are a highly advantaged group with a long history of personal success. Perhaps it is not surprising, under these circumstances, to find that the self-image is so highly stable. We simply may not have enough variance in the independent variables to demonstrate very large effects, even if, in the broader population, they are crucial influences on adult well-being. Moreover, it has been suggested that positive self-concepts are more resistant to change over time (Epstein, 1973:411). Only future longitudinal studies, including persons in less advantaged circumstances, as well as women, can resolve this question of generalizability.

While this research is not without its limitations, confirmatory factor analysis has provided very precise estimates of self-concept stability. Our analytic strategy has also enabled an examination of the effects of several important independent variables over a relatively long period of time. On the whole, this research provides an impressive confirmation of previous studies by accentuating the stability of the self-concept; it also supports the findings of long-term developmental studies of personality, mental health, and life adjustment.

ACKNOWLEDGMENT

This research was supported by grants from the Center for Studies of Metropolitan Problems of the National Institute of Mental Health (MH 26421), the National Science Foundation (NSF SOC 75-21098), and the University of Minnesota Computer Center. The authors would like to thank Melvin Kohn, David Mangen, Geoffrey Maruyama, Morris Rosenberg, Roberta G. Simmons, and Irving Tallman for their helpful criticisms and suggestions; Ronald Schoenberg for providing us with the LISREL program; Gerald Gurin for use of the Michigan Student Study data; and Donald Kumka and Joan Dreyer for technical assistance.

NOTES

1. To assess the degree of sampling bias, the 1976 respondents were compared with the non-respondents, using the senior year data. The two groups were almost identical in family background, college grade point average, and senior year career choice.

2. Tangri (1974) followed up a sample of women in the Michigan study three years following their college graduation. Her analysis focuses on the determinants of the women's post-graduate aspirations and experiences relating to education and work.

3. Since this last item loaded on both the well-being and competence dimensions in the exploratory factor analysis, it was used previously as an indicator of competence (Mortimer and Lorence, 1979b).

4. The three measures of satisfaction are: "All things considered, how satisfied are you with your job as a whole?"; "All in all, how satisfied are you with your marriage?"; and "Consider how your life is going now. Would you like it to continue in much the same way, or would you like it to change?"

5. Listwise deletion was used in all measurement models except that of well-being. N's ranged from 399 to 404. Pairwise deletion (after removing cases for which information was not obtained at all three time periods) was used in estimating the variance-covariance matrix for the well-being construct. In calculating the significance levels for the measurement model, the smallest N (410) was used. Because the causal analysis included a fairly large number of variables, listwise deletion would have excessively limited the number of cases in the analysis.

6. No correlated errors were estimated between variables in the freshman year and variables in the 1976 survey.

7. Parameters that were twice their standard errors were considered to be statistically significant.

8. Though these are self-reports, their validity as indicators of parent-son relationships is supported by their relation to the transmission of occupational values (Mortimer, 1976). In the family relations constructs, the indicators are ordered as follows: father understands, father close, mother understands, mother close.

9. This strategy is made tenable by the assumption that variables from the earlier time period affect 1976 well-being only indirectly through senior well-being. College grade point average is expected to influence 1976 educational attainment. However, it would only be necessary to include grade point average in estimating the "selection effect" from senior well-being to 1976 educational attainment if this measure of academic achievement were significantly related to well-being in the senior year.

10. The measurement parameters of the family relations constructs were also estimated previously and fixed. The measurement parameters for family socio-economic status and college social activity were, however, freely estimated.

11. As noted earlier, the path from well-being in the freshman year to family relations in the senior year was fixed at zero. Examination of the appropriate first-order partial derivative indicated that the assumption that there would be no significant effect of earlier well-being on family relations at this time was justified.

12. As in Figure 3, the measurement parameters of the well-being and family relations constructs have been fixed at the values obtained before, and the model has been estimated as specified.

13. As in the previous model, there is no evidence of a causal path from the senior sense of well-being to 1976 family relations, due to the extremely small partial derivative.

14. However, as discussed earlier, an item tapping 1976 marital satisfaction was positively correlated with a scale representing 1976 well-being (.256).

REFERENCES

Allport, Gordon (1955), *Becoming*. New Haven: Yale University Press.

Bachman, Jerald G., Patrick M. O'Malley, and Jerome Johnston (1978), *Adolescence to Adulthood—Change and Stability in the Lives of Young Men,* Youth in Transition, Volume VI. Ann Arbor: Institute for Social Research.

Becker, Howard S., Blanche Geer, and Everett C. Hughes (1968), *Making the Grade: The Academic Side of College Life.* New York: John Wiley.

Block, Jack, and Norma Haan (1971), *Lives Through Time*. Berkeley: Bancroft.

Bloom, Benjamin S. (1964), *Stability and Change in Human Characteristics*. New York: Wiley.

Bradburn, Norman M. (1969), *The Structure of Psychological Well-Being*. Chicago: Aldine.

Breytspraak, Linda K. and Linda K. George (forthcoming), "Self-concept and self-esteem," in D. J. Mangen, W. A. Peterson, and R. Sanders (eds.), *Handbook of Research Instruments in Adult Development and Aging*. Minneapolis: University of Minnesota Press.

Brim, Orville G. Jr. (1970), "Personality development as role-learning," pp. 158–169 in W. Richard Scott (ed.), *Social Processes and Social Structures*. New York: Holt.

———— (1976), "Life span development of the theory of oneself: Implications for child development." Pp. 241–251 in *Advances in Child Development and Behavior*, Volume 11. New York: Academic Press.

Buben, Judith (1975), "Adolescent and young adult Rorschach responses," pp. 127–149 in Daniel Offer and Judith B. Offer (eds.), *From Teenage to Young Manhood*. New York: Basic Books.

Carlson, Rae (1963), "Identification and personality structure in preadolescents," *Journal of Abnormal and Social Psychology* 67(December):566–573.

Cohn, Richard M. (1978), "The effect of employment status change on self-attitudes," *Social Psychology* 41(June):81–93.

Cooley, Charles Horton (1902), *Human Nature and the Social Order*. New York: Scribners.

Cottrell, Leonard S. (1969), "Interpersonal interaction and the development of the self," pp. 543–570 in David A. Goslin (ed.), *Handbook of Socialization Theory and Research*. Chicago: Rand McNally.

Cox, Rachel D. (1970), *Youth into Maturity*. New York: Mental Health Materials Center.

Crandall, Virginia C. (1972), "The Fels study: Some contributions to personality development and achievement in childhood and adulthood," *Seminars in Psychiatry* 4(November):383–398.

Elder, Glen (1974), *Children of the Great Depression*. Chicago: University of Chicago Press.

Engel, Mary (1959), "The stability of the self-concept in adolescence," *Journal of Abnormal and Social Psychology* 58(March):211–215.

Epstein, Seymour (1973), "The self-concept revisited: or a theory of a theory," *American Psychologist* 28(May):404–416.

Erikson, Erik H. (1959), "The problem of ego identity," *Psychological Issues* 1:101–164.

Feldman, Kenneth A. and Theodore M. Newcomb (1969), *The Impact of College on Students*, Volume 1, *An Analysis of Four Decades of Research*. San Francisco: Jossey-Bass.

Fischer, Anita Kassen, James Marton, E. Joel Millman and Leo Srole (1979), "Long-range influence on adult mental health: The Midtown Manhattan Longitudinal Study, 1954–1974," pp. 305–333 in Roberta G. Simmons (ed.), *Research in Community and Mental Health: An Annual Compilation of Research*, Volume 1. Greenwich, Connecticut: JAI Press, Inc.

Franks, David D. and Joseph Marolla (1976), "Efficacious action and social approval as interacting dimensions of self-esteem: A tentative formulation through construct validation," *Sociometry* 39(December):324–341.

French, John R.P., Jr. (1968), "The conceptualization and measurement of mental health in terms of self-identity theory," pp. 135–159 in S. B. Sells (ed.), *The Definition and Measurement of Mental Health*. Washington, D.C.: Department of Health, Education, and Welfare.

Gergen, Kenneth (1972), "Multiple identity. The healthy, happy human being wears many masks," *Psychology Today* 6(May):31–35, 64, 66.

Glenn, Norval D. (1975), "The contribution of marriage to the psychological well-being of males and females," *Journal of Marriage and the Family* 37(August):594–600.

Golden, Jules, Nathan Mandel, Bernard C. Glueck, Jr., and Zetta F. Feder (1962), "A summary description of fifty 'normal' white males," *American Journal of Psychiatry* 119(July):48–56.

Grinker, R. R. (1962), "Mentally healthy young males (homoclites)," *Archives of General Psychiatry* 6:405–453.

Gurin, Gerald (1971), *A Study of Students in a Multiversity*. Ann Arbor, Michigan: Survey Research Center.

Gurin, Gerald and Patricia Gurin (1976), "Personal efficacy and the ideology of individual responsibility," pp. 131–157 in Burkhard Strumpel (ed.), *Economic Means for Human Needs*. Ann Arbor: Institute for Social Research.

Gurin, Gerald, Joseph Veroff, and Sheila Feld (1960), *Americans View their Mental Health*. New York: Basic.

Haan, Norma (1964), "The relationship of ego functioning and intelligence to social status and social mobility," *Journal of Abnormal and Social Psychology* 69(December):594–605.

——— (1972), "Personality development from adolescence to adulthood in the Oakland Growth and Guidance Studies," *Seminars in Psychiatry* 4(November):399–414.

Heath, Douglas H. (1968), *Growing Up in College*. San Francisco: Jossey-Bass.

——— (1976), "Adolescent and adult predictors of vocational adaptation," *Journal of Vocational Behavior* 9:1–19.

Hunt, Jane V. and Dorothy H. Eichorn (1972), "Maternal and child behaviors: A review of data from the Berkeley Growth Study," *Seminars in Psychiatry* 4(November):367–381.

Jacques, Jeffrey M. and Karen J. Chason (1977), "Self-esteem and low status groups: A changing scene?", *Sociological Quarterly* 18(Summer):399–412.

James, William (1892), *Psychology. Briefer Course*. New York: Henry Holt and Co.

Jones, Mary C., Nancy Bayley, Jean W. Macfarlane, and Marjorie P. Honzik (1971), *The Course of Human Development*. Waltham, Mass.: Xerox.

Jöreskog, Karl G. (1973), "A general method for estimating a linear structural equation system," pp. 85–112 in Arthur S. Goldberger and Otis Dudley Duncan (eds.), *Structural Equation Models in the Social Sciences*. New York: Seminar Press.

Jöreskog, Karl G. and Dag Sörbom (1977), "Statistical models and methods for analysis of longitudinal data," pp. 285–325 in Dennis J. Aigner and Arthur S. Goldberger (eds.), *Latent Variables in Socio-economic Models*. Amsterdam: North-Holland Publishing Co.

Jöreskog, Karl G. and Marielle van Thillo (1972), "LISREL: A general computer program for estimating a linear structural equation system involving multiple indicators of unmeasured variables," Research Bulletin 72-56. Princeton, N.J.: Educational Testing Service.

Kagan, Jerome and Howard A. Moss (1962), *Birth to Maturity*. New York: Wiley.

Kaplan, Howard B. and Alex D. Porkorny (1969), "Self-derogation and psychosocial adjustment," *Journal of Nervous and Mental Disease* 149(November):421–434.

Katz, Joseph (1968), "Four years of growth, conflict and compliance," pp. 3–73 in Joseph Katz and associates, *No Time for Youth*. San Francisco: Jossey-Bass.

Kelly, E. Lowell (1955), "Consistency of the adult personality," *American Psychologist* 10:659–681.

King, Stanley H. (1972), "Coping and growth in adolescence," *Seminars in Psychiatry* 4(November):355–366.

——— (1973), *Five Lives at Harvard: Personality Change during College*. Cambridge: Harvard University Press.

Kohn, Melvin L. (1977), *Class and Conformity: A Study in Values* (second edition). Chicago: University of Chicago Press.

Kohn, Melvin L. and Eleanor E. Carroll (1960), "Social class and the allocation of parental responsibilities," *Sociometry* 23:372–392.

Kohn, Melvin L. and Carmi Schooler (1973), "Occupational experience and psychological functioning: An assessment of reciprocal effects," *American Sociological Review* 38(February):97–118.

——— (1974), "Follow-up survey on occupational conditions and psychological functioning." Washington, D.C.: National Institute of Mental Health.

——— (1978), "The reciprocal effects of the substantive complexity of work and intellectual flexibility: A longitudinal assessment," *American Journal of Sociology* 84(May):24–52.

Korman, Abraham K. (1970), "Toward an hypothesis of work behavior," *Journal of Applied Psychology* 54(February):31–41.

Korn, Harold A. (1968a), "Careers: choice, chance or inertia?", pp. 207–238 in Joseph Katz and associates, *No Time for Youth*. San Francisco: Jossey-Bass.

───── (1968b), "Personality scale changes from the freshman year to the senior year," pp. 162–184 in Joseph Katz and associates, *No Time for Youth,* San Francisco: Jossey-Bass.

Kuhlen, Raymond G. (1964), "Personality change with age," pp. 524–555 in Philip Worchel and Donn Byrne (eds.), *Personality Change*. New York: Wiley.

Lecky, Prescott (1945), *Self-consistency. A Theory of Personality*. New York: Island.

Lidz, Theodore (1968), *The Person*. New York: Basic Books.

Luborsky, Lester and H. Bachrach (1974), "Factors influencing clinicians' judgements of mental health," *Archives of General Psychiatry* 31(September):292–299.

Luborsky, Lester and Jean Schimek (1964), "Psychoanalytic theories of therapeutic and developmental change: Implications for assessment," pp. 73–99 in Philip Worchel and Donn Byrne (eds.), *Personality Change*. New York: Wiley.

Luck, Patrick W. and Jerold Heiss (1972), "Social determinants of self-esteem in adult males," *Sociology and Social Research* 57(October):69–84.

Monge, Rolf H. (1973), "Developmental trends in factors of adolescent self-concept," *Developmental Psychology* 8(May):382–393.

Mortimer, Jeylan T. (1976), "Social class, work and the family: Some implications of the father's occupation for familial relationships and sons' career decisions," *Journal of Marriage and the Family* 38(May):241–256.

Mortimer, Jeylan T. and Jon Lorence (1979a), "Work experience and occupational value socialization: A longitudinal study," *American Journal of Sociology* 84(May):1361–1385.

───── (1979b), "Occupational experience and the self-concept: A longitudinal study," *Social Psychology Quarterly* 42(December):307–323.

Moss, Howard A. and Jerome Kagan (1972), "Report on personality consistency and change from the Fels Longitudinal Study," pp. 21–28 in David R. Heise (ed.), *Personality and Socialization*. Chicago: Rand McNally.

Oden, Melita H. (1968), "The fulfilment of promise: 40-year follow-up of the Terman Gifted Group," *Genetic Psychology Monographs* 77(February):3–93.

Offer, Daniel and Judith B. Offer (1975), *From Teenage to Young Manhood*. New York: Basic Books.

Osgood, Charles E., George J. Suci, and Percy H. Tannenbaum (1957), *The Measurement of Meaning*. Urbana: University of Illinois Press.

Pearlin, Leonard I. and J. S. Johnson (1977), "Marital status, life strains, and depression," *American Sociological Review* 42(October):704–715.

Pearlin, Leonard I. and Carmi Schooler (1978), "The Structure of coping," *Journal of Health and Social Behavior* 19(March):2–21.

Peskin, Harvey and Norman Livson (1972), "Pre- and postpubertal personality and adult psychologic functioning," *Seminars in Psychiatry* 4(November):343–353.

Purkey, William W. (1970), *Self Concept and School Achievement*. Englewood Cliffs, New Jersey: Prentice-Hall.

Rosenberg, Morris (1965), *Society and the Adolescent Self-image*. Princeton: Princeton University Press.

───── (1979), *Conceiving The Self*. New York: Basic Books.

Shaver, Philip (1969), "Measurement of self-esteem and related constructs," Pp. 45–160 in John P. Robinson and Philip R. Shaver (eds.), *Measures of Social Psychological Attitudes*. Ann Arbor: Survey Research Center, Institute for Social Research.

Siegelman, Ellen, Jack Block, Jeanne Block, and Anna von der Lippe (1970), "Antecedents of optimal psychological adjustment," *Journal of Consulting and Clinical Psychology* 35(December):283–289.

Smith, M. Brewster (1968), "Competence and socialization," pp. 270-320 in John A. Clausen (ed.), *Socialization and Society*. Boston: Little Brown.

Sörbom, Dag (1975), "Detection of correlated errors in longitudinal data," *British Journal of Mathematical and Statistical Psychology* 28:138-151.

Symonds, Percival M. (1961), *From Adolescent to Adult*. New York: Columbia University Press.

Tangri, Sandra S. (1974), "Effects of Background, Personality, College and Post-college Experiences on Women's Post-graduate Employment," Final Report, Grant number 91-34-71-02. U.S. Department of Labor, Manpower Administration.

Tuddenham, Read D. (1971), "The constancy of personality ratings over two decades," pp. 395-403 in Mary C. Jones, Nancy Bayley, Jean W. MacFarlane, and Marjorie P. Honzik (eds.), *The Course of Human Development*. Waltham, Massachusetts: Xerox.

Vaillant, George E. (1974), "Natural history of male psychological health, II. Some antecedents of healthy adult adjustment," *Archives of General Psychiatry* 31(July):15-22.

―――― (1976), "Natural history of male psychological health, V. The relation of choice of ego mechanisms of defense to adult adjustment," *Archives of General Psychiatry* 33(April):535-545.

―――― (1977), *Adaptation to Life*. Boston: Little, Brown.

―――― and Charles C. McArthur (1972), "Natural history of male psychologic health, I. The adult life cycle from 18-50," *Seminars in Psychiatry* 4(November):415-427.

Van Maanen, John (1976), "Breaking-in: Socialization to work," pp. 67-130 in R. Dubin (ed.), *Handbook of Work, Organization, and Society*. Chicago: Rand McNally.

Wells, L. Edward and Gerald Marwell (1976), *Self-Esteem: Its Conceptualization and Measurement*. Beverly Hills: Sage.

Werts, Charles E., Karl G. Jöreskog, and Robert L. Linn (1973), "Identification and estimation in path analysis with unmeasured variables," *American Journal of Sociology* 78(May):1469-1484.

Wessman, Alden E. and David F. Ricks (1966), *Mood and Personality*. New York: Holt, Rinehart, and Winston.

Wheaton, Blair, Bengt Muthen, Duane F. Alwin, and Gene F. Summers (1977), "Assessing reliability and stability in panel models," pp. 84-136 in David R. Heise (ed.), *Sociological Methodology*. San Francisco: Jossey-Bass.

White, R. W. (1973), "The concept of healthy personality: What do we really mean?", *The Counseling Psychologist* 4,2:3-12.

Yarrow, Leon J. and Marion Radke Yarrow (1964), "Personality continuity and change in the family context," pp. 489-523 in Philip Worchel and Donn Byrne (eds.), *Personality Change*. New York: John Wiley.

APPENDIX A

Figure A-1. Measurement Model of Self-Doubt Construct.

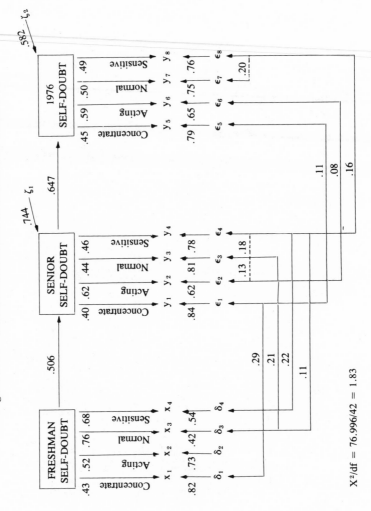

$X^2/df = 76.996/42 = 1.83$

39

Figure A-2. Measurement Model of Sociability Construct.

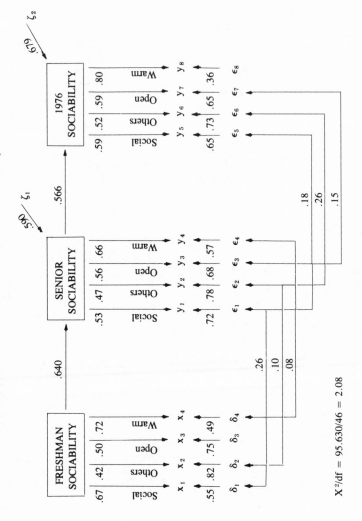

$X^2/df = 95.630/46 = 2.08$

40

Figure A-3. Measurement Model of Competence Construct.

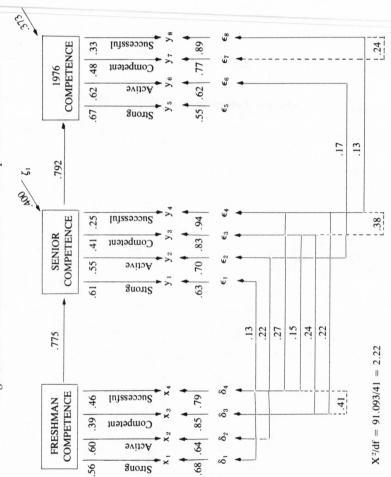

$X^2/df = 91.093/41 = 2.22$

41

Figure A-4. Measurement Model of Unconventionality Construct.

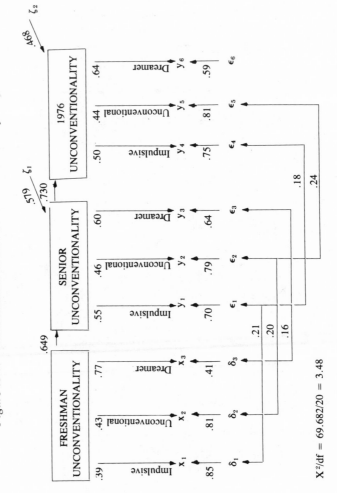

$X^2/df = 69.682/20 = 3.48$

THE EFFECTS OF PHYSICAL DEVELOPMENT ON SELF-IMAGE AND SATISFACTION WITH BODY-IMAGE FOR EARLY ADOLESCENT MALES

Dale A. Blyth, Roberta G. Simmons, Richard Bulcroft, Debbie Felt, Edward F. Van Cleave, and Diane Mitsch Bush

INTRODUCTION

Puberty and related aspects of physiological change have long been recognized as important for understanding adolescent development. All textbooks on adoles-

Research in Community and Mental Health, Volume 2, pages 43–73

cence include one or more chapters discussing biological changes which take place in this period of human development, and a number of popular and theoretical statements have been made concerning the relationship of physical change to social and psychological changes at this age. Clausen (1975), for example, discusses three ways in which physical development may influence the social and psychological development of adolescents. He notes first, that relative maturity, size, and type of physique directly affect the individual's actual performance capabilities; second, that physical maturation influences the way in which one is seen by others and the expectations that are held by these others; and finally, that the self-image of the adolescent is influenced both by these increased or decreased performance capabilities and by the responses of others to his changing physical appearance (Clausen, 1975:26-27). Still another way in which the changes taking place around puberty could affect an individual is through hormonal changes. All of these mechanisms by which physical development can affect an individual are extremely complex and difficult to specify. This difficulty is further enhanced when one considers the complexity of what we mean by physical development itself.

Work by Nicolson (1953), Stolz and Stolz (1951), Tanner (1962), Reynolds and Wines (1948), Faust (1977), and Roche (1979), among others, has served to increase our awareness of the tremendous complexity of the physiological changes which are taking place during adolescence. In addition to the increase in height and weight, there are related changes: alterations in the distribution of fat, an increase in strength, development of secondary sexual characteristics, and changes in body proportion such as shoulder and hip width and leg length. As if this complexity were not enough, there is also the issue of differential rates of change and the asynchrony of these changes to be coped with. Hence, it is not only that an individual is changing in many dimensions simultaneously, but that the onset of these changes and their coordination can vary considerably from one individual to another. Given this variety, it is not surprising that we know relatively little about the effects of particular aspects of physical development on specific aspects of social and psychological development during the early adolescent time period.

In this article, we shall first review previous research relating specific aspects of physical development in the adolescent male to social and psychological factors with a focus on satisfaction with one's physical appearance and on the self-image. Our own research data will then be presented, and we shall relate specific dimensions of a boy's physical status to his satisfaction with those dimensions and to his self-image in early adolescence. In this way, it is hoped that the present analysis can contribute new information about the relationship among physical characteristics, satisfaction with certain body-image dimensions, and self-image at a particular developmental point.

PREVIOUS RESEARCH

Early versus Late Development

In the literature, one frequent way of dealing with the complexity of physical development involves the classification of individuals as either early or late developers. This classification has typically been accomplished in one of three ways. First, investigators have looked at the skeletal age of individuals at given chronological ages (Jones and Bayley, 1950; Jones, 1957; and Peskin, 1967). This technique attempts to identify the extreme groups of early maturers, who are defined as having a skeletal age greater than the average at a particular chronological point in individuals' lives. A second technique is that used by Mussen and Boutourline-Young (1964) which involved observational ratings of boys over a four- or five-year period. Individuals who were consistently rated as younger or older than the rest of the persons in the sample were so classified. Finally, there is the approach used by Stolz and Stolz (1951) in which they found the point of most rapid height growth for the adolescent and then classified him as early or late on the basis of where that maximum growth spurt occurred chronologically in comparison to others in the sample.

Although all of these techniques are somewhat different, they share a number of common features which are subject to two major criticisms. A primary criticism of these techniques is that they have usually been used to separate individuals into extreme groups of early versus late maturers, rather than to explore the entire continuum of early to late maturation. This use of extreme groups can introduce severe methodological problems. For example, other theoretically relevant factors may be either causing or related to the differences in physical development and hence introduce spurious relationships.

Furthermore, it is unfortunate that once a classification as to early versus late is made, the chronology of these differences and the relationship to other physical characteristics is usually ignored. In the few cases where early and late developers have been compared on other physical status characteristics, important differences have been noted. Jones (1957), for example, noted significant differences in height and weight from ages 12 to 17. The early maturing boys were taller and heavier on the average than the later maturers. This difference peaked at around age 13 and 14. It should also be noted that the early maturing boys were stronger and rated as having a more attractive physique. As support for his classification of early and late maturers, Peskin (1967) noted the earlier age of maximum growth (13 years versus 15 years) and the earlier onset and termination of the development of secondary sexual characteristics. While these findings serve to validate differences between extremely early and extremely late maturers, they neither enable one to talk about the effects of these other physical characteristics at any particular point in time, nor provide clear explanations for the effects of early or late maturation. In order to draw these types of conclusions, one would need to look at the actual physical characteristics of a sample of individuals and relate them to given social and psychological dimensions for those same individuals at the same point in time.

The second criticism of the three techniques used to define early versus late maturation is that they either have utilized knowledge from many points throughout the entire adolescent time frame or from a point late in adolescence. While it is extremely helpful to be able to have a long-term longitudinal data set on adolescents in order to see their entire growth pattern, it would also be useful to have an indicator of early and late development that could actually be used while the individual is in early adolescence. Without modifying the above measures, it becomes difficult to classify an individual while he is still in the early or even the middle stage of adolescence. This timing is problematic if one wishes to diagnose or predict likely handicaps or advantages a child will face during the first four or five years of the second decade of life. A different approach would utilize the individuals' standing on a number of physical characteristics during the early, middle, and late adolescent time periods. It is this latter approach which will be illustrated in this article, using data from the early adolescent time period.

Given these methodological criticisms, what are the social and psychological correlates of early and late development as reported in the literature? Since a number of excellent summaries of this literature already exist (see Clausen, 1975; Dwyer and Mayer, 1968; and Eichorn, 1963), only the highlights will be noted here. Early maturing boys have generally been found to be more poised, relaxed, socially advanced, and more respected in their peer group. These differences tend to be more important in the high school than in the junior high school age range. Late maturing boys, on the other hand, have been found to be expressive, dynamic, and buoyant, but also tenser and more concerned with their physical appearance. Peskin (1967) has looked at these findings in both a social learning and a psychodynamic theoretical context. In the psychodynamic context, he compares individuals at common points in the developmental cycles even though their chronological ages are quite different. This difference in approach aside, he finds that early developers may indeed have a number of advantages socially, but may be "escaping into adulthood" prematurely and hence have a number of late psychological adjustment problems. Peskin concludes that "the early maturer is now seen to pay a psychological price for his social prominence by clinging rigidly to early success patterns" (Peskin, 1967:3). The late maturer on the other hand is viewed as having a longer period of time to adjust to adult status and hence while he may be "gradually learning to cope with and compensate for his adverse social status," he is also gradually developing a psychological maturity which will stay with him for many years. Peskin essentially concludes that the difference between early and late maturers in terms of mental health may be minimal and that the real difference will be with respect to their interpersonal versus intrapersonal orientations.

In summary, early development appears to have some initial advantages for males. It must be remembered, however, that most studies cited used small groups (usually less than 20) whose members show extreme developmental patterns, and frequently developmental patterns are defined at the end of adolescence. As a result, the studies do not provide as rich an understanding as they might, of the effects of several correlated physical characteristics on normal youth at different points during the adolescent development cycle. Furthermore, these studies also tend to ignore the potential effects of differences in the composition of one's peer group and possible differences in peer group values. The single notable exception to this is a study by Mussen and Boutourline-Young (1964) which did find significant differences between the effects of early and late maturation in American versus Italian cultures. Whether these differences might not also exist as a function of different subcultures at different periods in adolescence is an interesting, but as yet unanswered question.

In response to these criticisms, this paper will concentrate on one point in time, that of early adolescence, but will investigate a large randomly selected sample of normal youth rather than selected extreme groups. Furthermore, the effects of several key physical characteristics will be investigated, including early development. In addition, we will explore whether or not there are any significant differences due to students being located in two contrasting school contexts with different peer composition. Before doing this, however, we should also note that the physical characteristics to be examined other than pubertal development also have a history in prior research.

Effects of Body Type and Weight

Another approach of prior research to the problem of the effects of physical development in adolescence involves weight and body type. Here, the attempt is to focus on a single aspect of physical development which is believed to be significant in terms of social and psychological development. It is important to make a distinction between body type and weight, since their effects for boys may be opposite in direction. Weight generally refers to an individual's absolute mass without regard for the distribution of the weight or a sense of being over- or underweight. Body type, on the other hand, refers to the combination of weight and its distribution. The customary classification differentiates among "endomorphic" body types (a fat or well-rounded body build), "mesomorphic" body types (an athletic or muscular body build), and "ectomorphic" body types (thin or lean body build). Body type is generally established using either observer ratings or the ponderal index of body leanness which is the ratio of height to the cube root of weight (Hendry and Gillies, 1978).

The distinction between weight and body type or body leanness may be particularly important for boys. Although there is a dramatic increase in weight for boys during the pubertal period, this gain in weight is not significantly correlated with a gain in subcutaneous tissue (or fat) for boys (Faust, 1977). If anything, Stolz and Stolz (1951) have shown that boys actually experience a decrease in the amount of fatty tissue during the pubertal period. This fact is not true for girls. The importance of this difference is further highlighted by the work of Huenemann et al., (1966), who found that boys felt it was advantageous to gain weight since they attributed excess weight to bone and muscle components rather than to fat. Hence, a gain in sheer mass or bulk was seen to be advantageous rather than problematic.

Several studies of body type have shown that in both childhood (Staffieri, 1967) and in adolescence (Dwyer and Mayer, 1968) there is a strong preference for a mesomorphic body type for males. This preference existed for both males and females when rating silhouettes of males. Hendry and Gillies (1978) argue that the reactions to and expectations of different body types become incorporated into the individual's own body concept and as Staffieri notes "thus provide a framework for his body concept which becomes a significant part of the total self concept." In testing this relationship, Hendry and Gillies find that overweight individuals at age 15 and 16 were, in fact, the least physically fit and had the lowest body esteem of the groups studied. They found no differences in body esteem for average or thin individuals. They also noted that both same and opposite sex friendship were related to the ponderal index in that the underweight body type was positively related to the number of same sex friends, while the average body type was positively related to the number of opposite sex friends. Clausen (1975) further noted that mesomorphic body type was more important in the working class than in the middle class. In particular, working class people saw mesomorphs as more aggressive and evaluated ectomorphs negatively. In a self-report inventory used in both junior and senior high schools, Clausen found that working class boys who were high in mesomorphy were significantly more likely to see themselves as social leaders and athletes than were those who were low in mesomorphy (1975:42).

Another interesting distinction in body type is the effect it has on peer ratings at different ages. Clausen found that endomorphic physiques were most devalued by preadolescents, but by the junior high age these relationships were quite weak. Other work by Stolz and Stolz (1944) and Dwyer and Mayer (1968) point out that one of the effects of body type in middle and late adolescence has to do with the "sex-appropriateness" of the distribution of the weight. By this, they are referring to whether or not there is an excessive build-up of weight in the hips, waist, and chest of males. Such differential fat distribution is seen by individuals as being inappropriate for males and more like what one would expect for females. Thus, Dwyer and Mayer conclude that "unless the obesity is very marked, those disturbances which do exist over body weight and fatness in adolescence generally occur in early puberty and concern body fat laid down in what the boys consider to be a sex-inappropriate manner'' (1968:378).

In summary, it is probably important when dealing with male physical development to distinguish between sheer weight and the distribution of that weight in terms of leanness or body type. This distinction seems important because of the value placed on increased mass attributed to bone and muscle development, as opposed to the negative evaluation of excess fat which may be inappropriately distributed.

Height

Another physical characteristic which has been examined in relation to social and psychological development on a few occasions is height. For boys in particular, there are a number of reasons why being tall might be considered an important dimension. It is generally believed that taller boys are more often chosen to be leaders in a group, particularly if the group is made up of strangers. Many of the popular team sports at school (such as basketball) tend to emphasize height. Stolz and Stolz (1944) found that short boys were under-represented in the athletic activities that were most popular among adolescents. For some boys, the lack of height can be a particularly embarrassing problem, in terms of relations with girls. It is generally assumed that both boys and girls prefer that the male be taller. Despite all these positive aspects of being tall, Stolz and Stolz (1944) found only two groups that were upset about their height. These were the extremely thin or ectomorphic boys who were quite tall (in excess of 6' 3") and those early maturing boys who were growing when no one else around them was growing. It is interesting to speculate about the comparison group early adolescents use to determine if they are too tall. Is it their close friends, their age mates at school, or some composite of the entire school population? If it is the last of these, we should be able to detect differences in satisfaction with height as a function of school composition.

Clausen (1975) cites data from the Oakland Growth Study in which students were rated by their peers on a number of characteristics. The study found that the tallest boys were regarded by their peers as the least friendly and least assured. While these findings are puzzling in light of the positive aspects of being tall, the peers ratings were considerably more influenced by a mesomorphic body type than by height, per se.

In a study by Jourard and Secord (1954), the relationship between several body measurements and satisfaction with those body measurements (referred to as body-cathexis by the authors) was discussed for late adolescence. Among undergraduate males, they discovered that increased measurements were positively correlated with increased satisfaction with that dimension. This held for height, shoulders, chest (both relaxed and expanded) and muscular strength. Thus, as one would have suspected, increased height is related to increased satisfaction with one's height. This was the only study for males which directly examined satisfaction with one's body in relationship to the actual dimensions of the body.

In summary, before we move to the next section, it is appropriate to note that the literature has seriously examined four dimensions of physical characteristics in relationship to social and psychological development in the adolescent time period. The first of these involves early or late maturation. Although this characteristic can be assessed in several ways as noted above, it is a general summary of a number of changes which are occurring together but at varying rates. The second and third dimensions of physical development which were discussed had to do with sheer weight (or bulk) and body type (or leanness). It was discovered that this distinction between absolute weight and weight relative to its distribution in terms of height was probably important. Finally, we have noted that height itself for boys is a significant factor which can affect how the individual feels about himself and his body. Having thus delineated four aspects of physical development which are important, we now turn to the issue of which aspects of psychological development we shall examine in greater detail.

STATEMENT OF PROBLEM

The rest of this chapter explores the effects of these four dimensions of physical development on early adolescents' *satisfaction* with different aspects of their physical development and on the development of their *self-image*. In the pioneering work of Secord and Jourard (1953), the relationship between body satisfaction and self-image is firmly established for older adolescents (college undergraduates). They find a correlation of .58 for males between body-cathexis (satisfaction with one's body) and what they described as self-cathexis (satisfaction with the self). This study serves to demonstrate that feelings toward the body can play a significant part in the mental health of adolescents. Lerner and Brackney (1978) and Klein and Simmons (1978) show similar findings, the latter with different measures. However, using a somewhat different approach, Musa and Roach (1973) reported that an individual's self-evaluation of his personal appearance relative to other students was not significantly related to his total self-concept. In only one of the studies cited above was the relationship between *actual body size* and satisfaction with body image or self-image explored directly. Thus, while it is a generally accepted notion in social psychology that specific aspects of one's physical appearance such as body type, height, and weight can significantly affect *both* one's satisfaction with one's appearance and one's total self-image, this assertion requires more testing.

Furthermore, there has been little or no examination of the consequences of a given set of physical characteristics for individuals when those individuals are in significantly different school environments for the early adolescent time period. Here, we are specifically referring to different age groupings of early adolescents which place them in contexts where they are either the oldest or the youngest in relationship to their school peers. Stolz and Stolz (1944) note the potential importance of different school environments when they say, "The nicknames and the thoughtless derogatory comments which, before the adolescent period, may cause the fat boy or girl only rather vague discomfort or no discomfort at all, take on a new penetrative quality for the physically self-conscious and socially sensitive juvenile in the less friendly atmosphere of the junior high school" (1944:90).

All these issues will be explored in this paper, using three dimensions of satisfaction with body-image: satisfaction with height, satisfaction with weight, and satisfaction with muscle development. That is, the four dimensions of physical development (height, weight, body leanness, and pubertal onset) will be related first to the above three aspects of satisfaction with one's body. Then, we shall investigate the impact of these same physical characteristics and of body-image satisfaction upon the total self-image. In delineating the aspects of the total self-image which might be affected by either physical characteristics directly or by satisfaction with those characteristics, we shall discuss: (1) the overall evaluation of self in terms of self-esteem; (2) one's degree of sensitivity to others in terms of self-consciousness; and (3) one's general sense of a constant identity (the stability of the self).

METHOD

Sample

The data for the analysis in this paper come from the first two years of a five-year longitudinal study being conducted in the Milwaukee Public Schools (see Simmons *et al.*, 1978, 1979; Blyth *et al.*, 1978, 1980; Bush *et al.*, 1978). In this study, students were followed from the sixth grade through the tenth grade within the public school system. The initial design of the study involved comparing (1) schools which were kindergarten through eighth grade and fed into four-year high schools to (2) schools which were kindergarten through sixth grade and fed first into three-year junior highs and then into three-year senior highs. (For the purposes of the current analyses, we will use only those students who were in directly comparable school types as defined in Blyth *et al.*, 1978; that is, in predominantly white schools. There were no predominantly black K-8 schools in Milwaukee.) After schools had been categorized either as K-8 or as K-6 feeding into a three-year junior high, we invited all of the K-8 schools and a stratified random sample of the K-6 schools to particiate. All but one of the seven K-8 schools participated. In selecting eight K-6 schools which would be as comparable as possible to the K-8 schools, we used a constrained, stratified, random sampling procedure (see Simmons *et al.*, 1979). The two stratifying variables were the percentage of minority students in the school (0 to 20 percent versus 21 percent to 42 percent) and the size of the sixth-grade class within each school.

These factors were used because of their high association with such other school variables as achievement scores and social behaviors. A comparison of the schools selected with those in the entire Milwaukee school population from which they were drawn indicates a high degree of comparability along a number of social and educational variables such as family income, mean achievement levels and experience levels of teachers (see Blyth, 1977). Along the same characteristics, the K-8 and comparable K-6 schools were shown to be very similar (see Blyth, 1977). Furthermore, a comparison of father's education, occupation, and marital status revealed no statistically significant differences between our sample of students in the two types of schools.

Within each of the 14 schools so selected, all sixth-grade students were asked to participate in the study. This gave every student within each stratum of the sample an equal probability of being invited to participate. Parental permission was solicited from all sixth-graders in the sampled schools and was secured from 85 percent of the population. In the second year of the study, we were able to reinterview 88.5 percent of these students so that a total of 75 percent of the original population of sixth-graders in the 14 schools were followed over the two-year period under consideration. Thus, there are 622 students in the current sample (boys and girls). Furthermore, a comparison of the students we interviewed versus those we were unable to interview the first year indicates only a slight bias in terms of higher standard achievement scores and greater school attendance, with no difference in grade point average (Blyth *et al.*, 1978:153).

All students in the study participated in a one-hour personal interview conducted by professional survey research interviewers in their school. These interviews covered a wide range of topics dealing with self-image, perception of others' expectations, attitudes toward school, and several behavioral questions. Data on the individual's physical development were collected by a registered nurse every six months and involved both anthropometric measurements and a brief interview on attitudes toward recent growth.

For the purposes of this paper, we will be looking only at white males who are in comparable school types during the sixth and seventh grade and who were less than 13.5 years of age in sixth grade. This last condition affected only six students and was included in order to eliminate those students who were significantly below grade level for their age. It was felt these students could bias the relationship between physical characteristics and other dimensions since they were more than two years older than the majority of other students in the sample. Our total sample for this analysis is 274 boys.

Measurement

Physical Characteristics.   As mentioned earlier, we are interested primarily in measuring height, weight, early pubertal growth, and body leanness. Thus, for the purposes of current analyses, we will confine our interests to the absolute height (in inches), absolute weight (in pounds), the change in height between sixth and seventh grade (inches per year), and the ponderal index score for each student. The ponderal index is a measure of body leanness and is calculated by taking the ratio of height in inches to the cube root of weight in pounds (see Hendry and Gillies, 1978; or Tanner, 1964).

It should be noted that the height measurements were made using specially designed portable equipment similar to that used by Stolz and Stolz (1951). Students were asked to stand with their heels and back up against a vertical board while a perpendicular headpiece was lowered to the crown of the head with the student looking directly forward. The average of two measurements was used as the individual's height score to the nearest millimeter. Measurements were later changed to inches to facilitate the calculation of the ponderal index. Weight was measured on the available school scales to the nearest quarter of a pound. Each scale was calibrated using a certified 25-pound weight at the beginning of each day.

In order to validate the use of the ponderal index as calculated from height and weight measurements, we looked at the correlation between this index and the nurse's rating of the student in terms of how athletic his build was (.33) and in terms of whether he was thin or obese (.72). These two latter ratings were combined to create a categorical variable describing endomorphic, mesomorphic, and ectomorphic body builds.[1] The correlation between this created variable and the ponderal index was .61 (p < .001). Since the ponderal index of body leanness is a continuous variable rather than a categorical variable and an objective rather than a subjective indicator, we shall use it for the current analyses.

In calculating the change in height between sixth- and seventh-grade measurements, we took a simple difference score between heights and divided it by the number of days between measurements. This was then adjusted to reflect the change in inches per year. Since there was a correlation of .97 between height as measured in sixth grade and height as measured in seventh grade, we did not attempt to adjust for the small amount of unreliability. As in Simmons *et al.*, (1979), this measure can be used as an index of puberty. The very fast growers are likely to be in their growth spurt and thus be early maturers, while the slowest growers are unlikely to be pubertal as yet (see Stolz and Stolz, 1951).[2] Thus, for our purposes, we have adapted a previously used index of pubertal development. While the previous index required a longitudinal study and multiple measures of height throughout adolescence, the present index can be utilized in early adolescence. By using the norms developed with this prior index, we are able to identify boys as probably early and non-early developers in seventh grade at the onset of adolescence; we do not have to wait until adolescence is completed for classification.[3] It should be noted that this measure of puberty correlates with

Table 1.   Intercorrelations between Physical Characteristics
(White Males Only)

	Leanness	Rate of Height Growth	Weight
Height (inches)	−.06	.62*	.71*
Leanness (Height/Weight^{-3})		−.01	−.72*
Rate of Height Growth (inches/yr.)			.40*
Weight (pounds)			

N = 274
*p < .01

several less rigorous ones we collected. As reported in Simmons *et al.*, (1979):

> Among medium height boys, rate of height growth . . . correlates significantly (p < .05) with
> other indicators of puberty: presence of underarm hair (r = .19), self-reported rate of muscle
> growth (.11), degree of voice change (.17), presence of acne (.30), presence of lip hair (.23),
> nurse's rating of muscular build (.41), and nurse's overall rating of physical maturity (.44).

The intercorrelations between the four dimensions of physical development are indicated in Table 1. All of the correlations are quite high with the exception of the relationship between height and leanness. The correlations are as expected, given the fact that these are early adolescents, some of whom have begun to grow rapidly and are likely to be taller and somewhat heavier than their classmates. The correlations between rate of height growth and leanness and between absolute height and leanness are low, since the degree of excess fat need not be associated with how tall or how fast one is growing. It is interesting to note that when we asked the nurses to rate students as to whether they were younger looking or older looking than the other students at that grade level we found their judgments to be highly correlated with absolute height (.67) and weight (.60). This would suggest that those students who are both heavy (but not necessarily fat) and tall appear to an observer to be more physically mature than their age mates. Finally, the negative correlation between weight and leanness is a function of the direction of the ponderal index score where a high score indicates thinness or a more ectomorphic body type, while a low score indicates obesity or a more endomorphic body type.

Satisfaction With Body-Image.   The student's satisfaction with his body-image is measured for three different aspects of physical development: height, weight, and overall muscle development. In each of these areas the student was asked during the interview to respond to the following three questions:

> How happy are you with how tall you are? Are you very happy, somewhat happy, not very
> happy, or not at all happy with how tall you are?

How happy are you with how much you weigh?

How happy are you with your overall muscle development?

For each of the questions the same four-point scale was used. In order to facilitate the interpretation of the correlations, a score indicating high satisfaction on each of the questions received a four, with a low-satisfaction score receiving a one.

It is interesting to note that the correlations between the different dimensions of satisfaction with body type are significant at the .01 level, but not very large. The correlation between satisfaction with height and satisfaction with weight is only .16, as is the correlation between satisfaction with height and satisfaction with overall muscle development. The correlation between satisfaction with weight and one's satisfaction with muscle development is .20. The significant but low intercorrelation suggests that it is not advisable to build a single satisfaction with doby image scale, but rather to treat each aspect separately. This is in contrast to the procedure used by Jourard and Secord (1954). Unfortunately, Secord and Jourard do not report on the degree of internal consistency of their scales but only on the split-half reliability of the scale (.78 for males).

Self-Image Dimensions. As noted previously, this chapter shall look at three dimensions of self-image: self-esteem, self-consciousness, and the stability of the self-image. These dimensions of the self-image are of considerable importance theoretically in relation to changing physical development in the adolescent time period. In this chapter, we adopt Murphy's (1947) view of the self as "the individual as known to the individual." So conceived, the self-image can be viewed as one's attitude toward an object where the object is one's self. As a result, it can be broken down into several dimensions, as noted by Rosenberg (1965).

The first dimension of self-image to be considered is self-esteem or the individual's global positive or negative attitude toward himself. Wylie (1961) notes that probably more research has been devoted to this aspect of the self-image than to all others combined (see Rosenberg, 1979). Simmons *et al.,* (1973) believes this is "probably attributable to the great relevance of self-esteem for emotional disturbance." In order to measure self-esteem, we use the same scale as Simmons *et al.* (1973) which consists of six items adapted from the earlier Rosenberg scale (see Simmons *et al.,* 1973:567 for the complete list of items in this scale). This scale is a six-item Guttman scale with a coefficient of reproducibility of .927 and a coefficient of scalability of .765, a minimal marginal reproducibility of .690 and the percent of improvement is .237. These coefficients are comparable to those found by Simmons *et al.* (1973) in earlier research. A high score on the scale indicates that the person considers himself to be a person of worth, though not necessarily superior to others. On the other hand, a low score would seem to indicate some degree of self-rejection or dissatisfaction.

The second dimension of the self-image to be considered is self-consciousness and refers to the salience of the self to the individual. More specifically, it refers to the extent to which the individual is painfully aware of and bothered by the reactions of others to himself and his behavior. Given the degree of physical changes which are taking place during adolescence, it is theoretically important to know whether or not such changes have an effect on how self-conscious the individual is with regard to others' evaluations.

The self-consciousness scale used here is an adaptation of that used by Simmons et al. (1973) and Rosenberg (1979). The scale contains four items and is scored as a Guttman scale with a coefficient of reproducibility of .933, a coefficient of scalability of .620, a minimal marginal reproducibility of .824 and the percent improvement is .109. The four items used in the scale are as follows:

A young person said: "When I am with people I get nervous because I worry about how much they like me." Do you feel like this often*, sometimes, or never?

Let's say some grownup or adult visitors came into class and the teacher wanted them to know who you were, so she asked you to stand up and tell a little about yourself. Would you like that, not like it*, or wouldn't you care*?

If the teacher asked you to get up in front of the class and talk a little bit about your summer, would you be very nervous*, a little nervous, or not at all nervous?

If you did get up in front of the class and tell them about your summer, would you think a lot about how all the kids were looking at you*, a little bit about how all the kids were looking at you*, or wouldn't you think at all about the kids looking at you?

The responses with asterisks are those responses considered to reflect high self-consciousness on a scale scored such that a high value equals high self-consciousness.

The final dimension of self-image has to do with how stable the individual's attitude is toward himself. Theoretically, one could argue that a person undergoing rapid growth or other physical changes in adolescence might change how he feels about himself frequently and thus have an unstable self-image.

The stability of the self-image is measured with a four-item Guttman scale which has been adapted from the work of Simmons et al. (1973) and Rosenberg (1979). The scale has a coefficient of reproducibility of .901, a coefficient of scalability of .650, a minimal marginal reproducibility of .718 and a percent improvement of .184. The four items in the scale are as follows:

How sure are you that you know what kind of person you really are? Are you very sure, pretty sure, not very sure*, or not at all sure*?

How often do you feel mixed up about yourself, about what you are really like? Often*, sometimes*, or never.

A kid said: "Some days I am happy with the kind of person I am, other days I am not happy with the kind of person I am." Do your feelings change like this? Yes*, No.

A kid said: "Some days I think I am one kind of a person, other days, a different kind of person." Do your feelings change like this? Yes*, No.

Each of the responses marked with an asterisk indicate instability and the scale is scored such that a high value equals high stability.

All three of these dimensions assess different aspects of one's attitudes toward oneself. As such, it is interesting to note that the correlation between self-esteem and self-consciousness is $-.13$, as is the correlation between self-consciousness and stability. These correlations are negative because high self-esteem and high stability are negatively related to high self-consciousness. The correlation between self-esteem and stability is higher $(.35)$ and positive. All of these correlations are significant at the .01 level or better. Once again, we have a situation where the three dimensions of a theoretically important concept are not sufficiently highly correlated to permit building a single overall scale. Furthermore, greater clarity and specificity should be obtained by using these dimensions separately. (See Rosenberg, 1979, for a discussion of the importance of examining separate dimensions of the self-image.)

FINDINGS AND DISCUSSION

Satisfaction With Body-Image

Before we look at the various findings concerning satisfaction with body-image and different physical characteristics, it is important to note the possibility of curvilinear relationships in this area. That is, it is quite possible that short and tall people will be equally dissatisfied while average people are satisfied. Given the high possibility of such curvilinear relationships, the first step taken in the analysis was to test for the existence of curvilinearity by doing a one way analysis of variance using trichotomized physical characteristics.

To be consistent with earlier work (see Simmons *et al.*, 1979), rate of height growth was trichotomozed as discussed above. The other physical characteristics were trichotomized so as to create a roughly 20 percent-60 percent-20 percent split. This method was chosen as preferable since it also provided other information useful for substantive interpretation. The split was made at these points so as to look at groups which were, in general, more than a standard deviation away from the average value for the sample.

When the relationship between satisfaction with a body-image dimension and a physical characteristic is found to be nonlinear, we used an analysis of variance

Table 2.   Mean Satisfaction with Height as a Function of Physical Characteristics
(White Males Only)

				With Covariates		
	F-Test for Linearity	Oneway Analysis of Variance	Height	Leanness	Rate of Height Growth	Weight
Height						
Short		2.59	—	2.59	2.67	2.68
Average		3.20	—	3.20	3.21	3.21
Tall		3.43	—	3.44	3.34	3.33
F-Value	5.22**	23.04**	—	23.02*	12.05*	10.69*
Rate of Height Growth						
Slow		2.94	3.14	2.94	—	3.00
Medium		3.13	3.10	3.13	—	3.13
Fast		3.43	3.18	3.43	—	3.34
F-Value	.27	11.72*	.26	11.67*	—	5.13*
Leanness						
Fat		3.32	3.22	—	3.31	2.91
Average		3.03	3.09	—	3.03	3.09
Thin		3.28	3.21	—	3.29	3.43
F-Value	9.43*	4.72*	1.15	—	5.15*	6.97*
Weight						
Light		2.74	3.08	2.61	2.83	—
Medium		3.18	3.17	3.15	3.17	—
Heavy		3.44	3.12	3.69	3.37	—
F-Value	1.24	14.53*	.37	21.94*	7.53*	—

Grand Mean = 3.14
N = 274
*p < .01
**p < .05

and covariance framework to explore the nature of the relationship, both directly and controlling for other physical characteristics. If the relationship was found to be linear, we used a correlational procedure with zero-order and partial correlations to explore the relationship. This latter method took advantage of the full range of our independent variables.

Satisfaction With Height.   Table 2 summarizes the basic findings with regard to the relationship of satisfaction with height to the different physical characteristics under study. When we look at the first set of rows in the table we find that there is a significant relationship between satisfaction with height and actual height. As one would expect, short individuals are significantly more dissatisfied with their height than are either average or tall individuals (compare the mean satisfaction of 2.59 to 3.20 and to 3.43). Furthermore, this relationship persists even when we take out the variance due to leanness, rate of height growth or weight.

From the rest of the table, it would appear at first as if other physical characteristics also affect satisfaction with height. In particular, fast growers (i.e., those who may be entering puberty) and those who weigh more appear significantly more satisfied with their height. However, as we recall from Table 1, tall youngsters are more likely to be fast growers and heavier. One would therefore presume that it is their greater height, rather than their fast growth or weight, that is affecting their satisfaction with height; and, in fact, when height is controlled, neither rate of height growth nor weight nor leanness remains significantly associated with satisfaction with height.

In summary, as one might have expected, an individual's satisfaction with his height is largely a function of his actual height; those who are shortest are least satisfied; those who are tallest are most satisfied. This effect of height on satisfaction with height holds in both K-8 and junior high schools. One might expect the relationship to be stronger in a junior high school, where there are many more older and taller boys with whom to compare oneself. However, a two-way analysis of variance exploring the impact of school type and height on satisfaction with height reveals no significant interaction—there is no significant difference between school types in the effect of height on satisfaction with height.

The interaction between rate of height growth and school type, however, was found to be significant. Those boys who were rapidly growing in the junior high school were considerably more satisfied with their height than those in the K-8 school. However, those individuals who were slow growers in the K-8 were the most dissatisfied, even more than the comparable slow growers in the junior high school. While we cannot explain the latter effect, it is possible that the rapid growers in the junior high school are pleased to be catching up to older boys in the school. Although the number of cases begins to get small when we examine the effects of school type and then try to introduce a control variable, the introduction of height as a covariate does reduce these differences.

Satisfaction With Weight. Table 3 contains the findings with regard to satisfaction with weight as a function of physical characteristics. Perhaps the first thing to note is that the overall level of satisfaction with weight is less than the satisfaction with height. Since the relationship between satisfaction with weight and most physical characteristics is curvilinear, we will once again use an analysis of variance and covariance framework.

At first, it appears that tall persons are significantly less satisfied with their weight than their shorter peers. This reaction, however, is not due to the height of the tall boys but to the fact that many of them are, in reality, heavy. When weight is controlled, no significant relationship between height and satisfaction with weight remains.

When we look at the effect of different degrees of leanness in relation to

Table 3.   Mean Satisfaction with Weight as a Function of
Physical Characteristics (White Males Only)

	F-Test for Linearity	Oneway Analysis of Variance	With Covariates			
			Weight	Leanness	Rate of Height Growth	Weight
Height						
Short		2.88	—	2.86	3.01	2.66
Average		2.93	—	2.92	2.95	2.91
Tall		2.61	—	2.64	2.46	2.86
F-Value	4.21**	4.23**	—	3.51**	8.33*	2.06
Rate of Height Growth						
Slow		2.89	2.82	2.90	—	2.80
Medium		2.73	2.74	2.71	—	2.73
Fast		2.90	2.99	2.91	—	3.02
F-Value	2.79***	1.40	2.04	1.97	—	3.60**
Leanness						
Fat		2.40	2.41	—	2.39	2.55
Average		2.99	2.98	—	2.99	2.96
Thin		2.86	2.86	—	2.86	2.80
F-Value	17.77*	13.69*	12.52*	—	13.71*	5.05*
Weight						
Light		2.84	2.87	2.78	2.91	—
Medium		3.01	3.01	3.00	3.00	—
Heavy		2.35	2.32	2.46	2.31	—
F-Value	24.10*	18.26*	17.08*	9.84*	19.85*	—

Grand Mean = 2.85
N = 274
*p < .01
**p < .05
***p < .10

satisfaction with weight, we find exactly what one would predict. Those boys who are obese tend to be most dissatisfied with their weight, while those who are quite thin for their height are slightly more dissatisfied than those who are average. This relationship persists when we control for height, rate of growth, and weight. In addition, when we examine the last row of the table, there are similar significant differences for weight which do not disappear when we adjust for leanness; that is, boys who weigh most are most dissatisfied with their weight. Furthermore, despite the general value placed on being thin in our society, both our thinner- and lighter-than-average boys were less satisfied with their weight than were boys of average leanness or weight.

With respect to different rates of height growth, we find no overall differences in satisfaction with weight which reach a significant level until we control for the student's actual weight. When weight is introduced as a covariate, we find that rapidly growing boys are somewhat more satisfied with their weight than are the medium and slow growing boys. This finding could be due to the different nature of the weight for rapidly growing or pubertal boys versus slow-growing or pre-pubertal youth. At the same level of weight, pubertal boys may be developing muscle, while slow-growing, pre-pubertal youth still find themselves with a distribution in body-fat which is definable as sexually inappropriate (see Stolz and Stolz, 1944). Unfortunately, neither the measure of weight nor leanness captured this distinction in the components of weight directly. This issue is discussed further when we examine boys' satisfaction with their muscle development. If this reasoning is accurate, we would expect fast-growing boys to be more satisfied with their muscular development.

In summary then, an individual's satisfaction with his weight is largely a function of his actual weight and the distribution of that weight with respect to his height. Both heavy and light boys were more dissatisfied than medium weight boys and the more obese boys were particularly dissatisfied when compared to their leaner counterparts.

When we ran checks to explore whether one's satisfaction with weight was in any way altered by being in different types of schools with differing numbers of older and younger peers, we found no main effects or interactions. This would suggest that one's satisfaction with his weight is not as affected by those around him as it is by a more generally accepted or societally defined standard.

Satisfaction with Overall Muscle Development. In our sample of white males, we find that they are generally satisfied with their overall level of muscle development, though not quite as satisfied as they are with height. In testing for nonlinearity, we find that all of the relationships are linear so that it is possible to switch to a correlational analysis.

If it is true, as we suggested above, that fast growers are entering puberty early and therefore becoming more muscular, then one would expect fast-growing boys to be more satisfied with their muscle development. In fact, Table 4 shows a significant correlation of .14 at the zero-order level between rate of height growth and satisfaction with muscles; this correlation persists when controls for height, leanness, and weight are introduced. Thus, as predicted, those individuals who are growing most rapidly are more satisfied with their level of muscle development.

At the zero-order level, taller, less lean, and heavier boys also appear slightly more satisfied with their muscle development. Most of these factors lose significance when any other physical factor is controlled, however. Unfortunately, none of our measures directly taps muscularity—that is, the body weight of heavier and less lean boys may be due to either increased muscle, or fat, or both.

In summary then, we found that satisfaction with muscle development is most

Table 4.   Correlations of Satisfaction with Muscle Development with Physical Characteristics (White Males Only)

	F-Test for Linearity	Zero-order Correlation	Controlling for ...			
			Height	Leanness	Rate of Height Growth	Weight
Height	1.14	.08***	—	.07	−.01	.01
Rate of Height Growth	.62	.14*	.12**	.14*	—	.11**
Leanness	.05	−.08***	−.07	—	−.08***	−.02
Weight	1.40	.10***	.06	.05	.04	—

Grand Mean = 3.02
N = 274
*p < .01
**p < .05
***p < .10

affected by one's rate of height growth, which is an indicator of boys' early development. The effects for height, leanness, and weight are significant but are not particularly strong.

In order to test for the possible effects of differences in school types with respect to satisfaction with muscular development, we ran a dummy variable regression including a school type and a school type by physical characteristic interaction term. The only significant interaction with respect to satisfaction with muscular development occurred for leanness. When we explored this finding further, we discovered that the relationship between leanness and satisfaction with muscle development was significantly negative only in the junior high school (−.16, p < .05) and near 0 in the K-8 school. These data suggest that being thin in junior high school was particularly disadvantageous with respect to how satisfied a boy was with his muscular build. This finding may reflect a different comparison group in junior high school, given the higher proportion of physically mature and muscular youth.

Effects on Self-Image

In the next series of tables we shall be exploring the relationship between physical characteristics and the different dimensions of self-image noted above. In doing this, we will report only the correlational analysis since the relationships are linear.

Self-Esteem.   Table 5 contains the basic analysis with respect to self-esteem. An adolescent's physical characteristics appear to be significantly but mildly related to his global positive or negative view of himself. However, the relationships are complex. Several of the body-type characteristics that go together affect the self-esteem in opposite directions, thus acting as "suppressor variables" and "spurious antecedent variables" (see Rosenberg, 1968) for each other. Thus, as noted above, among tall boys there are many who are also fast growers; that is, who have reached their pubertal growth spurt earlier than their peers and are considered early maturers. Also among tall children, there are many very heavy youths. However, greater height, early maturing, and increased weight do not all affect the self-esteem in the same direction.

As Table 5 shows, heavier and more obese youth have significantly lower self-esteem; the zero-order correlation between weight and self-esteem is $-.15$ and the correlation between leanness and self-esteem is $.12$.[4] It also appears at first glance that tall boys have slightly lower self-esteem than short boys (Table V: $r = -.08$, $p < .10$). This result is surprising, given the earlier finding that tall boys are more satisfied with their height. In fact, the negative relationship between self-esteem and height is a spurious one due to the association of greater height with greater weight. That is, because tall boys are more likely to be heavy and heavy boys tend to have low self-esteem, it appears as if height itself is disadvantageous for self-esteem. But when weight is controlled, the relationship between height and self-esteem disappears (partial $r = .04$). Thus, at this age, we have many tall, heavy boys whose self-esteem is lower than that of their peers— but this is a result of their heaviness not of their height.

What about the effect of early maturity or rapid height growth on self-esteem? (See Simmons *et al.*, 1979.) The zero-order correlation indicates no relationship ($r = .04$). However, the real relationship appears to be suppressed by the association of rapid height growth with greater weight and height. When either weight or height is controlled, a positive, significant relationship (partial $r = .11$, $p < .05$) between rate of height growth and self-esteem emerges; that is, while heavy, tall children have lower self-esteem, fast growing youths have higher

Table 5. Correlations of Self-esteem with Physical Characteristics
(White Males Only)

	F-Test For Linearity	Zero-order Correlation	Controlling for . . .			
			Height	Leanness	Rate of Height Growth	Weight
Height	.07	$-.08$***	—	$-.08$***	$-.14$*	.04
Height Growth	1.15	.04	.11**	.04	—	.11**
Leanness	2.46	.12**	.12**	—	.12**	.01
Weight	.39	$-.15$*	$-.14$*	$-.10$**	$-.19$*	—

N = 273
*p < .01
**p < .05
***p < .10

self-esteem. This effect of fast growth is hidden because so many fast growing youngsters are also heavy and suffer in self-esteem due to this heaviness.[5] It is likely that the increasing muscularity and absence of "baby fat" associated with the rapid growth of puberty is beneficial to self-esteem, while heaviness itself is detrimental.

In summary, we find that self-esteem is most closely related to the weight of these adolescent boys. The findings suggest that tall, heavy, fat boys have the lowest self-esteem, while early developers (the fast growers) have higher self-esteem. The effects of heaviness and those of early puberty mask each other to some extent.

Does one's evaluation of himself depend in part upon the setting and particularly the peer group which is used as a reference point? In order to explore this, we looked at the relationships in a linear regression model using school type and the interaction of school type with each physical characteristic as independent variables. In doing this, we found only one significant interaction and that had to do with leanness. When we ran zero-order correlations for the relationship between self-esteem and leanness for K-8 students separately from junior high students, we found no significant relation among the K-8 students ($-.05$), but a strong positive relationship in the junior high school ($.22$, $p < .01$). It is interesting to note that the effect of weight on self-esteem is also considerably stronger in the junior high school than in the K-8 school ($-.21$ vs. $-.05$), although the interaction term does not quite reach statistical significance. These findings suggest that those individuals who are learner or less heavy in appearance have a strong self-esteem advantage in the junion high school, where more and more of the older youths have lost their prepubertal "baby fat." In the K-8 schools, where there are fewer individuals in this advanced state of physical maturity, it is possible that being lean and athletic is somewhat less important and hence has less effect on how one evaluates oneself.

Self-Consciousness. The relationship between self-consciousness and the physical characteristics measured are again only moderate ones (see Table 6), very similar in many ways to the relationships of these characteristics with self-esteem. Being heavy or fat is detrimental to yet another aspect of the self-picture. Heavier males ($r = .16$, $p < .01$) are more self-conscious as are more obese males ($r = -.14$, $p < .01$).[6] Once again, tall youths, at first glance, appear slightly but significantly more self-conscious ($r = .08$, $p < .10$). However, this increased self-consciousness is probably due to their heaviness, since the relationship drops below the level of statistical significance and is in the opposite direction when weight is controlled. Early development or rapid height growth appears unrelated to self-consciousness, although it had favorable effects for self-esteem.

In summary, heavy children are most likely to be self-conscious. When we

Table 6. Correlation of Self-consciousness with Physical Characteristics
(White Males Only)

	F-Test for Linearity	Zero-order Correlation	Controlling for . . .			
			Height	Leanness	Rate of Height Growth	Weight
Height	.01	.08***	—	.06	.06	−.07
Height Growth	.91	.04	−.01	.04	—	−.03
Leanness	.54	−.14*	−.15*	—	−.15*	−.04
Weight	.34	.16*	.16*	.09***	.16*	—

N = 274
*p < .01
**p < .05
***p < .10

looked at differences in self-consciousness in the junior high school as opposed to the K-8 school, we found no significant interaction terms.

Stability of Self. When we look at the effects of different physical characteristics on how stable one perceives his self-image, virtually none of the correlations are significant (see Table 7). Only when we look at weight do we find even a slight, significant correlation and this occurs only when we introduce rate of growth as a control variable. Here, once again the relationship suggests that being heavy has negative consequences for the self-image. Those individuals who are heavier in absolute weight have a slightly less stable view of themselves, particularly when the variance due to rate of height growth is removed. Thus, rate of height growth has acted as a mild suppressor variable.

This effect of weight on stability is no different in junior high than in the K-8 school. The only significant interaction for self-stability using school type involves height. It turns out that height has a negative effect on the stability of the self-image only in the K-8 schools and either no effect or a slight positive effect in the junior high schools (−.10 vs. .97). This would suggest that being tall in an environment that has few tall people may cause uncertainty about oneself.

Summary. Of the four physical characteristics measured here—height, rate of height growth (an indicator of early pubertal development), leanness, and actual weight—actual weight has the greatest effects on early adolescent boys' satisfaction with their body image and on the self-image in general. Being heavy or fat carries with it many negative consequences. Heavy and fat boys are least satisfied with their weight (although average boys are more satisfied than those who are thinner than average.) Compared to their peers, heavy boys also have the

Table 7.   Correlation of Stability of Self-image with Physical Characteristics
(White Males Only)

	F-Test for Linearity	Zero-order Correlation	Controlling for...			
			Height	Leanness	Rate of Height Growth	Weight
Height	.95	−.04	—	−.04	−.07	.01
Height Growth	1.31	.02	.06	.02	—	.05
Leanness	2.47	.04	.04	—	.04	−.02
Weight	.04	−.07	−.06	−.06	−.09***	—

N = 272
*p < .01
**p < .05
***p < .10

lowest self-esteem, are the most painfully self-conscious, and show the least stable self-image.

Being taller than average is an advantage only in terms of satisfaction with height itself. It has little effect on other aspects of the self-image when the remaining physical characteristics (weight, height growth, and leanness) are controlled.

Early pubertal development, as indexed by rate of height growth, appears to be an advantage when weight and height are controlled. In seventh grade, early developing boys are more satisfied with their weight and their muscular development and show higher self-esteem than do other boys. We have suggested that these advantages reflect the pubertal boy's satisfaction with his greater muscularity and with his loss of the "baby fat" possessed by many of his less developed fellow students.

Unfortunately, we have no objective indicator of muscularity to verify this hypothesis. The concept of leanness was introduced to deal with the fact that some children will weigh more than others due to height not body mass. However, in neither the measure of leanness nor body weight can we distinguish between body mass due to fat and due to muscle. Furthermore, it is difficult to conceptualize why some relationships between leanness and dimensions of the self-image disappear when weight is controlled. It should, however, be noted that leanness was more highly correlated to a nurse's rating of obesity than was weight (.72 versus −.64) and that weight was more highly correlated to the nurse's rating of athleticness (−.54 versus .33). It is probably more important to note that at a zero-order level, heavy body weight and being less lean than average are both disadvantageous, and that the above negative effects of weight persist when all other variables including leanness are controlled.

In addition, it should be noted that at this age, early development, height, and heaviness are correlated; that is, there are many fast growing, tall, heavy boys. For such boys, their fast growth is an advantage, while their weight is a disadvantage. These contrary effects tend to mask one another and also lead to erroneous first conclusions. Thus, for example, it appears that taller boys are less satisfied with their weight and have lower self-esteem than do other boys. Yet, their height itself has little effect on these variables; it is their increased weight that has the negative effect. Finally, comparison of the effects of these variables in a K-8 versus a junior high school environment revealed only a few significant differences.

Relationship between Self-Image Dimensions and Satisfaction with Body-Image

We have found evidence that the adolescents' basic physical characteristics affect both his satisfaction with his body and his self-image. We now turn to an exploration of whether these latter two constructs are related; whether the dimensions of the self-image studied here are themselves directly affected by body-image satisfiaction. In particular, given the work of Secord and Jourard (1953), which indicated a high relationship between satisfaction with one's body and satisfaction with one's self-image, one would expect to find a strong relationship.

Table 8 summarizes the correlations between the three self-image dimensions and the three satisfaction dimensions for each school type separately and for the entire population. First of all, satisfaction with height appears to have few significant, consistent effects. Adolescents' satisfaction with height has no effect on self-esteem, a positive effect on self-consciousness only in K-8 schools, and contrary effects on stability depending on school type. While the overall relationship between satisfaction with height and stability is virtually zero, the relationship for students in K-8 schools is strongly negative, while in junior high schools it is strongly positive ($-.20$ versus $.20$). This suggests that in K-8 schools, the more one is satisfied with one's height, the less stable is one's self-image. This might be due to the fact that those individuals who are satisfied with their height are most likely taller and hence stick out more in a K-8 environment. Because they deviate from the norm, they may be treated inconsistently. In the junior high environment, with the larger number of physically more mature individuals, the more satisfied a youth is with his height (and the taller he is), the more reassured he would be that he fits in.

However, satisfaction with weight is positively and significantly correlated with all three dimensions of the self-image. Those more satisfied with their weight show higher self-esteem, less self-consciousness, and greater stability of the self-picture in both K-8 and junior high schools.

Finally, satisfaction with muscular development has significant effects on the self-image only in junior high school. In junior high school, those more satisfied with their muscle development have higher self-esteem ($r = .20$), lower self-consciousness ($r = -.10$) and greater stability of the self-picture ($r = .17$). In K-8 schools, satisfaction with muscular development has no effect upon the global

Table 8. Correlations between Self-image Dimensions and Satisfaction with Body-image Dimensions by School Type (White Males Only)

| | Satisfaction with . . . | | | | | | | | |
| | Height | | | Weight | | | Muscle Development | | |
	K-8	7-9	Total	K-8	7-9	Total	K-8	7-9	Total
Self-Esteem	-.03	.04	.01	.19**	.31*	.26*	-.04	.20*	.10**
Self-Consciousness	-.12***	-.01	-.05	-.14***	-.13**	-.13**	.00	-.10***	-.06
Stability of Self-Image	-.20**	.20*	.04	.22*	.19*	.20*	-.01	.17*	.09***

N for K-8 schools equals 111.
N for Junior Highs (7-9) equals 163.
*p < .01
**p < .05
***p < .10

self-image. Perhaps muscular development becomes more important in an environment where more boys are older and the norms for muscularity are more advanced.

In summary then, we find that satisfaction with weight, more than any other characteristic, is related to the three self-image dimensions. This relationship persists at a significant level for both school types; satisfaction with weight is always advantageous for the self-image.

While being satisfied with one's muscle development has vitually no effect in the K-8 schools, it has a consistent positive effect on all the self-image dimensions in the junior high schools.

CONCLUSION

A stratified random sample of 274 white boys from the Milwaukee public school system was studied in seventh grade in order to determine the effects of puberty and objective physical characteristics upon early adolescents' self-image in general and upon satisfaction with their bodies in particular. Earlier studies investigating some of these phenomena have tended to deal with small extreme groups (rather than with an entire representative sample), use fewer physical characteristics and fewer differentiated dimensions of both body-image satisfaction and self-image. The early studies also tended to concentrate less on the early adolescent time period.

The effects of height, weight, body leanness, and pubertal development (as indexed by annual rate of height growth) were investigated. The major finding from this study is that being heavy (as measured by weight or body leanness) and being dissatisfied with one's weight had the most consistent and largest negative effects upon several dimensions of the self-image. Heavy boys and those dissatisfied with their weight had lower self-esteem, higher levels of self-consciousness, and less stable self-images than their peers.

In contrast, while a boy's being tall led to increased satisfaction with height itself, neither greater height nor satisfaction with height had consistent effects upon the overall self-image of the early adolescent.

Early pubertal development did seem to have some positive effects for the seventh-grade boys. Those boys who were growing the fastest (and therefore most likely to be pubertal) had the highest levels of self-esteem, once weight or height were controlled. On the basis of prior studies (Stolz and Stolz, 1951; Faust, 1977; Huenemann *et al.*, 1966) which indicate that pubertal development involves increased muscularity and decreased fatty tissue, we speculated that the advantage of early puberty for the self-esteem was due to feelings of satisfaction evoked by a muscular body. In fact, early developers (or fast growers) are the ones most satisfied both with their muscular development and their weight. And in certain environmental contexts, namely junior high school, boys who are more satisfied with their muscularity show higher self-esteem, lower self-consciousness, and greater stability of the self-picture than their fellow students.

The fact that school context conditions the effect of puberty on the self-image in this way is interesting. In an environment like the junior high school, where there are many more pubertal and, therefore, muscular boys, satisfaction with muscularity benefits the global self-image; in a context with more younger boys, such as the K-8 school, satisfaction with muscularity has little effect upon the dimensions of the self-image. Thus, the effects of a specific element of one's body image for the global self-picture can depend upon the context in which one finds oneself.

The general findings in our study concerning the effects of height, weight, and early development are consistent with the literature reported at the beginning of this paper, although our study asked a somewhat different set of questions and measured different variables than earlier work. The negative consequences of being fat, the positive consequences of muscularity, the positive effects of early development at the onset of adolescence, and the unclear effects of height for boys seem to fit with many prior research findings. The overwhelming disadvantage of being too fat should not be underestimated. In fact, studies of Richardson et al. (1961, 1968), which present subjects with photographs to rate, indicate that distaste for obese people is often greater than prejudice against racial minorities and than prejudice against the physically disabled.

There are many questions unanswered by this research, some of which we hope to answer by following these same boys further into adolescence. First of all, is early development merely a temporary advantage for early adolescent boys as some studies indicate (Peskin, 1967)? Will the self-esteem of late developers be higher in later years? Does the advantage of being muscular early disappear after everyone arrives at puberty and has greater muscular development? Secondly, will height assume more importance for the self-image once it finalizes? Perhaps, in early adolescence, relative height changes too frequently for youngsters to be affected by it. Perhaps the children are aware that being tall early does not necessarily correlate with one's final height relative to peers. Third, what are the effects of changing environmental contexts—changing school types—on the relationship between physical development and the self-image in middle and later adolescence? Finally, in later adolescence is there still a group of heavy, tall, early developing boys, for whom the advantages of muscularity and the disadvantages of weight counteract and mask one another? A future study either of this or later age groups should utilize a better, objective index of muscularity than the current study. It is important not only to control for height as we did when comparing children of different weights, but also to be able to distinguish between heavyset, muscular children and heavy, fat youngsters.

Finally, another set of questions revolves around the reasons early development or puberty affects a boy's self-image. We have speculated one cause to be satisfaction with a muscular-looking body. However, hormonal factors may also play a role. In addition, the important issue may be less the boy's pleasure at the way his body looks, than his satisfaction at being able to do well in athletic activities because of increased muscularity. Teasing out the causal linkages remains the work of future research.

In the interim, this study and others point to the importance of physical development and physical appearance for several dimensions of the global self-picture.

ACKNOWLEDGMENTS

The work of Blyth and Felt is primarily supported by the Boys Town Center for the Study of Youth Development. Simmons, Bulcroft, and Van Cleave are at the University of Minnesota, Department of Sociology. Bush is at the University of Arizona. The work of the second author is currently supported by a Research Development Award from the National Institute of Mental Health #2 KO2 MH-41688. The research for this article was made possible by NIMH Grant RO1 MH-30739 and a grant from the William T. Grant Foundation. Special gratitude is given to Dwight Rowe and the students and staff of the Milwaukee Public Schools who have made this study possible.

NOTES

1. The categorical body type variable was created by classifying as endomorphic those individuals who were rated as fat or chubby and not rated as very athletic looking; mesomorphs were those who were rated average in weight and at least a little athletic looking or were either chubby or thin but rated as very athletic looking; finally, ectomorphs were those who were rated either as average in weight but not athletic looking or thin but less than very athletic looking.

2. In this paper, this variable is treated as continuous for the most part. When it is trichotomized, the cutoff points are derived from Stolz and Stolz (1951) so that the slowest growing group is almost certainly nonpubertal (40 percent), and the fastest growing group is almost certainly pubertal (31 percent), with the middle group (29 percent) unclear. Boys whose yearly growth ranged from 25.4 millimeters to 49.9 millimeters (40 percent of the sample) were growing less fast than any pubertal boys in Stolz and Stolz' series, and hence are termed slow growing or nonpubertal here. At the other extreme, boys were classified as fast growing or within their pubertal growth spurt if, at the minimum, their height growth was not more than one standard deviation below Stolz and Stolz' mean for pubertal boys. In our sample, these fast growers (31 percent of the sample) grew between 67.7 and 134.6 millimeters the past year. (See Simmons *et al.,* 1979, for more details.)

3. In fact, our study is longitudinal and will follow the boys from sixth to tenth grade. Thus, we will be able to validate our adaptation of this indicator by seeing if the boys classified as early developers in seventh grade would be so classified once we had several more years of information on their rate of height growth.

4. The relationship between leanness and self-esteem disappears, however, when weight is controlled. The relationship of leanness and self-esteem did not disappear when we controlled for athleticness (.11).

5. Simmons *et al.,* (1979) also find that fast growth is beneficial for boys' self-esteem once height is controlled. In that article, however, the effects of height are eliminated by looking only at "medium height boys."

6. As in the case of self-esteem, the relationship between self-consciousness and leanness disap-

pears when weight is controlled. However, substantively it is difficult to disentangle the meanings of weight and leanness above and beyond the control for height which is built into the ponderal index for leanness.

REFERENCES

Blyth, D. (1977) *Continuities and Discontinuities During the Transition into Adolescence: A Longitudinal Comparison of Two School Structures.* Ph.D. Doctoral Dissertation, University of Minnesota.

Blyth, D., R. G. Simmons, and D. Bush (1978), ''The transition into early adolescence: A longitudinal comparison of youth in two educational contexts.'' *Sociology of Education,* 51(3):149–162.

Blyth, D., K. Smith Thiel, D. Mitsch Bush, and R. G. Simmons (1980) ''Another look at school crime: Student as victim,'' *Youth and Society,* March.

Bush, D. E., R. G. Simmons, B. Hutchinson, and D. A. Blyth (1978), ''Adolescent perception of sex roles in 1968 and 1975.'' *Public Opinion Quarterly,* Winter 41(4):459–474.

Clausen, J. A. (1975), ''The social meaning of differential physical and sexual maturation,'' in Dragastin, S. E. and G. H. Edler, Jr. (Eds.), *Adolescence in the Life Cycle: Psychological Change and Social Context.* New York: Halsted Press.

Dwyer, J., and J. Mayer (1968), ''Psychological effects of variations in physical appearance during adolescence,'' *Adolescence* 3:353–380.

Eichorn, D. (1963), ''Biological correlates of behavior,'' in *Child Psychology,* Part I. Chicago: National Society for the Study of Education.

Faust, M. S. (1977), *Somatic Development of Adolescent Girls.* Monographs of the Society for Research in Child Development (Serial No. 169).

Hendry, L. B., and P. Gillies (1978), ''Body type, body esteem, school and leisure: A study of overweight, average, and underweight adolescents,'' *Journal of Youth and Adolescence* 7:181–195.

Huenemann, R. L., L. R. Shaping, M. D. Hampton, and B. W. Mitchell (1966), ''A lonitudinal study of gross body composition and body conformation and association with food and activity in a teenage population: Views of teenage subjects on body conformation, food and activity,'' *American Journal of Clinical Nutrition* 18:323–338.

Jones, M. C. (1957), ''The late careers of boys who were early or late maturing boys,'' *Child Development* 28:118–128.

Jones, M. C., and Bayley, N. (1950), ''Physical maturing among boys as related to behavior,'' *The Journal of Educational Psychology* 42:129–148.

Jourard, S. M., and P. F. Secord (1954), ''Body size and body cathexis,'' *Journal of Consulting Psychology* 18:184.

Klein, S. D., and R. G. Simmons (1979), ''Chronic diseases and childhood development: Kidney disease and transplantations,'' *Research in Community and Mental Health* 1:21–59.

Lerner, R. M., and B. E. Brackney (1978), ''The importance of inner and outer body parts attitudes in the self-concept of late adolescents,'' *Sex Roles* 4:225–231.

Murphy, G. (1947) *Personality.* New York: Harper.

Musa, K. E., and M. E. Roach (1973), ''Adolescent appearance and self-concept,'' *Adolescence* 8:385–393.

Mussen, P., and H. Boutourline-Young (1964), ''Relationships between rate of physical maturity and personality among boys of Italian descent,'' *Vita Humana* 70:186–200.

Nicolson, A. B., and C. Hanley (1953), ''Indices of physiological maturity: Derivation and interrelationships,'' *Child Development* 24:3–28.

Peskin, H. (1967), ''Pubertal onset and ego functioning,'' *Journal of Abnormal Psychology* 72:1–15.

Reynolds, E. L., and J. V. Wines (1948), ''Individual differences in physical changes associated with adolescence in girls,'' *American Journal of Diseases in Childhood* 75:1–22.

Richardson, S. A., A. H. Hastorf, N. Goodman, and S. M. Dornbusch (1961), "Cultural uniformity in reaction to physical disabilities," *American Sociological Review* 26:241–247.

Richardson, S. A., and J. Royce (1968), "Race and physical handicap in children's preference for other children." *Child Development,* 39(2):467–480.

Roche, A. F. (1979), *Secular Trends in Human Growth, Maturation, and Development,* Monographs of the Society for Research in Child Development (Serial No. 179).

Rosenberg, M. (1979), *Conceiving the Self.* New York: Basic Books, Inc.

Rosenberg, M. (1968). *The Logic of Survey Analysis.* New York: Basic Books, Inc.

Rosenberg, M. (1965), *Society and the Adolescent Self-Image.* New Jersey: Princeton University Press.

Secord, P. F., and S. M. Jourard (1953), "The appraisal of body-cathexis: Body-cathexis and the self," *Journal of Consulting Psychology* 17:343–347.

Simmons, R. G., D. A. Blyth, E. F. Van Cleave, and D. Mitsch Bush (1979), "Entry into early adolescence: The impact of school structure, puberty, and early dating on self-esteem." *American Sociological Review,* 44(6):948–967.

Simmons, R. G., L. Brown, D. Bush, and D. A. Blyth (1978), "Self-esteem and achievement of black and white early adolescents." *Social Problems,* 26(1):86–96.

Simmons, R. G., F. Rosenberg, and M. Rosenberg (1973), "Disturbance in the self-image at adolescence." *American Sociological Review,* 38(5):553–568.

Staffieri, J. R. (1967), "A study of social stereotype of body image in children," *Journal of Personality and Social Psychology* 7:101–104.

Stolz, H. R., and L. M. Stolz (1951), *Somatic Development of Adolescent Boys.* New York: Macmillan.

Stolz, H. R., and L. M. Stolz (1944), "Adolescent problems related to somatic variations," in H. B. Henry (Ed.) *The 43rd Yearbook of the National Society for the Study of Education: Part I. Adolescence.* Chicago: University of Chicago Press.

Tanner, J. M. (1964), *The Physique of the Olympic Athlete.* London: Allen and Unwin.

Tanner, J. M. (1962), *Growth at Adolescence.* Oxford: Blackwell Scientific Publications.

Wylie, R. C. (1961) *The Self Concept,* Vol. 1, Revised Edition. Lincoln, NE: University of Nebraska Press.

Section B

EFFECTS UPON DEPRESSION AND SUICIDE

THE EPIDEMIOLOGICAL
SIGNIFICANCE OF SOCIAL
SUPPORT SYSTEMS IN DEPRESSION

Alfred Dean, Nan Lin, and Walter M. Ensel

INTRODUCTION

Recently the National Institute of Mental Health (1973) reported that the prevalence of depression in the United States had become a major health problem, and that from two to four of every 100 Americans require treatment each year. Weissman and Klerman (1977) estimate that 8 to 18 percent of the population may suffer symptoms of depression at any one time. It is believed that rates of depression have increased strikingly over the past quarter-century (Paykel, 1976). The increased incidence and seriousness of depression among adolescents and young adults is particularly notable and may portend even more serious trends (Schwab et al., 1979). Thus, Klerman (1979) has aptly asked, "Is this the age of melancholy?"

Reviews of the research literature reveal that our knowledge about the possible

Research in Community and Mental Health, Volume 2, pages 77–109
Copyright © 1981 by JAI Press, Inc.
All rights of reproduction in any form reserved.
ISBN: 0-89232-152-0

role of sociological factors in depression is substantially undeveloped (Bart, 1974; Becker, 1974; Schwab et al., 1979). The thrust of much of the epidemiological literature has been in several areas: (1) developing applicable measures of depression; (2) describing the sociodemographic correlates of depression, such as age, sex, social class; and (3) examining the influence of stressful life events on the occurrence of depression. Recently, the role of social support systems has been attracting considerable interest in social epidemiology as well as applied mental health programs.

The view that social support systems may have powerful epidemiological significance is associated with two major concepts: (1) that social support may buffer the impact of stressful life events; and (2) that social support may directly influence the occurrence of various disorders. Probably the most prominent current interest in social support systems is the first mentioned and has been stimulated by accumulated studies demonstrating the influence of life events on the occurrence of depression, suicide, and other psychiatric and physical disorders, and which may be mediated by social support.

The appeal of these views is grounded in a wide variety of suggestive evidence and theory as exemplified in a number of reviews (Cassel, 1976; Dean and Lin, 1977; Dohrenwend and Dohrenwend, 1978a; Kaplan et al., 1977). There are additional reasons for this compelling interest. It is expected that the *joint* examination of stress and social support may clarify the differential vulnerability of individuals to life events. Moreover, the most influential events, such as death of a spouse, may clearly reflect disturbances in social support. Thus, social support, like stressors, may be implicated in a wide variety of diseases or disorders. Finally, the concept has pragmatic appeal—implying possibilities for prevention; that is, social support may be modifiable in contrast to genetic or constitutional factors and the occurrence of certain inevitable stressors.

These conceptions are nonetheless largely hypothetical and empirically controversial. There is a relative paucity of relevant research; serious problems in theory and method; and competing causal models of the relationships among stressful life events, social support, and illness (Dean and Lin, 1977).

The present study attempts to contribute to the resolution of a number of problems which have limited present knowledge. The nature of these problems and our approaches to them are discussed next.

ISSUES AND APPROACHES

Sample

This study was conducted with a representative, random sample (N = 99) of adults aged 20 and over in the Albany-Troy-Schenectady area of New York State as defined by the U.S. Census SMSA area. The detailed description of the sample and the scale properties of these measures have been reported elsewhere

(Lin, Dean, and Ensel, 1979). Here, we will briefly recapitulate the psychometric details essential to this paper. We will also extend our examination of the conceptual and empirical properties of these scales and their pertinence to the epidemiology of depression.

Measuring Social Support

One of the most serious obstacles in determining the epidemiological significance of social support has been the limited status of appropriate measures. Ideally, such measures should meet several requirements: (1) they should be subjected to scaling techniques to establish their dimensions; (2) they should be reliable and valid; and (3) they should be theoretically significant and phenomenologically revealing and detailed. These properties should encourage their use in replicational or convergent studies and thus promote the development of cumulative knowledge.

There remains a need for the systematic development of such social support scales. In general, the application of existing scales has been predicated on their face validity and several have exhibited some predictive validity (Medalie and Goldbourt, 1976; Nuckolls et al., 1972; Gore, 1978; Lowenthal and Haven, 1968). Some studies utilize surrogate indicators such as marital status or other sociodemographic variables (Myers et al., 1975; Pearlin and Johnson, 1977). Few studies using the same social support indicators have been reported and these were not designed for scale development (Moriwaki, 1973; Berle et al., 1952; Holmes et al., 1961).

As will be detailed, our approach to the above objectives has been to assess the scale properties of certain measures which (1) empirically have shown suggestive relationships to depression or other disorders (Lowenthal and Haven, 1968; Medalie and Goldbourt, 1976); (2) have been proposed but untested (Kaplan, 1975); and (3) are based on our own conceptualizations of instrumental and expressive support (Dean and Lin, 1977; Lin, Dean, and Ensel, 1979). The scale properties of these measures, along with other variables examined in this paper, were subjected to an empirical test in this study.

Types of Social Support

The nature of the scales applied here will be best appreciated in the context of a number of theoretical and empirical issues. The term "social support" has wide intuitive acceptance as a primitive concept. However, a concept with too much meaning is in danger of having no meaning at all. Thus, there is the need for further conceptual as well as operational specification of social support. In part, this implies the need to differentiate types of social support and to examine the ways in which their epidemiologic functions may vary in theory and in fact.

Confidant Support. It is interesting that some of the pioneering work on social support has had reference to depression. Lowenthal and Haven's study

(1968) served as a harbinger and stimulus to the study of social support. Investigating the processes of aging, they noted that the presence or absence of a "confidant"—someone with whom the elderly person could talk intimately about themselves or their problems—was associated with the risk of depression. Specifically, the presence of a confidant reduced the risk of depression associated with role losses, widowhood, and other problems of aging.

Later, Moriwaki (1973) found that the number of confidants reported by retired individuals was correlated with their emotional well-being as indicated by Washburn's Affective Balance Scale. Recently, Brown and Harris (1978), in a carefully conceived strategy for discerning factors associated with the differential susceptibility of women to depression under conditions of stressful life events, observed that the presence or absence of a confiding relationship with their husband, boyfriend, or other male was the most important factor.

However, there is need to elaborate our understanding of the nature of confidant relationships and their possible functions. Thus, Kaplan (1975) has proposed that the following properties of confidant relationships be examined:

1. *Durability* - number of years respondent has known the confidant.
2. *Frequency* - frequency of contact with the confidant.
3. *Density* - how often the respondent has talked over problems with the confidant.
4. *Directedness* - how often the confidant has talked over problems with the respondent.
5. *Reachability* - how easy it has been for the respondent to get hold of the confidant.
6. *Content* - how freely the respondent has been able to talk about things with the confidant.
7. *Intensity* - how important the confidant is to the respondent.

These properties, combined with the basic Lowenthal-Haven (1968) items dealing with the number of confidants, the relationship of the respondent to the confidant, and the change in the relationship with a confidant, make up a battery of 11 items dealing with confidant characteristics (Appendix C).

Item-total correlation among the items ranged from .279 to .822.

Among the inter-item correlations, 12 of the 21 coefficients were not significant. Obviously, these items do not constitute a unidimensional scale. The decision was to examine the relationships between these items and the dependent variables individually. Hopefully, such analysis would identify specific confidant characteristics which contribute to the prediction of the dependent variables.

Family Support.   As Lowenthal and Haven (1968) correctly note, the study of confidant relationships is an integral although limited effort to study intimate relationships in general. In sociology, an interest in close relationships and interactions has been an important tradition stemming from the work of Cooley on primary groups. Despite their apparent importance, the study of such relationships has been neglected. Previously, we have reviewed the nature and functions of primary relationships and indicated how they may be implicated in stress reduction and induction in the light of stress research in man and infra-human animals (Dean and Lin, 1977). In epidemiological research, there have been some attempts to ascertain the strength of certain primary relationships basically and broadly conceived as providing emotional support. In particular, attention has been focused on the status of certain family relationships, most notably relationships to spouse and other family members. Usually, the focus has been on the buffering or risk-reducing function of social support.

There are several compelling justifications for examining the family as a support system. First, it is typically defined normatively as the group in which members have mutual obligations to provide a broad range of emotional and material support—routinely as well as particularly at times of crises or threatening events. It may distinctly communicate three types of support functions identified by Cobb (1976): affection and caring; self-esteem; and group solidarity. Many of the stressful life events associated with depression and other disorders represent losses or disturbances in family relationships (Brown and Harris, 1978; Myers, 1971, 1972; Paykel et al., 1969).

Regarding the epidemiological functions of these hypothetical supports in the context of potentially stressful events, an example is the well-recognized study by Nuckolls, Kaplan, and Cassell (1972). They found some evidence that the relationships of pregnant women to their husbands and other family members influenced the risk of complications of pregnancy. Similarly, Gore (1978) found that affective changes and other symptoms among men who were laid off due to a plant closing were related to the relationships they had with their wives.

Available descriptions of the instruments applied by these investigators indicate that they are comprised of diverse items apparently tapping psychological, interpersonal and situational factors. To our knowledge, the scale or subscale properties of these instruments have not been reported. By contrast, Medalie and Goldbourt applied a more homogenous set of items focused upon relationships within the conjugal family. In a prospective study of cardiovascular disorders in 10,000 men, they found that those who reported favorable love relationships with their wives were significantly less likely to present symptoms of angina pectoris even in the presence of biological risk factors (1976).

With regard to the considerations discussed, we decided to examine the scale properties of the Medalie-Goldbourt instrument and its relationship to depression in a community population. These items focus on family problems: (1) problems in the past; (2) problems at present; (3) effects of spouse/children not listening or opposing; and (4) whether spouse shows his/her love (Appendix C).

The Medalie-Goldbourt scale of family problems consisted of four items. (Appendix C presents the exact wording of items and their response categories.) The total scale score (created by summing the responses to the four items) was then correlated with the individual items. All items correlated highly (between .590 and .756) with the total score. All inter-item correlations were in the positive direction and all, except two of the correlation coefficients, were significant at the .05 level. The fourth item (spouse not showing love) seems to have a slightly weaker relationship with the total score, as compared with other items. As most of these items concerned married persons, only 57 of the 99 respondents qualified to respond to these items.

Community and Neighborhood Support.   Sociological theories about the nature and social-psychological consequences of various types of communities are as old as sociology itself. Early American sociology, stimulated by the profound societal changes associated with industrialization and urbanization, evidenced considerable interest in community cohesion, stability, and change. Psychiatrically-oriented sociology and social psychiatry displayed a similar interest. Illustrative examples include the early work of Faris and Dunham (1939), the later work of Hollingshead and Redlich (1958), and the more recent investigations of Alexander Leighton and his associates (A. Leighton, 1959; D. Leighton, 1963). In essence, numerous epidemiological studies have had a community dimension. Thus, there is something vaguely familiar and yet different in the current concepts of the community as a support system. Klerman (1979) has recently stated:

> In modern life, the main forces that initiate depressive responses are more often threats to the psychosocial integrity of the individual—to the sense of self, which is enhanced by our attachment to work, family, friends, and community—than to our physical well-being and survival.

However, there have apparently been relatively limited attempts to study the epidemiological significance of community support elements. Certainly, this is an area deserving substantial empirical and theoretical investment. In this paper, we will be limited to some partial results of our efforts in this direction.

Lin et al. (1979), in a study of Chinese Americans in Washington, D.C., examined the effects of stressors and social support on the incidence of psychiatric symptomatology. Among the items comprising the social support scale were: satisfaction with neighborhood and community, both of which were significantly related to each other; the other support items (satisfaction with job, involvement in Chinese activities and associations, getting together with friends from the old country, having close friends in the immediate area, etc.); and the total social support scale itself. In the current study, we attempted to build upon their work by including community and neighborhood satisfaction as social support indicators (Appendix C).

The community-neighborhood satisfaction scale consisted of two items: satisfaction with community and satisfaction with neighborhood. The means and standard deviations of the two items were consistent ($\bar{X}$ = 1.57 and 1.59, respectively; S.D. = .90 and .89, respectively) and responses to both items were concentrated in the positive direction. Since the zero order correlation between them was .67, the decision was made to combine the two items into a summated scale.

It should be clear that social support systems may serve both instrumental and expressive functions. Existing scales appear to mix these functions (Gore, 1978; Andrews et al., 1978a). At the same time, interest in the possible buffering functions of support appears to have focused attention largely on expressive support. The importance of "exits from the social field" on one hand (Paykel et al., 1969) and job loss on the other (Gore, 1978) illustrate that these events may reflect disturbances in either expressive or instrumental functioning (or both). We have also felt there is a need to elaborate the instrumental and expressive variables involved. These considerations led us to develop new measures of expressive and instrumental support which will now be described.

Instrumental-Expressive Support Items. We operationalized a set of 26 items which we felt would reflect the instrumental or expressive support available to the respondent. One objective in constructing these items was to make them capable of describing the various modes of support despite differences that might be attributable to sociodemographic characteristics (e.g., marital status, employment status). In other words, we wanted to make the items applicable across demographic subsets, and status and role characteristics of respondents. Following a general introduction (Would you tell me how often you have been bothered by these problems over the past 12 months?), a list of 26 items were asked of each respondent. (The specific wording of the items and the response categories can be found in Appendix C.) The set of 26 instrumental expressive support items was subjected to a factor analysis (orthogonal solution, varimax rotation, with a limiting eigenvalue of one or more) resulting in five identified factors: (1) monetary problems; (2) lack of companionship; (3) demands: (4) communication problems; and (5) not having children. (The factors and associated items are presented in Appendix A.)

It should be noted that the labelling of these items is somewhat arbitrary rather than definitive; that is, the labels do not necessarily represent all of the items. For example, under the factor "demands," three of the four items reflect excessive demands, while the fourth—unsatisfactory sex life—may or may not fit under this typology. The same is true with regard to the "lack of companionship" factor and the item, "too dependent on others," which is subsumed under it.

The items constituting each factor were summated, resulting in five constructed social support variables tapping the instrumental and expressive support factors. It seemed clear that monetary problems and demands were instrumental dimensions; and lack of companionship, communication problems, and problems with not having children were expressive dimensions. The decision was to use these five constructed instrumental-expressive support scales either separately or in the functional groups (instrumental versus expressive).

Incorporating other Relevant Variables

Previous studies have established that certain sociodemographic variables are related to depression and other psychiatric disturbances (Schwab et al., 1979;

Silverman, 1968). Some of these variables, such as sex, marital status, and socio-economic status, have shown rather consistent relationships to depression. Others, such as age, appear to be inconsistent or may be changing. In any case, these variables require incorporation into empirical and analytic models.

While such variables may be useful in identifying populations at risk, they are crude and have had limited explanatory value. They require the identification of "underlying" or intervening variables with which they are associated and which may explain their relationship to depression or other disturbances. In this regard, an examination of their relationship to social supports is indicated.

As previously noted, the occurrence of stressful life events also requires its incorporation as an independent variable. In the present study, several instruments were combined. Specifically, our strategy was as follows: (1) include the original Holmes and Rahe (1967) items (excluding Christmas) so that we could replicate the original findings; (2) add items recently proposed by Rahe (1975) along with items used by Myers and others (1972); and (3) expand certain items to reflect positive or negative effects. While stressful life events were tapped for each respondent for two time periods (last six months and the six months prior to that), the most recent time period will be used here. The measure was derived by summing all the events occurring to the individual in the last six months. The rationale for this procedure can be found elsewhere (Lin, Dean, and Ensel, 1979).

Of special interest in such studies are the functions of prior history of illness. This factor may influence both current social support (Dean, 1976; Dean et al., 1967; Weissman and Paykel, 1974) and vulnerability to further illness. Indeed, some have argued that only individuals who are predisposed to illness will manifest illness under ordinary stressors (Dohrenwend and Dohrenwend, 1978a; Hinkle, 1974). Similarly, it is important to monitor disorders which may be proximal to or concurrent with depression. It is well known that psychiatric disturbances may be associated with physical illness (Crandall and Dohrenwend, 1967; Neff et al., 1978; Schwab et al., 1978; Warheit et al., 1973). It is specifically useful here to be able to distinguish depression which may be associated with physical illness (secondary depression) from primary depression.

In brief, the role of the history of illness or recent illness is unclear in the literature because it is not generally accounted for. It has also been noted that life event schedules contain illness events as well as items which may be associated with illness, thus confounding illness as an independent and dependent variable (Dohrenwend and Dohrenwend, 1978; Mueller et al., 1978; Rabkin and Struening, 1976).

In this study, the presence of identified disorders is monitored for the antecedent year as well as during the past month. This was documented with a substantially revised version of the Cornell Medical Index (Lowe, 1975). Finally, depression, the ultimate dependent variable here, was measured by the Center for Epidemiologic Studies Depression (CES-D) Scale (Radloff, 1977), which consists of 20 items, each of which contained four point responses (ranging from "none of the time" to "all of the time"), based on the last week prior to the interview. The CES-D Scale has been validated and applied in a number of studies (Husaini and Neff, 1979; Markush and Favero, 1974; Myers et al., 1979).

RESULTS

The Significance of Social Support in the Epidemiology of Depression

Given the previous discussion, the question becomes: to what degree are these sociodemographic factors and social supports related to (and possible predictors of) psychiatric symptomatology? In addition, to what degree do prior history of illness and stressful life events contribute to the explanation of variations in depression?

Marital status is collapsed here into two categories: not married (0) and married (1). Income was operationalized by categories ranging from $0-$999 to $50,000 and over. Number of dependent children refers to the number of children still living at home. Employment status was dichotomized into two categories: employed (part-time or full-time = 1) and not employed (retired, laid off, disabled, keeping house, in school = 0). Age ranged from 18–80, while sex was coded 0-males, 1-females. Prior history of illness refers to the total number of identified illnesses the respondent reported as existing prior to the current year.[1]

Table 1 presents the zero order correlations between the selected independent variables and the dependent variable, depression. Among the sociodemographic factors selected, only marital status and income were significantly correlated with depression (not married people and those of a lower income level evidencing more psychiatric symptomatology). Stressful life events occurring to the respondent in the last six months were significantly related to depression (the more stress, the more depressive symptoms evidenced). Prior history of illness was also found to be significantly and positively related to depression, with an increase in illness associated with an increase in depression.

Among the social support items, all the instrumental-expressive support scales (with the exception of "not having children") were significantly related to depression, with correlations ranging from .32 to .46. Those who were more satisfied with their community and neighborhood were less likely to become depressed than those who were more dissatisfied. Additionally, for those who were married, the Medalie-Goldbourt scale measuring presence of family problems was positively related to depression (r = .42). The general trend here is: the lower the level of social support that was manifested (reflected in an increase in money problems, increase in demands, in communication problems, lack of companionship, and dissatisfaction with community and with neighborhood, and

Table 1.   Zero-Order Correlations between Selected Independent Variables and
the Dependent Variable (CES-D Scale)

INDEPENDENT VARIABLES	Coefficient (N)	P
Sociodemographic Variables		
Sex (Male (0), Female (1))	.08 (99)	n.s.
Age	−.02 (98)	n.s.
*Marital status (not married (0) vs. married (1))	−.21 (98)	.02
*Family Income	−.45 (78)	.001
Employment Status (not employed (0), employed (1))	−.07 (99)	n.s.
Number Dependent Children	−.01 (99)	n.s.
*Prior History of Illness	.35 (99)	.001
Stressful Life Events		
*To self, last 6 months	.31 (99)	.001
Social Support Scales		
The Medalie-Goldbourt Scale of Family Problems	.42 (57)	.001
Community and neighborhood satisfaction	−.38 (97)	.001
The instrumental-expressive support scales		
*(a) Monetary problems	.46 (97)	.001
*(b) Demands	.43 (90)	.001
*(c) Lack of companions	.32 (68)	.004
*(d) Communication problems	.37 (69)	.001
*(e) No children	.03 (64)	n.s.
Confidant characteristics		
Durability of confidant	−.11 (84)	n.s.
Directedness with confidant	−.22 (84)	.02

*Scales and items retained for regression analysis; see text.

the presence of family problems), the higher the level of depressive symptomatology.

Finally, of the 11 confidant characteristics identified by Lowenthal and Haven (1968) and Kaplan (1975), only directedness in the confidant relationship was significantly related to depression (the more directedness—that is, the more the confidant confided in the respondent—the lower the level of depression). We next examined the extent to which these characteristics jointly contribute to—and act as significant predictors of—depressive symptomatology.

The first step was to regress depression on all the independent variables that were significantly correlated with it (see items with asterisks in Table 1). The procedure involved the construction of a regression model for depression with the various independent variables treated as predictor variables. The model was further refined after the independent variables that did not exceed a regression coefficient of .10 were dropped from the model and the regression equation recalculated. It became necessary to eliminate some independent variables so as to minimize problems of multicollinearity. The final regression model is presented in Table 2.

As can be seen in the table, three indicators of social support (monetary problems, demands, and community and neighborhood satisfaction) were inversely related to depression (more support, less depression). In addition, family income, stressful life events, and prior history of illness were all independently related to depression. Specifically, the lower the income, the more stressful life events, and the more prior illness experienced by the respondents, the greater the resultant level of depression. In terms of contributions to explanation of depression, the six factors explained a total of 46 percent of the variance in depression. By and large, the best predictors of depressive symptoms were monetary problems and family income accounting for 33.9 percent of the variance in depression. The other social support variables (demands, community-neighborhood satisfaction) explain 5 percent and 3 percent additional variance. Stressful life events and physical illness respectively explained only 2.7 percent and 1.0 percent variance additional to that explained by the other four variables.

Thus, the social support scales explained more variance than stressful life events. Specifically, the findings suggest that when the other variables in Table 2 are controlled, the instrumental nature of social support (reflected in money problems and too many demands) has a substantially greater direct effect on depressive symptomatology than do stressful life events.

However, part of the original, total relationship between stressful life events and depression may be mediated by the incorporation of social support into the

Table 2.   Ordinary Least Squares Estimates for Depression as
Dependent Variable

	*Metric Coefficients**	*Standard Coefficients*	R^2 *Change*	*Cumulative* R^2
Monetary Problems	.220	.120**	.208	.208
	(.219)			
Family Income	−.839	−.335	.131	.339
	(.251)			
Demands	.493	.214	.054	.393
	(.243)			
Comm-Neigh Satisfaction	−.978	−.183	.031	.424
	(.526)			
Stressful Life Events	.532	.180	.027	.451
	(.289)			
Prior Illness	.496	.104	.009	.460
	(.485)			
Constant	39.85			
Error of Estimate	6.66			
R^2	.459			

*Metric coefficients appear on the first line, standard errors appear underneath in parentheses.

**Due to the high correlation between demands and monetary problems (see Table 3), demands is repressing part of the β_1 in monetary problems. This may be due to a certain amount of redundancy between the two instrumental support variables.

model (Lin, Dean, and Ensel, 1979). Also, because of the wording of the questions, we expect that social support affects the level of depression;[2] however, it is possible that part of the association reported in Table 1 between these variables reflects the reciprocal impact of a person's depression on the level of support he perceives and receives. We will return to some of these issues in the discussion section.

Patterns of Social Support

Having discerned the significance of the different types of social support to depression, a number of relevant questions concerning the interrelationships among types of support may be addressed. This is of substantive as well as methodological interest. For example, are instrumental and expressive support related? Similarly, if the Medalie-Goldbourt scale measures expressive relationships in the family, what is the strength of its relationship to our more general measures of expressive support? Thus, the relationships among types of social support are briefly explored (Table 3).

It may be seen that there is a high degree of consistency within both the instrumental (money problems and too many demands) and the expressive (communication and companionship problems) support scales (r = .583 and .597, respectively). Further, the instrumental and expressive support scales were significantly related to each other, with correlations ranging from .404 to .535. These findings suggest that instrumental and expressive problems overlap to a significant degree, and they both showed significant relationships with depression (see Table 1). Therefore, in the regression analysis (see Table 2), the multicollinearity of instrumental and expressive support scales did not permit the retention of the expressive support scales in the final model.

Similarly, the Medalie-Goldbourt scale, ostensibly measuring general family problems and relationships, was significantly related to both the instrumental and the expressive social support scales. (The more family problems faced by the respondent, the more money problems, demands, communication problems, and companionship problems faced by the respondent; r = .635, .560, .656 and .614, respectively). However, it must be kept in mind here that due to the nature of the Medalie-Goldbourt scale, relationships reported with regard to it refer only to the married segment of the sample. Family support (Medalie-Goldbourt) is also related directly to confidant directedness. This suggests that for some respondents, family members served as their confidants.

Community and neighborhood satisfaction, which related to family support and having a durable confidant, appears to be more related to instrumental rather than expressive support.

Among the confidant items, durability was positively related to community-neighborhood satisfaction and directedness was negatively related to the Medalie-Goldbourt scale. Neither was related to any of the instrumental and expressive support scales.

Table 3. Zero Order Correlations among Social Support Scales

Social Support	Money Problems	Demands	Communications Problems	Lack of Companions	Medalie-Goldbourt	Comm.-Neigh. Satisfaction	Durability Confidant	Directedness Confidant
Money Problems	1.000 —	.583** (90)	.481** (69)	.404** (68)	.635** (57)	-.324** (95)	.073 (82)	-.111 (82)
Demands		1.000 —	.535** (67)	.415** (66)	.506** (56)	-.195* (88)	.034 (77)	-.029 (77)
Communications Problems			1.000 —	.597** (54)	.656** (46)	-.122 (69)	-.079 (58)	-.114 (58)
Lack of Companions				1.000 —	.614** (53)	-.069 (66)	.089 (59)	-.073 (59)
Medalie-Goldbourt					1.000 —	-.393** (56)	-.039 (52)	-.272* (52)
Comm.-Neigh. Satisfaction						1.000 —	.183* (82)	-.058 (82)
Durability of Confidant							1.000 —	.069 (84)
Directedness of Confidant								1.000

*p ≤ .05
**p ≤ .01

89

The examination of the inter-relations among the social support scales helped clarify some of the results of the regression analysis. For one thing, expressive support seems to remain an important aspect of social support even though the scales did not appear in the final regression equation for depression. Their significant zero-order correlations with depression and substantial overlap with instrumental support scales suggest their potential substantive relations with depression. The Medalie-Goldbourt family problems scale also overlapped extensively with other social support scales. It remains legitimate to examine its contribution to depression, although its confinement to married persons reduces its general applicability. Finally, the non-significant linear contribution from confidant items to depression has been reinforced by their lack of linear relationships with other social support scales. As they are currently formulated and worded, the confidant items probably do not have any linear effects on depression. Whether they are curvilinearly related to depression remains to be examined. At this point, there is a lack of conceptual analysis to guide empirical explorations.

Sociodemographic Correlates of Support

However, questions may be raised about the support scales: are there objective, structural factors associated with social support? That is, what factors

Table 4. Zero Order Correlations of Sociodemographic Characteristics and Illness with Measures of Social Support

Social Support	Sex	Age	Marital Status	Family Income	No. Depend. Children	Employ. Status	Prior Hist. of Illness
Money Problems	−.033 (97)	−.328** (96)	.084 (96)	−.209* (76)	.346** (96)	.279** (96)	.322** (97)
Demands	−.179* (90)	−.301** (90)	.017 (89)	−.047 (72)	.295** (89)	.281** (89)	.293** (90)
Communic. Problems	.129 (69)	−.469** (69)	.132 (69)	.008 (57)	.279** (69)	.103 (69)	.143 (69)
Lack of Companions	.049 (68)	−.295** (68)	−.126 (67)	−.059 (55)	.158 (68)	.026 (68)	.095 (68)
Medalie-Goldbourt	.059 (57)	−.439** (57)	— —	−.153 (47)	.427** (57)	.257* (57)	.315** (57)
Comm.-Neigh. Satisfaction	−.089 (97)	.069 (96)	.183* (96)	.254* (76)	−.061 (96)	−.061 (96)	−.131 (97)
Durability of Confidant	−.243** (84)	.521** (83)	−.038 (84)	−.311** (67)	−.176 (83)	−.159 (83)	−.174 (84)
Directedness of Confidant	.085 (84)	.025 (83)	−.026 (84)	−.254* (67)	.125 (83)	−.074 (83)	.248** (84)

*p ≤ .05
**p ≤ .01

influence social support? To explore these questions, we felt it would be useful to examine the sociodemographic correlates of social support. We thus examined age, sex, marital status, family income, number of dependent children, and employment status, as well as prior history of illness, and assessed their effects on the various social support scales.

First, we examined the correlations among sociodemographic factors, prior illness, and the various types of social support. Then, we regressed each of the support items on the sociodemographic variables and prior illness to determine which of these factors, in combination, affected each of the social support scales.

Table 4 presents the results of the correlation analysis, while the results of the regression analysis can be found in Appendix B. The findings with regard to level of support maintained in each of the specific support systems can be summarized as follows:

1. Younger people, those with lower income, those with more dependent children, the employed, and those with more of a prior history of illness are likely to manifest lower levels of instrumental social support (i.e., more money problems and more demands) than that of their counterparts. These five variables taken together explain almost 50 percent of the variance in money problems. Also, excluding family income, these five variables explain 27 percent of the variance in demands.

2. Younger people and those with more dependent children are likely to manifest lower levels of expressive social support than that of their counterparts. While the number of children drops out in the regression analysis, age remains a significant predictor, explaining 9 percent of the variance in lack of companionship and more than 21 percent of the variance in demands.

3. Males, older people, and those with higher incomes are likely to have a more durable relationship with a confidant they can trust and talk to than their counterparts, while those with lower income and more history of illness are likely to have a more directed relationship with their confidant. Income and prior history of illness explain approximately 10 percent of the variance in directedness, while age, sex, and income combine to explain 35 percent of the variance in durability.

4. Those married and making more money tend to be more satisfied with their community and neighborhood. While marital status drops out of the regression analysis, income remains, explaining 6 percent of the variance in community-neighborhood satisfaction.

5. Finally, younger people, those employed, those with more dependent children, and those with more of a prior history of illness are likely to have more family problems. These four variables taken together explain more than 40 percent of the variance in the Medalie-Goldbourt scale.

These findings suggest that sociodemographic factors and a prior history of illness are effective factors in predicting and explaining levels of social support maintained by individuals. Clearly, the most consistent finding is that instrumental support—or, rather, the lack of it—as well as family support, is a function of the number of children, employment status, and prior history of illness. Expressive social support seems to be more a function of age. Community-neighborhood satisfaction appears to be a function of socioeconomic status, while durability of relationships with confidants appears to be a function of sex, age, and income.

Directedness with a confidant (reciprocity) is a function of prior history of illness.

Several patterns may be seen in the data which illuminate the previously posed questions. First, instrumental role failures are associated with objective conditions of instrumental demands (number of children, being employed, having a prior history of illness). It is interesting to note that age is consistently inversely related to level of demands and monetary problems (as well as expressive support problems). It may be suggested that early stages of the life cycle are particularly demanding and problematic. Also of interest is the fact that men experience more instrumental disturbances. This is the only social support factor related to sex.

The two instrumental scales are quite similar to each other in their relationship to these factors. However, the expressive support scales clearly exhibit a different pattern of relationship to the sociodemographic factors. For example, a prior history of illness is related to instrumental, but not expressive problems. Interestingly, while the number of dependent children is related to communication problems, it is not related to companionship. These findings give some support to the idea that instrumental-expressive scales are distinguishable, consistent with their conceptualization, and related to objective, external social conditions.

DISCUSSION

It is apparent that depression in a community population is associated with social support problems of the following nature: (1) inability to satisfy monetary wants or needs; (2) the inability to master other instrumental functions (demands); (3) interpersonal conflicts (communication problems); (4) inadequate primary relationships (companionship problems); and (5) dissatisfaction with the community. It is also clear in this community population that when both social support variables of this nature and life-event variables are in the same regression equation, the problems in social support appear to have greater direct consequences on depression than does the extent of recent exposure to stressful life events.

Some of the further implications of these findings will be briefly discussed.

The present study suggests that the extent to which the social systems in which individuals are located fulfill routine adaptive and adjustive functions (i.e., provide *active social support*) is of distinct epidemiological significance in depression. This active support concept is consistent with the structural-functional frameworks of several investigators (Dean and Lin, 1977; Kaplan, Wilson, and Leighton, 1976; Henderson, 1977, 1978). Other studies have also discerned the independent effects of active social support rather than its interactive effects with life events (Myers et al., 1975; Andrews et al., 1978a).

By contrast, interest in the buffering functions of social support has tended to focus upon *reactive* social support. For example, Husani and Neff (1978) studied the supports which were available to help individuals cope with their specific life events. The availability of such supports reduced the risk of depression significantly, though modestly. Of course, the active social support system may be regarded as the system which will be reactive in the context of life events—the approach essentially taken by some investigators (Gore, 1978; Nuckolls et al., 1972).

However, it is important to clearly keep these two types of systems analytically distinct. As suggested earlier, life events may reflect problems in the active support systems (e.g., economic conditions). In a prior analysis, we discerned that the influence of life events on depression was both direct and through social support (Lin, Dean, and Ensel, 1979). Future studies will need to jointly relate types of life events and types of social support to disorders. In any case, the present study suggests that, in a community population, active social supports may ordinarily be of distinct epidemiological significance.

The finding that social support factors contribute more to explaining depression than stressful life events when both are in the same equation does not imply that life events are unimportant. Rather, it shows that social support makes a larger direct and independent contribution to explaining depressive symptomatology than stressful life events. In a separate paper (Lin, Dean, and Ensel, 1979), we found that approximately one-third of the effect of stressful life events is mediated through social support and also, in an analysis of Chinese Americans in Washington, D.C. (Lin, Simeone, Ensel, and Kuo, 1979), the possibility of a mediating or reactive role played by social support. The true test of this proposition will come with a longitudinal design of panel data which we are in the process of gathering.

A related issue is the extent to which depression is a function of fairly chronic conditions, or life changes. The present study does not allow for the careful examination of this question. However, it would appear that the factors of support and income, as well as some of the sociodemographic factors, are more persistent than life events. This is an important theoretical and empirical question which will require longitudinal investigation.

Prospective studies will also be required to determine the extent to which social support systems and life events lead to identifiable disorders in contrast to transient symptomatic states. It is noteworthy that Brown and Harris (1978) found that women in a community population had a fairly chronic history of depression. Moreover, they found that serious life events, confidant support, and other factors functioned similarly in the occurrence of clinical depression, borderline depression, and nonclinical depressive symptoms.

The functions of income merit innovative investigation in future studies, given its established relationship to psychiatric disturbances. Our analysis to date indicates a direct effect on depression. The factors associated with income and their relationship to psychiatric disturbances have not been established. Similarly, monetary problems were not adequately explained by income. It would seem that depression may partly reflect problems of status and self-esteem attached to success in our "open-class" society. However, this is speculative and would require examination in related research.

Future research will also be needed to discern the ways in which expressive and instrumental support are a function of environmental or sociological variables in contrast to personality or constitutional factors. The proposed scales should prove useful in discerning the ways in which instrumental and expressive functioning is associated with specific sociocultural conditions known to have epidemiological significance, such as sex roles, poverty or migration. Obviously, the role of instrumental support merits increased attention.

This study also indicates that susceptibility to depression is significantly related to a history of identified illness (see Simmons et al., 1977). However, this does not contribute substantially to the prediction of depression in a community population when the other variables are controlled. More generally, however, crucial questions still remain concerning the causal sequences of stressful life events, social support, and illness and depression. One-way reciprocal and interactive causal relationships need to be examined more closely. In the final analysis, these causal issues will require prospective investigation. We are presently completing data collection for the first benchmark of a panel study. Hopefully, in the future, we may be able to present data pertinent to these significant questions.

ACKNOWLEDGMENTS

The work reported here was supported by a grant from the Center for Epidemiological Studies, the National Institute of Mental Health (MH 30301). We wish to acknowledge the participation of Ronald Simeone and Irene Farrell in data collection and analysis.

NOTES

1. It should be noted that since the correlation between prior history of illness and recent illness was very high (r = .84), we decided to employ prior history of illness as our measure so as to avoid problems of multicollinearity.

2. Note depression is measured for the week before the interview while perceived social support is measured usually for the past 12 months.

REFERENCES

Andrews, G., C. Tennant, D. M. Hewson, and G. E. Vaillant (1978a), "Life event stress, social support, coping style and risk of psychological impairment," *Journal of Nervous and Mental Disease* 166(5):307-316.

Andrews, B., C. Tennant, D. Hewson, and M. Schonell (1978b), "The relations of social factors to physical and psychiatric illness," *American Journal of Epidemiology* 108:27-35.

Bart, P. B. (1974), "The sociology of depression," pp. 139-157 in P. M. Ro-an and H. M. Trice (eds.), *Explorations in Psychiatric Sociology*. Philadelphia: F. A. Davis Company.

Bart, P. B. (1970), "Mother Portnoy's complaint," *Transaction* 8:69-74.

Bart, P. B. (1969), "Why women's status changes in middle age," *Sociological Symposium* 3:1-18.

Beck, J. C., and K. Worthen (1972), "Precipitating stress, crisis theory, and hospitalization in schizophrenia and depression," *Archives of General Psychiatry* 26:123-129.

Becker, J. (1974), "Psychosocial research on depression," pp. 121-132 in J. Becker (ed.), *Depression: Theory and Research*. Washington, D.C.: V. H. Winston and Sons.

Berle, B., R. Pinsky, S. Wolf, and H. Wolf (1952), "Berle index: A clinical guide to prognosis in stress disease," *Journal of the American Medical Association* 149:1624-1628.

Bibring, E. (1953), "The mechanism of depression," pp. 13-48 in Phyllis Greenacre (ed.), *Affective Disorders*. New York: International Universities Press.

Bloom, B., S. Asher, and S. White (1978), "Marital disruption as a stressor, review and analysis," *Psychological Bulletin* 85:867-894.

Brown, G. W., and T. Harris (1978), *Social Origins of Depression: A Study of Psychiatric Disorder in Women*. New York: The Free Press.

Brown, G. W., T. Harris, and J. Copeland (1977), "Depression and loss," *British Journal of Psychiatry* 130:1-18.

Brown, G. W., M. N. Bhrolchain, and T. Harris (1975), "Social class and psychiatric disturbance among women in an urban population," *Sociology* 9:225-254.

Brown, G. W. (1974a), "Life events and the onset of depression and schizophrenic conditions," pp. 164-188 in E. K. Gunderson and R. H. Rahe (eds.), *Life Stress and Psychiatric Illness*. Springfield, Ill.: Charles C. Thomas.

Brown, G. W., T. Harris, and J. Peto (1973b), "Life events and psychiatric disorders—Part 2: Nature of causal link," *Psychological Medicine* 3:159-176.

Brown, G. W., F. Sklair, T. Harris, and J. L. T. Birley (1973a), "Life events and psychiatric disorders-Part 1: Some methodological issues," *Psychological Medicine* 3:74-87.

Brown, G. W., and J. L. T. Birley (1968), "Crises and life changes and the onset of schizophrenia," *Journal of Health and Social Behavior* 9:203-214.

Caplan, G., and M. Killilea (eds.) (1976), *Support Systems and Mutual Help: Multidisciplinary Explorations*. New York: Grune and Stratton, Inc.

Caplan, G. (1974b), *Support Systems and Community Mental Health*. New York: Behavioral Publications.

Carroll, B. J., J. M. Fielding, and T. G. Blashki (1973), "Depression rating scales: A critical review," *Archives of General Psychiatry* 28(3, March):361-366.

Cassel, J. (1976), "The contribution of the social environment to host resistance," *American Journal of Epidemiology* 104(2):107-123.

Cassel, J. (1974b), "An epidemiological perspective of psychosocial factors in disease etiology," *American Journal of Public Health* 64:1040-1043.

Cassel, J. (1974a), "Psychosocial processes and "stress": Theoretical formulation," *International Journal of Health Services* 4:471-482.

Catalano, R., and C. D. Dooley (1977), "Economic predictors of depressed mood and stressful life events in a metropolitan community," *Journal of Health and Social Behavior* 18:292-307.

Cobb, S. (1976), "Social support as a moderator of life stress," *Psychosomatic Medicine* 38:300-314.

Cohen, Y. A. (1961), "The sociological relevance of schizophrenia and depression," pp. 477-485 in Yehudi A. Cohen (ed.), *Social Structure and Personality*. New York: Holt, Rinehart and Winston.

Comstock, G. W., and K. J. Helsing (1976), "Symptoms of depression in two communities," *Psychological Medicine* 6 (4, November):551-563.

Cooley, C. H. (1902), *Human Nature and the Social Order*. New York: Scribner.

Craig, T. J., and P. A. van Natta (1976a), "Presence and persistence of depressive symptoms in patient and community populations," *American Journal of Psychiatry* 133(12, December):1426-1429.

Crandall, D. L., and B. P. Dohrenwend (1967), "Some relations among psychiatric symptoms, organic illness and social class," American Journal of Psychiatry 123(No.12):1527-1538.

Dean, A., and N. Lin (1977), "The stress-buffering role of social support: Problems and prospects for systematic investigation," *Journal of Nervous and Mental Disease* 165:403-417.

Dean, A. (1976), "Mental illness and family homeostasis," pp. 247-262 in A. Dean, A. Kraft and M. Pepper (eds.), *The Social Setting of Mental Health*. New York: Basic Books.

Dean, A., R. F. Klein, and M. D. Bogdonoff (1967), "The impact of illness upon the spouse," *Journal of Chronic Disease* 20:241-248.

Dohrenwend, B. S., L. Krassnoff, A. Askenasy, and B. P. Dohrenwend (1978b), "Exemplification of a method for scaling life events—Peri life events scale," *Journal of Health and Social Behavior* 19:205-229.

Dohrenwend, B. S., and B. P. Dohrenwend (1978a), "Some issues in research on stressful life events," *Journal of Nervous and Mental Disease* 166:7-15.

Dohrenwend, B. P. (1970), "Psychiatric disorder in general populations: Problem of the untreated 'case'," *American Journal of Public Health* 60(June 6):1052-1064.

Eaton, W. (1978), "Life events, social supports and psychiatric symptoms: A re-analysis of the New Haven data," *Journal of Health and Social Behavior* 19:230-234.

Faris, R. E. L., and H. W. Dunham (1939), *Mental Disorders in Urban Areas*. Chicago: University of Chicago Press.

Finlayson, A. (1976), "Social networks as coping resources: Lay help and consultation patterns used by women in husband's post-infarction career," *Social Science and Medicine* 10:97-103.

Freud, S. (1956), "Mourning and Melancholia," pp. 152-169 in James Strachey (ed.), *Collected Papers, 5*. London: The Hogarth Press.

Fried, M. A. (1965), "Transitional functions of working class communities: Implications for forced relocation," pp. 123-165 in Mildred B. Kantor (ed.), *Mobility and Mental Health*. Springfield, Ill.: Charles C. Thomas.

Gersten, J., T. Langner, J. Eisenberg, and O. Simcha-Fagan (1977), "An evaluation of the etiologic role of stressful life-change events in psychological disorders," *Journal of Health and Social Behavior* 18:228-244.

Gore, S. (1978), "The effect of social support in moderating the health consequences of unemployment," *Journal of Health and Social Behavior* 19:157-165.

Gove, W. R. (1978), "Sex differences in mental illness among adult men and women: An evaluation of four questions raised regarding the evidence on the higher rates of women," *Social Science and Medicine—Medical Anthropology* 12(3B, July):187-198.

Gove, W. R., and J. F. Tudor (1973), "Adult sex roles and mental illness," *American Journal of Sociology* 78:812-835.

Gove, W. R. (1972), "The relationship between sex roles, marital status, and mental illness," *Social Forces* 5:34-44.

Hagnell, O. (1966), *A Prospective Study of the Incidence of Mental Disorder*. Lund, Sweden: Scandinavian University Books.

Henderson, S., P. Duncan-Jones, H. McAuley, and K. Ritchie (1978), "The patient's primary group," *British Journal of Psychiatry* 132:74-86.

Henderson, S. (1977), "The social network, support and neurosis: The function of attachment in adult life," *British Journal of Psychiatry* 131:185-191.

Hinkle, L. E., Jr. (1974), "The effect of exposure to cultural change, social change, and changes in interpersonal relationships on health," Pp. 9-44 in B. S. Dohrenwend and B. P. Dohrenwend (eds.), *Stressful Life Events: Their Nature and Effects*. New York: John Wiley and Sons.

Hollingshead, A. B., and F. C. Redlich (1958), *Social Class and Mental Illness: A Community Study*. New York: John Wiley and Sons.

Holmes, T., J. Joffe, and J. Ketcham (1961), "Experimental study of prognosis," *Journal of Psychosomatic Research* 5:235-252.

Hudgens, R. W., E. Robins and W. B. Delong (1970), "The reporting of recent stress in the lives of psychiatric patients," *British Journal of Psychiatry* 117:635-643.

Hudgens, R. W., J. R. Morrison, and R. Barchha (1967), "Life events and onset of primary affective disorders," *Archives of General Psychiatry* 16:134-145.

Husaini, B. A., and J. A. Neff (1979), "Depression in rural communities: Establishing CES-D cutting points," *Mental Health Project, Tennessee State University*, (Feb.)

Husaini, B. A., and J. A. Neff (1978), "Characteristics of life events and psychiatric impairment in rural communities," Paper based upon presentation at the Annual Meeting of the American Public Health Association. Los Angeles, October 16.

Husaini, B. A., J. A. Neff, and R. Stone (1978), "Correlates of psychiatric impairment in rural middle Tennessee," Mental Health Project, Tennessee State University, paper presented at the Second National Conference on Need Assessment in Health and Human Services, Louisville, Kentucky.

Husaini, B. A., and J. A. Neff (1977), "The mental health needs of a rural middle Tennessee community: A preliminary report," Mental Health Project, Tennessee State University, July.

Ilfeld, F. W. (1977), "Current social stressors and symptoms of depression," *American Journal of Psychiatry* 134:161-166.

Ilfeld, F. (1976c), "Methodological issues in relating psychiatric symptoms to social stressors," *Psychological Reports* 39:1251-1258.

Ilfeld, F. (1976b), "Characteristics of current social stressors," *Psychological Reports* 39:1231-1247.

Ilfeld, F. (1976a), "Further validations of a psychiatric symptom index in a normal population," *Psychological Reports* 39:1215-1228.

Jacobs, S. C., B. A. Prusoff, and E. S. Paykel (1974), "Recent life events in schizophrenia and depression," *Psychological Medicine* 4:444-453.

Kaplan, B. H., J. C. Cassel, and S. Gore (1977), "Social support and health" *Medical Care* 15:47-58.

Kaplan, B. H., R. M. Wilson, and A. H. Leighton (Eds.) (1976), *Further Explorations in Social Psychiatry*. New York: Basic Books.

Kaplan, B. (1975), "Toward further research on family and health," pp. 89-106 in B. Kaplan and J. Cassel (eds.), *Family and Health: An Epidemiological Approach*. Chapel Hill, N.C.: Institute for Research in Social Science, University of North Carolina.

Kasl, S. V., S. Gore, and S. Cobb (1975), "The experience of losing a job: Reported changes in health, symptoms and illness behavior," *Psychosomatic Medicine* 37(2):106-121.

Katz, M. M. (1971), "The classification of depression: Normal, clinical and ethnocultural variations." pp. 31-40 in Ronald R. Fieve (ed.), *Depression in the 1970's: Modern Theory and Research*. Proceedings of the Symposium New York, New York, October. Amsterdam: Excerpta Medica.

Klerman, G. L. (1979), "The age of melancholy," *Psychology Today* 12(11):37-42.

Kramer, M., E. S. Pollack, R. W. Redick, and B. Locke (1972), *Mental Disorders/Suicide*. Cambridge: Harvard University Press.

Langner, T. S., and S. T. Michael (1963), *Life Stress and Mental Health*. New York: The Free Press of Glencoe.

Leff, M. J., J. F. Roatch, and W. F. Bunney (1970), "Environmental factors preceding the onset of severe depressions," *Psychiatry* 33.

Leighton, A. H. (1959), *My Name is Legion*. New York: Basic Books, Inc.

Leighton, D., J. Harding, D. Macklin, A. MacMillian, and A. Leighton (1963), *The Character of Danger*. New York: Basic Books.

Liem, R., and J. Liem (1978), "Social class and mental illness reconsidered: Role of economic stress and social support," *Journal of Health and Social Behavior* 19:139-156.

Lin, N., R. Simeone, W. M. Ensel, and W. Kuo (1979), "Social support, stressful life events and illness: A model and an empirical test," *Journal of Health and Social Behavior* 20:108-120.

Lin, N., A. Dean, and W. M. Ensel (1979), *Development of Social Support Scales*. Paper presented at the Third Biennial Conference on Health Survey Research Methods (May), Reston, Virginia.

Lowe, D. J. (compiled) (1975), *The Cornell Indices, A Bibliography of Health Questionnaires*. New York: The Cornell Medical College Library.

Lowenthal, M. F., and C. Haven (1968), "Interaction and adaptation: Intimacy as a critical variable," *American Sociological Review* 33:20-30.

Lynch, J. (1977), *The Broken Heart*. New York: Basic Books, Inc.

Markush, R., and R. Favero (1974), "Epidemiologic assessment of stressful life events, depressed mood and psychophysiological symptoms: A preliminary report," pp. 171-190 in B. S. Dohrenwend and B. P. Dohrenwend (eds.), *Stressful Life Events: Their Nature and Effects*. New York: Wiley.

Medalie, J. H., and U. Goldbourt (1976), "Angina Pectoris among 10,000 men II. Psychosocial and other risk factors as evidenced by a multivariate analysis of a five year incidence study," *The American Journal of Medicine* 60:910-921.

Miller, P., J. G. Ingham, and S. Davidson (1976), "Life events, symptoms and social support," *Journal of Psychosomatic Research* 20:516-522.

Mitchell, C. (ed.) (1969), *Social Networks in Urban Situations*. Manchester, England: University of Manchester Press.

Moriwaki, S. Y. (1973), "Self disclosure, significant others and psychological well being in old age," *Journal of Health and Social Behavior* 14(3):226-232.

Mueller, D., D. Edwards, and R. Yarvis (1978), "Stressful life events and community mental health center patients," *Journal of Nervous and Mental Disease* 166:16-24.

Mueller, D. D. Edwards, and R. Yarvis (1977), "Stressful life events and psychiatric symptomatology: Change or undesirability?" *Journal of Health and Social Behavior* 18:307-317.

Muhlin, G. L. (1978), *Cultural Isolation and the Mental Hospitalization Patterns of the Foreign Born in New York City*. Paper presented at the Annual Meeting of the Eastern Sociological Society at Philadelphia, PA. (April).

Murphy, J. M. (1976), "Social causes: The independent variables," pp. 386-406 in B. H. Kaplan, R. N. Wilson and A. H. Leighton (eds.), *Further Explorations in Social Psychiatry*. New York: Basic Books.

Myers, J. K., M. Weissman, and D. Thompson (1979), *Screening for Depression in a Community Sample: The Use of Symptom Scale to Detect the Depressive Syndrome*. Paper delivered at the Annual Meetings of the Society for Edpidemiological Research. Yale University research.

Myers, J. (1976), *Future Research in Mental Disease*, Paper presented at the Annual Convention of the American Sociological Association, New York.

Myers, J. K., J. J. Lindenthal, and M. P. Pepper (1975), "Life events, social integration and psychiatric symptomatology," *Journal of Health and Social Behavior* 16:421-429.

Myers, J. K., J. J. Lindenthal, M. P. Pepper, and D. R. Ostrander (1972), "Life events and mental status: A longitudinal study," *Journal of Health and Social Behavior* 13:398-406.

Myers, J. K., J. J. Lindenthal, and M. P. Pepper (1971), "Life events and psychiatric impairment," *The Journal of Nervous and Mental Disease* 152:149-157.

National Institute of Mental Health. (1973), *Special Report; 1973, The Depressive Disorders*. Washington, D.C.: U.S. Government Printing Office.

Neff, J. A., B. A. Husaini, and J. McCorkel (1978), *Psychiatric and Medical Problems in Rural*

Communities. Prepared for presentation at the Annual Meeting of the American Public Health Association at Los Angeles, California (October 18).

Nuckolls, D., J. Cassel, and B. Kaplan (1972), "Psychosocial assets, life crisis and the prognosis of pregnancy," *American Journal of Epidemiology* 95:431–441.

Paykel, E. S. (1976), "Life stress, depression and attempted suicide," *Journal of Human Stress,* pp. 3–12, (September).

Paykel, E. S., B. A. Prusoff, and J. K. Myers (1975), "Suicide attempts and recent life events: A controlled comparison," *Archives of General Psychiatry* 32:327–333.

Paykel, E. S. (1974), "Life stress and psychiatric disorder: Applications of the clinical approach," pp. 135–149 in B. S. Dohrenwend and B. P. Dohrenwend (eds.), *Stressful Life Events: Their Nature and Effects*. New York: John Wiley & Sons.

Paykel, E. S., J. K. Myers, M. N. Dienelt, G. L. Klerman, J. J. Lindenthal, and M. Pepper (1969), "Life events and depression: A controlled study," *Archives of General Psychiatry* 21:753–760.

Pearlin, L., and C. Schooler (1978), "Structure of coping," *Journal of Health and Social Behavior* 19:2–21.

Pearlin, L., and J. S. Johnson (1977), "Marital status, life strains and depression," *American Sociological Review* 42:704–715.

Pitts, J. R. (1964), "The structural-functional approach," in H. T. Christensen (ed.), *The Handbook of Marriage and the Family*. Chicago: Rand McNally.

Rabkin, J., and E. Struening (1976), "Life events, stress and illness," *Science* 194:1013–1020.

Radloff, L. (1977), "The CES-D scale: A self-report depression scale for research in the general population," *Applied Psychological Measurement* 1:385–410.

Radloff, L. (1975), *Sex Differences in Depression. The Effects of Occupation and Marital Status* New York: Plenum Publishing Corporation.

Rahe, R. (1975), "Epidemiological studies of life change and illness," *International Journal of Psychiatry in Medicine* 6:133–146.

Ratcliffe, W. (1978), "Social networks and health: An initial report," *Connections Bulletin of the International Network for Social Network Analysis* 1:25–37.

"Report of the task panel on community support systems," (1978), submitted to the *President's Commission on Mental Health.*

Ross, C., and J. Mirowsky (1979), "A comparison of life event weighing schemes: Change, undesirability, and effect-proportional indices," June.

Schwab, J. J., R. A. Bell, G. J. Warheit, and R. B. Schwab (1979), *Social Order and Mental Health. The Florida Health Study*. New York: Brunner/Mazel, Publishers.

Schwab, J., N. Traven, and G. Warheit (1978), "Relationships between physical and mental illness," *Psychosomatics* 19:458–463.

Schwab, J. J. (1971), "Depressive illness: A sociomedical syndrome," *Psychosomatics* 12:385–389.

Sethi, B. B. (1964), "The relationship of separation to depression," *Archives of General Psychiatry* 10:486–496(May).

Silverman, C. (1968), *Epidemiology of Depression*. Baltimore: John Hopkins.

Simmons, R. G., S. D. Klein and R. L. Simmons (1977), *Gift of Life: The Social and Psychological Impact of Organ Transplantation*. New York: Wiley Interscience.

Tischler, G. L., J. E. Henisz, J. K. Myers, and P. C. Boswell (1975), "Utilization of mental health services. I. Patienthood and the prevalence of symptomatology in the community," *Archives of General Psychiatry* 32(4,April):411–415.

Tonks, C. M., E. S. Paykel, and C. L. Klerman (1970), "Clinical depressions among Negroes," *American Journal of Psychiatry* 127:329–335.

The U.S. Fact Book: The American Almanac. (1977) 97th Edition. New York: Grosset and Dunlap. p. 159.

Vinokur, A., and M. Selzer (1975), "Desirable versus undesirable life events: Their relationships to stress and mental distress," *Journal of Personality and Social Psychology* 32:329-337.

Warheit, G., C. Holzer, R. Bell, and S. Arey (1976), "Sex, marital status and mental health: A reappraisal," *Social Forces* 55:459-470.

Warheit, G. J., C. E. Holzer, and J. J. Schwab (1973), "An analysis of social class and racial differences in depressive symptomatology: A community study," *Journal of Health and Social Behavior* 14:291-299.

Weissman, M. M., and J. K. Myers (1978), "Rate and risks of depressive symptoms in a U.S. urban community," *ACTA Psychiatrica Scandinavica* 57(3):219-231.

Weissman, M., J. Myers, and P. Harding (1978), "Psychiatric disorders in the U.S. urban community, 1975-1976," *American Journal of Psychiatry* 135:459-462.

Weissman, M., D. Sholomskas, M. Pottenger, B. Prusoff, and B. Locke (1977), "Assessing depressive symptoms in five psychiatric populations: A validation study," *American Journal of Epidemiology* 106:203-214.

Weissman, M. M., M. Pottenger, H. Kleber, H. L. Ruben, D. Williams, and W. K. Thompson (1977), "Symptom patterns in primary and secondary depression: A comparison of primary depressives with depressed opiate addicts, alcoholics, and schizophrenics," *Archives of General Psychiatry* 34(7, July):854-862.

Weissman, M. M., and G. L. Klerman (1977), "Sex differences and the epidemiology of depression," *Archives of General Psychiatry* 34:98-111.

Weissman, M. M., and B. Z. Locke (1975), *Comparison of a Self-Report Symptom Rating Scale (CES-D) with Standardized Depression Rating Scales in Psychiatric Populations: A Preliminary Report.* Paper presented at Annual Meeting of the Society for Epidemiologic Research, Albany, New York (June 19).

Weissman, M. M., B. Prusoff, and C. Pincus (1975), "Symptom patterns in depressed patients and depressed normals," *Journal of Nervous and Mental Disease* 160(1, January):15-23.

Weissman, M. M., and E. S. Paykel (1974), *The Depressed Woman.* Chicago: The University of Chicago Press.

Wolfenstein, M. (1958), "Two types of Jewish mothers," pp. 520-534 in M. Sklare (ed.), *The Jews.* Glencoe, Ill.: The Free Press.

APPENDIX A. ITEM-TOTAL CORRELATIONS OF INSTRUMENTAL-EXPRESSIVE SUPPORT SALES

ITEMS	LOADING ON INSTRUMENTAL/EXPRESSIVE FACTORS*
MONETARY PROBLEMS	*Factor I*
Problems managing money	.809
Deciding how to spend money	.790
Not enough money to do things	.875
Not enough money to get by	.828
LACK OF COMPANIONSHIP	*Factor II*
No close companion	.720
Not happy with marital status	.834
Not enough close friends	.664
Problems with spouse/ex-spouse	.811
No one to show love/affection	.823
Too dependent on others	.543
DEMANDS	*Factor III*
Too many responsibilities	.833
No one to depend on	.782
Too many demands	.793
Unsatisfactory sex life	.722
COMMUNICATION PROBLEMS	*Factor IV*
Problems communicating	.627
Problems with children	.805
Unsatisfying job	.753
No one to understand problems	.738
Conflicts with those who are close	.781
NOT HAVING CHILDREN	*Factor V*
	.794

*All coefficients were significant at the .001 level

101

APPENDIX B. THE SOCIODEMOGRAPHIC CHARACTERISTICS OF SOCIAL SUPPORT

Social Support	Sex	Age	Marital Status	Family Income	No. Dep. Kids	Employ. Status	Prior Hist. of Illness	a	Error of Estimate
				Metric Coefficients*					
Monetary Problems	—	-.082 (.031)	— —	.690 (.146)	1.182 (.381)	2.80 (.955)	.740 (.237)	8.32	3.51
Demands	—	-.031 (.028)	—	—	.706 (.364)	1.78 (.896)	.857 (.218)	16.52	3.66
Communic. Problems	—	-.104 (.030)	—	—	.174 (.415)	—	—	15.87	3.71
Lack of Companions	—	-.072 (.029)	—	—	—	—	—	23.13	4.10
Medalie Goldbourt	—	-.027 (.013)	—	—	.435 (.173)	.316 (.424)	.383 (.103)	6.29	1.38
Comm.-Neigh. Satisfaction	—	—	.203 (.444)	.103 (.053)	—	—	—	4.09	1.59
Durability of Confidant	-.630 (.237)	.027 (.007)	—	-.038 (.035)	—	—	—	2.92	.84
Directedness of Confidant	—	—	—	.070 (.045)	—	—	.127 (.086)	1.54	1.21

Standardized Coefficients

								R^2
Monetary Problems	—	−.302	—	.504	.315	.296	.284	.488
Demands	—	−.128	—	—	.214	.212	.374	.270
Communic. Problems	—	−.467	—	—	—	—	—	.218
Lack of Companions	—	−.295	—	—	—	—	—	.087
Medalie Goldbourt	—	−.271	—	—	3.19	.091	.404	.406
Comm.-Neigh. Satisfaction	—	—	—	.254	—	—	—	.064
Durability of Confidant	−.275	.464	—	−.130	—	—	—	.349
Directedness of Confidant	—	—	—	−.194	—	—	.185	.095

*The unstandardized regression coefficients appear on the first line while their standard errors appear on the second.

APPENDIX C
SOCIAL SUPPORT SCALES

I. *Lowenthal-Haven-Kaplan Confidant Items*
    Now I would like to ask you some other questions about
    people you have contact with.

    1. During the past 12 months have you had anyone
        that you could trust and talk to?   _____
        1. Yes
        2. No (Skip to question #   )
        8. Don't know
        9. No answer

    2. How many people have you been able to trust and
        talk to?   _____
        _____ number of confidants
        8. Don't know
        9. No answer

    PROVIDE RESPONDENT WITH
    CARD AND PENCIL—CARD #10

    *Would you write down the names of these people on the
    card that I have given you. Don't list more than 3 people,
    and try to list them in order of those you have been most
    likely to talk with. This list is only for use in helping you
    answer the next several questions.*

    3. How many years have you known this (first,
        second, third) person?   1st _____
        _____ number of years   2nd _____
        98. Don't know   3rd _____
        99. No answer/not applicable
    SHOW CARD #11
    4. During this 12-month period, how often have you
        had contact with this (first, second, third) person?   1st _____
        RESPONSE SET A   2nd _____
        1. Most or all of the time (5–7 days a week)   3rd _____
        2. Occasionally or a moderate amount of time
            (3–4 days a week)
        3. Some or a little of the time (1–2 days a week)
        4. Rarely (less than once a week)
        5. Never
        8. Don't know
        9. No answer/not applicable

5. How often have you talked with this (first, second, third) person when you had a problem?

   RESPONSE SET B   1st _____
   1. Most or all of the time   2nd _____
   2. Occasionally or a moderate amount of time   3rd _____
   3. Some or a little of the time
   4. Rarely
   5. Never
   8. Don't know
   9. No answer/not applicable

6. How often has this (first, second, third) person talked over their problems with you?
   RESPONSE SET B   1st _____
   1. Most or all of the time   2nd _____
   2. Occasionally or a moderate amount of time   3rd _____
   3. Some or a little of the time
   4. Rarely
   5. Never
   8. Don't know
   9. No answer/not applicable

7. How easy has it been to get a hold of this (first, second, third) person? RESPONSE SET C   1st _____
   1. Very easy   2nd _____
   2. Easy   3rd _____
   3. Somewhat easy
   4. Not very easy
   5. Not easy at all
   8. Don't know
   9. No answer/not applicable

8. How freely have you been able to talk about anything you wished with this (first, second, third) person? RESPONSE SET D   1st _____
   1. Very freely   2nd _____
   2. Freely   3rd _____
   3. Somewhat freely
   4. Not very freely
   5. Not freely at all
   8. Don't know
   9. No answer/not applicable

9. How important would you say this (first, second, third) person is to you? RESPONSE SET E   1st _____

(continued)

APPENDIX C—(Continued)

1. Very important   2nd _____
2. Important   3rd _____
3. Somewhat important
4. Not very important
5. Not important at all
8. Don't know
9. No answer/not applicable

10. What is this (first, second, third) person's
    relationship to you?   1st _____
    1. Spouse (lover)   2nd _____
    2. Son/Daughter   3rd _____
    3. Mother/Father
    4. Brother/Sister
    5. In-laws
    6. Other relative
    7. Close friend
    8. Other acquaintance
    9. Neighbor
    10. Co-worker
    11. Helping professional
    12. Other (Specify) _____
    98. Don't know
    99. No answer/not applicable

11. At the present time, is this (first, second, third)
    person still someone you feel you can trust and
    talk to?   1st _____
    1. Yes   2nd _____
    2. No   3rd _____
    8. Don't know
    9. No answer/not applicable

II. *Medalie-Goldbourt Scale*
    IF MARRIED ASK NEXT 4 QUESTIONS
    *Now I would like to ask you a few questions about you
    and your family.* SHOW CARD #8
    1. Have you had any problems (conflicts) with your
       family at present? RESPONSE SET A   _____
       1. No problems at all
       2. No serious problems
       3. Yes, serious problems
       4. Yes, very serious problems

       8. Don't know

       9. No answer/not applicable

  2. Did you have any problems (conflicts) with your family in the past? RESPONSE SET A   _____

       1. No problems at all

       2. No serious problems

       3. Yes, serious problems

       4. Yes, very serious problems

       8. Don't know

       9. No answer/not applicable

  3. How does it affect you when your spouse or children do not listen to you or even oppose you? RESPONSE SET B   _____

       1. Never happens

       2. Does not affect me especially

       3. Upsets me quite a bit

       4. Upsets me very much

       8. Don't know

       9. No answer/not applicable

  4. Does your spouse show you his/her love? RESPONSE SET C   _____

       1. Loves me and shows it often

       2. Loves me and shows it occasionally

       3. Loves me but never shows it

       4. Does not love me

       8. Don't know

       9. No answer/not applicable

III. *Community-Neighborhood Satisfaction*

  1. In general, how satisfied are you with this neighborhood? SHOW CARD #1   _____

       1. Very satisfied

       2. Somewhat satisfied

       3. Somewhat dissatisfied

       4. Very dissatisfied

       8. Don't know

       9. No answer

  2. On the whole, how satisfied are you with living here in this community? SHOW CARD #1   _____

       1. Very satisfied

       2. Somewhat satisfied

       3. Somewhat dissatisfied

(*continued*)

APPENDIX C—(Continued)

4. Very dissatisfied
8. Don't know
9. No answer

IV. *Instrumental-Expressive Support*
*The following is a list of problems that people sometimes
have.* SHOW CARD #9
Would you tell me how often you have been bothered
by these problems over the past 12 months.
1. Most or all of the time
2. Occasionally or a moderate amount of time
3. Some or a little of the time
4. Rarely
5. Never
8. Don't know
9. No answer/not applicable

1. Having problems managing money . . . .   _____
2. Not having a close companion . . . .   _____
3. Having too many responsibilities . . . .   _____
4. Not having people you can depend on . . . .   _____
5. Too many demands on your time . . . .   _____
6. Not having a satisfactory sex life . . . .   _____
7. Having problems communicating with others . . .   _____
8. Not seeing enough of people you feel close to . .   _____
9. Deciding on how to spend money . . . .   _____
10. Not having enough responsibilities . . . .   _____
11. Having too little leisure time . . . .   _____
12. Not having enough money to do the things you want   _____
13. Problems with children . . . .   _____
14. Not having a satisfying job . . . .   _____
15. Feeling too controlled by others . . . .   _____
16. Not having enough money to get by on . . . .   _____
17. Dissatisfied with your marital status
     (single, married) . . . .   _____
18. Not having enough close friends . . . .   _____
19. Problems with spouse/ex-spouse . . . .   _____
20. Not having someone who shows you love and   _____
     affection . . . .
21. Feeling too dependent on others . . . .   _____
22. Not having children . . . .   _____
23. Problems with inlaws/relatives . . . .   _____

24. Not having someone who understands your problems .... _____
25. Having too much time on your hands .... _____
26. Conflicts with people who are close to you ..... _____
    Are there any other problems that I have not mentioned that really bother you?

_____

COMPONENTS OF THE SEX
DIFFERENCE IN DEPRESSION

Lenore Sawyer Radloff and Donald S. Rae

The goal of public health is the control and prevention of diseases and disorders even when their etiology is imperfectly understood. Even the simplest infectious disease is influenced by a combination of multiple causal factors. Intervention may be attempted at any point in the causal chain. The more we know about the necessary and sufficient conditions for the disease, the more efficient our interventions can be.

Epidemiology has developed strategies for the study of disorders of unknown (or imperfectly known) etiology. The first is simply to specify as clearly as possible the disorder being studied. This is important in obtaining a homogeneous dependent variable, and also in allowing research findings to be interpreted in the context of previous research and theory about the disorder. The more accurately the disorder can be defined and identified, the more homogeneous the study group can be, and therefore the more confidence we can place in the research findings. A second strategy is to make the distinction between susceptibility and precipitating factors. Each is a necessary but not sufficient condition

Research in Community and Mental Health, Volume 2, pages 111–137
Copyright © 1981 by JAI Press, Inc.
ISBN: 0-89232-152-0

for the occurrence of the disorder. The nature of the factors involved in susceptibility may be very different from those which are precipitants, but they should be related by mechanisms postulated by theory. The third strategy is to examine the multitude of empirical risk factors (which may relate to susceptibility as well as to precipitating factors) in order to seek empirical patterns and theoretical commonalities which lead to hypotheses regarding the ways underlying mechanisms might contribute to the disorder.

The purpose of the present paper is to describe an application of these strategies in the field of mental health. The disorder is specified as the depressive syndrome (described more fully below). This is more specific than "mental illness" in general, but not as specific as would be possible if sub-types of depression were distinguished. Risk factors for depression, with special emphasis on sex differences, will be examined in the context of a conceptual model which distinguishes susceptibility from precipitating factors. In terms of the sex difference in depression, data analyses will be presented regarding the relative contribution of male-female differences both in susceptibility and in exposure to precipitating factors.

Speculations regarding the sources and the mechanisms of these differences will be discussed in terms of current learning theories of depression.

Specification of the Disorder: The Depressive Syndrome

Depression has been defined in many ways, ranging from transient mood to psychotic illness. Current diagnostic practice identifies a variety of sub-types of depression. For example, DSM III (Spitzer *et al.*, 1978) lists seven diagnoses which have depressive features, and lists 11 non-exclusive sub-types of Major Depressive Disorder. For purposes of the *theoretical* discussion presented here, the disorder is specified as the depressive syndrome (as described by Beck, 1967). The syndrome includes symptoms of four types: *Cognitive* beliefs of helplessness and hopelessness; *Affective* feelings of sadness and lack of enjoyment; *Behavioral* manifestations of decreased activity and interest; and *Somatic* disturbances of appetite and sleep. (For brevity, the term depression will sometimes be used, but should be read as "the depressive syndrome.") As will be discussed in the conclusion, a theory which hypothesizes sequential causal relationships among the four types of symptoms can be developed (see Radloff and Rae, 1979; Radloff, in press.) Further research will be needed to determine whether in truth the four dimensions are related causally and therefore co-vary together or whether instead there are certain sub-types of depression (especially those which include schizophrenic features or manic episodes and those which are secondary to other disorders) for which the theory is not appropriate.

However, for the purpose of the empirical analysis in this paper, "the depressive syndrome" is treated as a unitary dependent variable. As will be described below, the level of the disorder is operationally defined by scores on a self-report scale of depressive symptomatology (the CES-D scale). This scale includes symptoms of the four types or dimensions of depression described above.

Sex Role and Depression

Sex is one of the most consistently confirmed risk factors in depression. Depression has been found to be more common in women than men in studies of treated cases and in household surveys using self-report symptom measures. Weissman & Klerman (1977) have reviewed the evidence and have concluded that this difference is not an artifact due to sex biases in diagnosis, symptom reporting, or help-seeking behavior. They also conclude that, although there is good evidence for biological factors in depression, there is no firm evidence for sex-linked biological factors which could explain all of the sex difference in depression.

The major issue to be dealt with in this paper involves the distinction between precipitating factors and susceptibility. On the one hand, females may be more likely than males to be exposed to *precipating* factors placing them at risk for depression (including disadvantaged social status and excess of other stressors). On the other hand, women may be more *susceptible;* that is, they may react more strongly with depression when exposed to the same degree of increasing risk. They may be more reactive to the same stressor, for example, because of so-cialization into learned helplessness or a "depressogenic" feminine sex role (Bart, 1975). There is clear evidence that women do experience some of these precipitating factors more than men, but the connection to depression has not been verified.

The distinction between susceptibility and precipitating factors has previously been made in analyses of the contribution of stress to general mental distress (see Langner and Michael, 1963) and in terms of depression in particular (see Beck, 1967; Brown and Harris, 1978). There are a variety of theories of depression to consider and we will not attempt to review them all (see Akiskal and McKinney, 1975, for one recent review). The types of causal factors suggested by these theories are biological (including genetic), intrapsychic, and environmental. In this analysis, we shall explore the impact of environmental precipitating factors, and shall assume that persons react differently to these precipitating factors depending on their susceptibility.

Environmental Precipitating Risk Factors for Depression

Risk factors for depression have been reviewed by Silverman (1968), and studied in several surveys since her review. Higher levels of depression have been found to be associated with having low socioeconomic status, being not-married, being non-white, living with children, lacking social support and activi-ties, being physically ill, and experiencing life changes (especially losses). Recent surveys (Benfari et al., 1972; Berkman, 1971) have found higher levels of depression in young respondents (ages 18 to 24), although previously depression was seen as a disorder of middle age. Results on urban/rural differences have been inconsistent.

In this study, we shall further investigate the impact of most of the above factors on depression (age, race, socioeconomic status, marital and family status, physical illness, life event losses, various types of activity-level). First, do our data also indicate similar effects upon depression for both men and women (see Radloff and Rae, 1979; Radloff, in press; Radloff, 1975)? And second, are females more likely than males to be exposed to those particular factors which appear to precipitate depression?

Sex-Role and Susceptibility

Whether or not females are exposed to the same levels of stressors as males, they may react more strongly to increasing stress. They may be more susceptible to stressors. Recently, Kessler (unpublished) has presented data suggesting that the sex difference in a global distress measure was due more to a sex difference in susceptibility than to differences in exposure to stressors. The mechanism by which sex might contribute to susceptibility has not been specified nor has the mechanism by which stress precipitates distress.

By specifying the disorder as the depressive syndrome, it may be possible to speculate about mechanisms. It is, of course, possible that females are biologically more susceptible to stressors than males through sex-linked genetic mechanisms. However, apart from genetics, there is some evidence in the literature to suggest that learned sex-role behavior will increase female susceptibility to depression (see Weissman and Klerman, 1977). Insofar as a person learns that behavior is ineffective in controlling outcomes, that one is helpless to alter events, then he or she should be more likely to develop the symptoms of depression (helplessness and hopelessness) and (if the other dimensions are causally related)[1] the full depressive syndrome. There is strong evidence (Radloff and Monroe, 1978) that women are more likely than men to experience the conditions that would produce such cognitions. From childhood on, females are less likely than males to learn that outcomes are contingent on their own actions.

At birth, according to one study, female babies were rated by their parents as smaller, weaker, and more in need of being taken care of than male babies of equal birth weight and health (Rubin et al., 1974). In another investigation, preschool teachers were more likely to react to boys' behavior and to ignore girls' actions (Serbin et al., 1973), so that boys may have learned that their actions produced results (whether positive or negative) and that they had control over their rewards and punishments. Dweck et al. (1978) found that elementary school teachers were likely to attribute failure by boys to lack of effort and urge them to try harder, while failure by girls was more attributed to lack of ability, with little encouragement of increased effort. Girls were seen as needing help and protection (Block, 1975). The differences between the childhoood socialization of boys and girls has been described by Bronfenbrenner: "With sons, socialization seems to focus primarily on directing and constraining the boy's impact on the environment. With daughters, the aim is rather to protect the girl from the impact of environment. The boy is being prepared to mold his world, the girl to be molded by it" (Bronfenbrenner, 1961, p. 260). Throughout childhood, the media reinforce this view (Sternglanz and Serbin, 1974; Hillman, 1974).

These patterns and attitudes appear to continue into adulthood. Assertive women and non-assertive men have been found to be considered deviates (Costrich et al., 1975). In mixed sex groups, women exhibited characteristics typical of low status (Unger, 1975): they contributed less in discussions (Alkire et al., 1968); their solutions to problems were devalued by the group (Wahrman and Pugh, 1974); they were less often chosen for leadership roles (Altemeyer and Jones, 1974); eventually, they tended to stop trying and became depressed (Wolman and Frank, 1975). It has also been reported (Feather and Simon, 1975) that women were likely to attribute success to the unstable factors of effort or luck rather than to competence, and to attribute failure to the stable factor of lack of competence, whereas men's attributions tended to be just the opposite (success because of competence, failure because of lack of effort or bad luck). With such attribution patterns, women would tend to view failure as more likely to continue into the future, while men would tend to expect success to continue.

In summary, there is evidence in the literature that females are more likely than males to learn the helpless cognitions that, according to our hypothesis, contribute to susceptibility to depression.[2]

In this analysis, we shall attempt to test whether females are more susceptible than males to the same environmental stressors: that is, whether they are more likely to react to an increasing source of stress with higher scores on the overall depression scale. In this paper, as mentioned above, the four dimensions of depression will not be treated separately. It should also be noted that some of the environmental precipitating factors or stressors could increase susceptibility to depression in their own right by similar mechanisms (e.g., low socio-economic status in childhood could also increase learned helplessness). However, in this analysis, these factors are considered as precipitants and stressors; focus is on the differential exposure and reaction of males and females to them.[3]

METHODS

Subjects

Data for present analyses were from a large household survey conducted in Kansas City, Missouri, in 1971-1972, and in Washington County, Maryland, in 1971-1973. Field work was done by local organizations[4] under contract with the

Center for Epidemiologic Studies (CES), National Institute of Mental Health. The survey covered representative samples of households in these communities, with one individual over age 18 randomly selected for interview from each household. The response rate in Kansas City was 74.8 percent, in Washington County, 80.1 percent, yielding responses from 1161 persons in Kansas City and 1671 in Washington County. For the present analyses, the data from the two sites were combined.

Measures

Depression. The survey questionnaire included the CES Depression Scale (CES-D Scale) which was designed to measure the level of depressive symptomatology in the general population. The 20 items in the scale (see Appendix) were chosen from several earlier depression scales (Minnesota Multiphasic Personality Inventory, Zung Self-Rating Depression Scale, Beck Depression Inventory). The criteria for selecting items were discriminatory power, validity, and representation of each of the major factors in the clinical syndrome of depression. Respondents were asked to report the frequency of each symptom during the past week, ranging from "never" (weight = 0) to "most or all of the time" (weight = 3). Response weights were reversed for the four positive items. The CES-D score is computed by adding the weights for the 20 items. The possible range of scores is zero to 60. The range of scores actually obtained was zero to 53, with an overall average of 9.43, and standard deviation of 8.70.

Properties of the CES-D Scale have been described in detail previously. High internal consistency and construct validity were found in a variety of demographic subgroups (Radloff, 1977). In a clinical validation study (Weissman et al., 1977) with a group of depressed outpatients, the CES-D correlated highly with other self-report scales and with clinical rating scales for depression (The Hamilton and the Raskin). CES-D scores decreased significantly as patients under treatment improved. In general, the scale correlates satisfactorily with clinical ratings of severity of depression, and discriminates well between depressed patients and normals.

In addition, the scale has good content validity as a measure of the syndrome of depression, since it includes symptoms of the four dimensions of depression described above (cognitive, affective, behavioral, and somatic manipulations). However, it cannot be expected to distinguish sub-types of depression, nor to distinguish primary from secondary depression. Therefore, the data analyses cannot be claimed to apply to a homogeneous diagnostic group. The data are relevant to the theory to the extent that the CES-D scale does indicate the presence (and level of severity) of the depressive syndrome, and to the extent that the theory applies to the syndrome across diagnostic sub-types and levels of severity. Further research, using recently developed structured diagnostic interviews, will make more refined analyses possible.

Risk Factors. The survey questionnaire also included measures of the risk factors for depression which have been found in previous studies. Urban/rural status was not significantly related to CES-D scores and was not used in the present analysis. The 30 variables used here, measuring six types of risk factors, are listed below. Each was scored so that the correlation with the CES-D scale was positive. The level associated with lowest depression was coded zero. Thus, in a regression analysis, the intercept (a) will have the same interpretation for every variable; i.e., the level of depression predicted by the best fitting regression line for a zero level or lowest stress-level of x.

Demographic
    Age
    Race
Socio-economic
    Education
    Household income
    Occupational status
    Number of persons supervised on job (zero if not employed)
    Know welfare (Does respondent know anyone currently receiving welfare?)
    Any welfare (Is respondent currently receiving welfare or unemployment?)
Physical problems
    Current illness
    Recent illness
    Handicap
Losses
    Early loss (Did respondent live with own parents through childhood?)
    Moved (past year)
    Life events losses (past year: broken friendship, family member left home, death of friend, income or property loss)
    Marital status loss (past year: widowed, divorced, separated)
Social support and activities
    Get together (with friends or neighbors)
    Religious activities
    Household activities (work around home, leave the house, spend money)
    Excessive bedrest (nap, stay in bed, oversleep)
    Leisure activities
Household status (combination of marital status, relationship to head of household, whether one lives with children, whether one lives with another adult; used as 10 binary ("dummy") variables, with each individual in one and only one category.)
  1. Married, no children present
  2. Married, with children present
  3. Never married, head of household
  4. Never married, not head of household
  5. Widowed, live with own children and no other adults
  6. Widowed, live alone
  7. Widowed, other
  8. Divorced/separated, live with own children and no other adult
  9. Divorced/separated, live alone
 10. Divorced/separated, other

The household status variables were handled this way because previous analyses of these data had shown that, with depression as the dependent variable, there were interactions between marital status, sex and relationship to head of household (Radloff, 1975). The measures indicating the presence of other people in the household (live with own children, live with other adult) also were confounded with marital status. A person who is married is, by definition, living with another adult. (Respondents who reported themselves as being married, but had no spouse living in the same household, were recorded as separated.) Very few of the never married were living with children.

It was therefore decided to create ten inclusive and mutually exclusive dummy variables reflecting various relevant combinations of these important variables. (In the multiple regression analysis, one of these variables was omitted to avoid a singular matrix.) Each respondent was coded yes (1) for the appropriate status and no (0) for the other nine. To keep the scoring of these 10 variables consistent with that of the other 20, it was decided that if the correlation of any item with CES-D was negative for both males and females then the item would be rescored so that yes = 0 and no = 1. (This was done for Married, no children; and Married, with children. Depression was lower for those in these two categories compared with all others.)

Three variables were found to have correlations of different signs for the two sexes (Never married, head; Widowed, other; and Widowed, alone). In all three cases, the correlations were positive for males and negative for females (i.e., males in these categories were more depressed than all others; females were less depressed). The scoring was based on the sign of the correlation with the largest absolute value (i.e., if the correlation between the variable and depression was higher for males than females, then the value indicating lowest stress for males was coded zero). By this criterion, only Widowed, other, was rescored so that yes = 0 and no = 1.

A Regression Model of Susceptibility and Precipitating Factors

The general model for susceptibility and precipitating factors can be represented by a simple linear regression, $y = a + bx$. (Note that a non-linear model would be more complex, but analogous.) The dependent variable, y, is the level of the disorder. In our application, the dependent variable, y, is the average level of the depression score in a group of respondents. The independent variable, x, represents the precipitating factor. In our application, there will be multiple x's, which are measures of a variety of sociodemographic risk factors for depression. The unstandardized regression coefficient, b, is the increase in depression which is associated with an increase in a precipitating factor. (The model assumes that each precipitating factor is coded so that its association with depression is positive, not negative.) It should be noted that we do not mean to assert causality, simply association. Note also that the susceptibility with which we are concerned is only that for *depression* associated with the precipitating factors, and does not include increases in *other* disorders which might also be associated with them. In our application, there will be a different regression coefficient, b, associated with each x. Our assumption here is that *one type* of susceptibility is the tendency to react to a precipitating factor with depression, so that b is an indicator of this type of susceptibility. (Let us call it *reactive* susceptibility, to distinguish it from individual differences in the disorder which are *not* associated with precipitating factors.) Group differences in reactive susceptibility (in this case, male-female differences) would be reflected in differences in the b's.

Thus, when we apply the regression model to the theory, the mean levels of empirical risk factors ($\bar{X}$'s) are seen as indicators of the probability of precipitating factors (stressors) and the regression coefficients (b's) as indices of the probability of depression *associated with* those precipitating factors. One can compare the $\bar{X}$'s for men and women to see which sex experiences the higher level of exposure to that precipitating factor. One can compare the b's to see which sex reacts more strongly with depression to that stressor (an index of reactive susceptibility).

Kessler (1979, unpublished) and Winsborough and Dickinson (1971), have described an arithmetic method to further explicate the contribution of differences in a, b, and x to the difference between the averages of the two groups on a dependent measure, y. The overall difference in y is decomposed into four components described below. This method will be used to estimate the relative contribution of differences in susceptibility and precipitating factors to the sex difference in depression.

Calculation of Decomposition Method

The multiple regression model for each sex is written as follows:

$$\bar{y}_M = a_M + \sum_i b_{iM}\bar{x}_{iM}$$

$$\tag{1}$$

$$\bar{y}_F = a_F + \sum_i b_{iF}\bar{x}_{iF}$$

where $\bar{y}_M$ and $\bar{y}_F$ are the average depression scores for males and females respectively: $\bar{x}_{iM}$ and $\bar{x}_{iF}$ are the average levels on the ith precipitating factor for males and females, respectively, and $\sum_i b_{iM}\bar{x}_{iM}$ and $\sum_i b_{iF}\bar{x}_{iF}$

are the sums over all precipitating factors of the product of the average on the ith precipitating factor and the susceptibility to that precipitating factor for males and females respectively.

It has been suggested previously (Winsborough and Dickinson, 1971; and Kessler, unpublished) that the difference can be decomposed into four components as follows:

$$\bar{y}_F - \bar{y}_M = \left[\sum_i b_{iM}(\bar{x}_{iF} - \bar{x}_{iM}) \right] + \left[\sum_i (b_{iF} - b_{iM})\bar{x}_{iM} \right] +$$
$$\left[\sum_i (b_{iF} - b_{iM})(\bar{x}_{iF} - \bar{x}_{iM}) \right] + [a_F - a_m] \qquad (2)$$

The components are calculated as follows:

1. The component attributable to differences in the $\bar{x}$'s, indicating *differential exposure to precipitating factors,* estimated by the difference between $\bar{y}_M$ and the $\hat{y}_M$ which would occur if the males had their own susceptibility (b's), but were exposed to the precipitating factors ($\bar{x}$'s) at the same level as the females:

$$\hat{y}_M - \bar{y}_M = \left(a_M + \sum_i b_{iM}\bar{x}_{iF} \right) - \left(a_M + \sum_i b_{iM}\bar{x}_{iM} \right) \qquad (3)$$

calculated by

$$= \left(\sum_i b_{iM}\bar{x}_{iF} \right) - \left(\sum_i b_{iM}\bar{x}_{iM} \right) \qquad (4)$$

2. The component attributable to differences in the b's, as an indicator of *differential susceptibility,* estimated by the difference between $\bar{y}_M$ and the $\hat{y}_M$ which occur if the males had their own $\bar{x}$'s but had the female b's.

$$\hat{y}_M - \bar{y}_M = \left(a_M + \sum_i b_{iF}\bar{x}_{iM} \right) - \left(a_M + \sum_i b_{iM}\bar{x}_{iM} \right) \qquad (5)$$

calculated by

$$= \left(\sum_i b_{iF}\bar{x}_{iM} \right) - \left(\sum_i b_{iM}\bar{x}_{iM} \right) \qquad (6)$$

3. The interaction, attributable to the additional effect of simultaneously changing both the $\bar{x}$'s and the b's:

$$= \sum_i (b_{iF} - b_{iM})(\bar{x}_{iF} - \bar{x}_{iM}) \qquad (7)$$

calculated by subtraction as indicated by equation (2).

4. The component attributable to a difference in *intercepts* (a's); i.e., $a_F - a_M$, calculated directly.

RESULTS

Variables Considered Singly

The precipitating factors were first analyzed separately as single variables, before being combined into multiple regression. The significance and linearity of the relationship of each variable to depression was tested for each sex, and the sexes were compared on the level of exposure to precipitating factors ($\bar{x}_M$ versus $\bar{x}_F$), on the strength of the relationship of the precipitating factors to depression (b_M versus b_F) and on the level of the intercepts (a_M versus a_F).

Relationships of Precipitating Factors to Depression. Two-way analyses of variance were done for each of the 30 variables by sex, with CES-D score as the dependent variable. Figure 1 shows graphically the average CES-D score for the levels of each variable, separately for men and women (tables available on request). There was a significant interaction of the variable by sex ($p < .01$) for two variables (Never married, head; and Widowed, alone). Twenty-five variables were significantly related to depression ($p < .01$, no interactions) in the direction expected from the literature. Three variables (Married, with children; Widowed, other; and Divorced/separated, alone) were not significantly related to depression. Thus, the majority of the risk factors related to depression significantly and in the same direction for both sexes (see also Radloff and Rae, 1979).

That is, in both the literature and in this study, higher levels of depression are manifested by non-whites, younger people, persons' lower in socioeconomic status (as measured by several variables), persons physically ill or handicapped, persons showing life-event losses, and persons lower in social activities. Also, in general, being single appears associated with depression.

Sex Difference in Exposure to Precipitating Factors ($\bar{x}'s$). Men and women were compared on the average level of each variable. (See Tables 1 and 2. Slight variations are due to missing data). Depending on the character of the variable, the significance of the sex difference was tested by Mann-Whitney U test of ranks, Chi-square test of the distributions, or t-test of the means. For 13 variables, the females had a significantly ($p < .05$) higher level (i.e., more exposure to the precipitating factor in the direction positively associated with depression); for six, the males had a significantly higher level, and for 11, there was no significant difference. In other words, overall the females had only slightly more exposure than males to the set of precipitating factors measured here. More specifically, however, women are clearly more exposed to a socioeconomic deficit than are males. They rank significantly lower in education, income, and occupational status; they are less likely to supervise others on the job and more likely to be receiving welfare. They are also more likely to be widowed and experience significantly more marital loss. In other areas, neither females nor males are at a clear disadvantage; the results differ according to the indicators.

Sex Difference in Susceptibility ($b's$). Regressions of the CES-D on each variable were calculated for males and females separately. Six regressions were significantly nonlinear (frequency of getting together with others and engaging in

Table 1.   Mean Differences in Precipitating Factors for
Males and Females

Precipitating Factor	Males $\bar{X}$	Females $\bar{X}$
Demographic		
Age	.37	.34
Race	.11	.12
Socioeconomic		
+ Education	3.27	3.42
+ Income	2.84	3.20
+ Occupational status	4.55	5.97
+ Number persons supervised	2.23	2.66
Know welfare	.50	.49
+ Any welfare	.04	.06
Physical Problems		
Current illness	.27	.30
+ Recent illness	1.11	1.19
+ Handicap	.09	.07
Losses		
Early loss	.24	.26
Moved	.12	.13
Life-events loss	.28	.32
+ Marital status loss	.03	.05
Social Support and Activities		
Get together	2.41	2.37
+ Religious activities	5.17	4.25
Household activities	3.78	3.79
+ Excessive bedrest	.67	.59
+ Leisure activities	5.28	5.68
Household Status		
+ Married, no children	.71	.79
+ Married, children	.54	.63
Never married, head	.05	.06
+ Never married, not head	.06	.04
+ Widowed, children	.003	.03
+ Widowed, alone	.03	.13
+ Widowed, other	.99	.97
+ Divorced/separated, children	.0045	.06
+ Divorced/separated, alone	.05	.04
Divorced/separated, other	.03	.03

Sex differences in $\bar{X}$ significant (p < .05) if marked +

religious activities for males; degree of recent illness and bedrest for both males and females). Further analyses were done using linear regression, which will give non-optimal estimates in these six cases. The linear regression coefficients of males and females were significantly different (p < .05) for only five variables. Three precipitating factors had higher coefficients for females (education,

Table 2. Multiple Regression and Decomposition of CES-D Score on 19 Variables Significant for Either Sex

Variable	Males b	Males $\bar{X}$	Females b	Females $\bar{X}$
Age	1.28	.37	1.22	.34
Race	1.71	.11	−.19	.12
Get together*	.035	2.41	.80	2.37
+ Religious activities	.33	5.17	.19	4.25
+ Income	.61	2.84	.13	3.20
+ Number supervised*	.04	2.23	.72	2.66
Current illness	2.57	.27	2.86	.30
+ Recent illness	.87	1.11	.99	1.19
Life events loss	1.35	.28	1.66	.32
+ Marital status loss	4.96	.03	2.68	.05
+ Bedrest	.86	.67	1.93	.59
+ Leisure activities	.26	5.28	.45	5.68
Married, with children	−2.10	.54	−1.15	.63
Never-married, head*	3.57	.05	−1.40	.06
+ Never-married, not head	1.59	.06	3.88	.04
+ Widowed, with children	12.07	.003	3.28	.03
+ Widowed, alone*	4.34	.03	.71	.13
+ Div/sep, with children	3.19	.0045	3.44	.06
Div/sep, other	1.41	.03	4.95	.03

a (Intercept)		.28	−1.67
R²		.2098	.1981
$\bar{Y}$ (CES-D)		8.05	10.05

Sex difference in intercepts (a's) not significant
Sex difference in overall regression (all b's) significant ($p < .05$)
Sex difference in individual b's significant ($p < .05$) if marked *
Sex difference in $\bar{X}$ significant ($p < .05$) if marked +

Decomposition Analysis
Component due to difference in b's   3.37
Component due to difference in $\bar{X}$'x   1.00
Component due to difference in intercepts   −1.95
Component due to interaction   − .42

$\bar{Y}_F - \bar{Y}_M$ 2.00

bedrest, leisure activities). Two had higher coefficients for males (Never married, head; and Widowed, alone). Ignoring the significance of the differences, the regression coefficients for males were higher for 13 variables, the coefficients for females were higher for 15, and the coefficients were equal to two decimal places for two variables. Thus, when variables were taken one at a time, there was only slight indication of higher b's, indexing higher susceptibility, for females.

Figure 1. Average CES-D Scores for Levels of Precipitating Factors by Sex

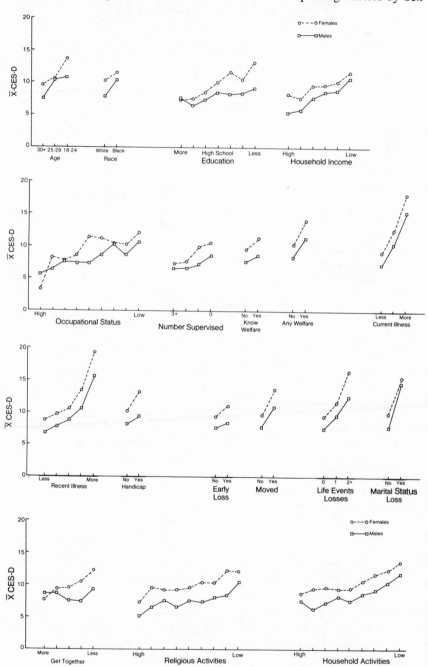

Figure 1—Continued

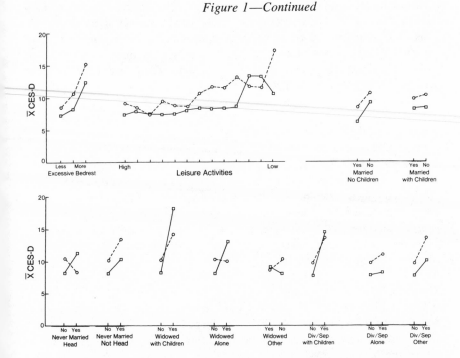

Sex Difference in "Residual" (a's).   The sexes differed significantly (p < .05) on the intercept, a, for 24 variables, with females higher in every case. The intercepts were not significantly different for six variables (get-together, education, occupational status, number supervised, leisure activities, and widowed, other). Note that the intercept is a predicted value, $\hat{y}_0$; i.e., the value of y predicted by the regression line for a zero value of x, or in this case for the lowest stress-level of the precipitating variable. The observed values ($\bar{y}_0$) for males and females at the zero level of each x were also compared by t-test (this was especially desirable for the variables for which the linear regression was not the optimal fit.) The t-test results agreed with the test of intercepts with only one exception.[5]

Considering the results of both types of tests, when the variables were considered singly, there was evidence of a higher baseline level of depression for females, even at the lowest level of the precipitating factors. Thus, when the precipitating factors were considered one at a time, there was no consistent sex difference in susceptibility. There was simply a higher level of depression for women across almost all conditions. This pattern is reflected in the higher intercepts (a's) in conjunction with the similarity of slopes (b's). It is illustrated in Figure 1, where the most typical pattern consists of two roughly parallel lines, with females higher than males.

In looking at exceptions, we note a tendency for the difference between males and females to disappear in certain cases when males are not married. In situations of marital loss, of being widowed and of being never-married head of households, males show depression equal to or greater than that of females. Other exceptions appear idiosyncratic and unpatterned. Usually, however, for each condition of each precipitating factor, females demonstrate more depression than males.

Multiple Variables Considered Jointly

Up until now, it would appear that neither differential exposure to precipitating factors nor differential susceptibility can explain male-female differences in depression. Females show more depression than males even when the level of each precipitating factor is controlled; thus, regardless of any differential exposure to stress, females usually remain more depressed. And analyzing each "b" separately, we do not find females to show greater susceptibility to the stressor.

However, it is possible that when sources of overall stress are cumulated or considered jointly, conclusions will differ.

Stress Score

The simplest way to include several precipitating factors simultaneously is to combine variables into a score. This was done, including only variables which were relatively objective measures and excluding the functioning items that may reflect the person's psychological state. Each of twelve variables (education, income, occupational status, any welfare, current illness, recent illness, handicap, moved, life events losses, marital status losses, age, and race) was dichotomized and scored as zero for the range of that variable which was judged to be *not* a precipitating factor, and otherwise scored as one. The total "Stress score" was the sum over the 12 variables, with a possible range of 0 to 12. Due to small numbers at the high end of the scale, categories above seven were combined, giving a range of 0-8. A score of zero on this scale should reflect a truly minimal exposure to precipitating factors for the average person.

The mean CES-D score for each value of the Stress score for males and females is shown in Figure 2. In the two-way analysis of variance, the main effect of the Stress score was highly significant ($p < .0001$), but the effect for sex was reduced to non-significance ($p = .13$), with no interaction. The correlation of sex with CES-D score was .12 ($p < .001$) and the partial correlation, controlling for Stress score, was .09 ($p < .001$).

In the regressions of CES-D scores on the Stress score, the quadratic coefficients were significantly greater than zero for both males and females. Using the regression model $y = a + bx^2$, there was a significant sex difference in the intercept (females higher), but not in b. Using the model $y = a + b_1x + b_2x^2$, there were no significant sex differences in a, b_1 or b_2. Using a linear model (which reduced the R^2 only slightly for each sex), there was no significant

Figure 2. Average CES-D Scores for Levels of Stress Score by Sex

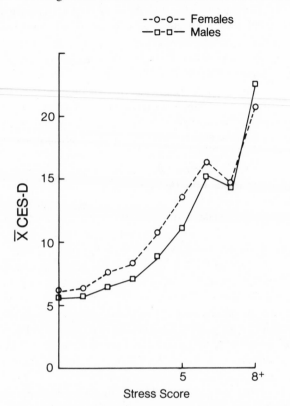

--o-o-- Females
—□-□— Males

Stress Score

difference in a, and a borderline difference (p < .06) in b (females higher). The t-test of male versus female CES-D score means in the groups with a Stress score of zero was non-significant.

Thus, combining risk factors into a score which reflects the number of risk factors present and has a reasonable zero point gave a very ambiguous picture of the sex difference. Depending on the model and test used, the sex difference in depression was eliminated altogether, remained only in the intercepts, or remained only in the strength of the relationship of depression to the Stress score.

Inspection of Figure 2 is interesting, however. It appears that females maintain higher levels of depression at low and medium levels of stress. But when stress is very high, the sex difference disappears. Confidence in this finding must be tempered by the small number of cases scoring at the high level of the Stress score (for a score of 8 or more, N = 23 with only five males).

Multiple Regression.   An alternative method of combining the x's is multiple regression. This method, using all 29 variables (one of the household status variables was omitted to avoid a singular matrix), was then examined for each sex. For both males and females, the R^2 was .21. The regression coefficients (b's) for ten variables were not significant for either sex. These were dropped, and the regressions calculated on the remaining 19 variables.

The R^2 using 19 variables was .21 for males, and .20 for females (confirming the superfluity of the ten omitted variables). Table 2 shows that the sex difference was significant for the overall regressions (all b's simultaneously), and for four individual b's (females had higher regressions for frequency of getting together with friends and for the number of persons supervised on the job; males had higher regressions for Never married, head, and Widowed, alone). The intercepts were not significantly different.

Thus, although there is a significant difference between the sex in the overall "b," one cannot conclude from this analysis that females are more susceptible than males to stressors, for the analysis of the component individual b's indicates that in some cases the female is more susceptible and, in some cases, the male.

Decomposition of the Sex Difference

In a final attempt to test for the effects of differential susceptibility and exposure, Kessler's (1978, 1979) decomposition method was applied to the regression analysis in Table 2. The sex difference in the depression score was about 2.00. This difference was "decomposed" into four parts. In all three analyses, the component due to the intercept (a) was negative. In other words, if all precipitating factors were zero or at the lowest stress level, the males would be predicted (by the regression equation) to score *higher* (more depressed) than the females on the CES-D scale.

In this analysis, the component attributable to the b's was much larger than the component attributable to the $\bar{x}$'s. In other words, there would be a larger increase in the CES-D scores of the males if they had the same b's as the females than there would be if they had the same $\bar{x}$'s as the females. Finally, the interaction term was trivially small, implying that the effects of changes in the $\bar{x}$'s and the b's can be estimated independently.

DISCUSSION

The purpose of the data analyses was to discover to what extent the sex difference in depression could be attributed to differences in exposure to risk factors (levels of x), to differences in the degree to which depression is associated with risk factors (b), and to differences in baseline level of depression independent of risk factors (a).

Findings indicate that the same environmental factors reported previously in the literature appear to be precipitants for depression, both for men and women; e.g., lower socioeconomic status, non-white status, physical illness and life losses, lower social support and activities, and many types of being non-married. Taking these precipitating factors one at a time, we find women more exposed to some (particularly low socioeconomic status and marital loss) and men more exposed to others. On balance, perhaps women suffer from somewhat more exposure to stress, although the pattern is not perfectly clear. However, differential exposure to any one source of stress does not appear to explain the male-female difference in stress.

When risk factors were considered singly, the sex difference in depression was apparent at every level of the risk factors, with a significant sex difference in the intercept, a, for 24 of the 30 variables. This would imply that women are simply more likely to be depressed than men, in almost all circumstances. The major exception involves marital loss. When widowed or after marital loss, men demonstrate depression equal or greater than that of women (also see Radloff, 1975).

However, it was possible that conclusions based on stressor variables considered singly would change if they were considered jointly. Two methods to combine stressor factors were used. One was simply to combine 12 of the risk factors into a "Stress score," so that an individual with a score of zero was exposed to no high level of stress on any of the 12 precipitating factors. The relationship of this score to depression was quadratic and results of different statistical tests were somewhat contradictory and therefore unclear. In general, when men and women were matched on this score, the sex difference in depression was considerably reduced and no longer significant according to some, but not all, tests. However, in absolute terms, the women still had somewhat higher scores at most levels of the stress score. It should be noted, however, that at the very highest level of stress, male-female differences in depression disappeared.

The second method of combining the effects of the multiple risk factors was multiple regression. Stressor variables that were non-significant for both sexes were omitted from the equation. The sexes no longer differed significantly in the intercept according to this analysis. But there was a significant overall difference in the regression coefficients (all b's simultaneously); however, given the fact that the individual b's were sometimes higher for women and sometimes higher for men, it would be difficult to conclude an overall greater susceptibility for women. Kessler's decomposition method tackled the issue more directly and indicated that the sex difference in depression was more due to differences in the b's than differences in the a's or the x̄'s.

Thus, different analyses presented in this paper lead to different conclusions about the relative roles of susceptibility and precipitating factors in causing depression. However, the decomposition method and the disappearance of a significant difference between the sexes in intercepts in the multiple regression analyses suggest that differential susceptibility may play an important role; that is, women may be more depressed than men because they are more susceptible. They may react more strongly with depression than do men to the total set of stressors in their lives, particularly if the total level of stress is not extremely high (see Figure 2). These conclusions remain tentative, however, due to the contradictions that stem from some of the other analyses presented.

There are a number of cautions that must be considered in the interpretation of the "decomposition" results. First, the "decomposition method" is an heuristic device, not a statistical test. It is like a standardized rate, really an imaginary number, based on "what if . . .". The calculations involve substitution of values from one group into a formula for another group. The amount of the mean difference in depression "attributable to" susceptibility is the amount that the mean difference would be reduced if the men had their own levels of precipitating factors but the women's susceptibility. In other words, if the men responded to precipitating factors as women do, then there would be a smaller sex difference in the symptom scores.

Interpretation of the intercepts (a's) should also be made with caution. The intercepts represent the level of depression at the point where all precipitating factors included in the regression are zero or at the lowest stress level, as predicted by the best fitting regression line. If the sex difference in depression were due to gender per se, and not explained solely by differences in susceptibility and/or by exposure to precipitating factors, and if we have included all relevant precipitating factors in our model, then there should be a sex difference in the intercepts. Results could change, however, if a significant precipitating factor were absent from the model. While it is impossible to be sure that all relevant precipitating factors have been included, we did measure almost all the risk factors found in previous studies.

In addition, the measures used here must be interpreted with caution. Some of the precipitating factors (x's) used in the present study may be confounded with susceptibility so that matching on these precipitating factors resulted in a *de facto* (though imperfect) match on susceptibility. The obvious examples are the socio-economic status indicators. A person high in the kind of susceptibility we are hypothesizing (likely to become depressed rather than to actively try to attain desired outcomes) would be unlikely to achieve high levels of education, occupation and income. In other words, high socio-economic status is a legitimate index of a current low-level precipitating factor, but may also reflect the consequences of low susceptibility. In the current study, this confounding can only be noted and accepted. It is hoped that in future studies, more direct measures of susceptibility can be included in the design. We would like to see research which uses measures of susceptibility relevant to specific theories of depression (including biological and psychosocial factors) and measures of precipitating factors appropriate to them. Then a clearer test could be made of whether men and women matched on both susceptibility and precipitating factors (measured independently of depression) will have similar levels of depression.

Caution in interpretation of susceptibility (as reflected in the b coefficients) is especially important. Our discussion of the data makes an assumption about the *nature* of susceptibility (a rise in depression *associated* with, though not necessarily directly caused by, the precipitating factors) but *not* about its *source*. Such susceptibility could be due to sex-linked biological factors as well as learned socio-cultural factors. Hopefully, future studies could investigate this issue.

Future studies might also be informed by a theory and analysis that separates and interrelates the four dimensions of depression which in this study are combined into a "depression syndrome." Current work of these authors attempts to develop such a theory (Radloff and Rae, 1979; Radloff, in press) by combining features of several "intra-psychic" theories of depression (the reinforcement model, Lewinsohn, 1975; the learned helplessness model, Seligman, 1975; the attribution model, Abramson, Seligman & Teasdale, 1978; the cognitive model, Beck, 1976; and the sequential model, McLean, 1976). Our model suggest that the four types of symptoms in the syndrome of depression (cognitive, behavioral, affective, and somatic) are logically linked together in a causal sequence. Furthermore, the symptoms are of such a nature that they reinforce each other so that the sequence can become a vicious cycle (see Beck, 1967).

First of all, the cognitive "symptoms" of depression could be considered the learned reactive susceptibility factors. The cognitive symptoms include beliefs such as "nothing I do matters" and "things will never get better, no matter what I do." This is the cognitive aspect of learned helplessness, which is defined as a generalized expectancy that rewards are *not* contingent on behavior. More informally, it can be called a belief in one's inability to cope with problems. It is here proposed that this expectancy is learned by cumulative experience that behavior does not control rewards. This past experience could involve uncontrollable situations (in which behavior has no effect) or conflict situations (in which behavior is both rewarded and punished). It could also be taught by direct instruction or come about because the individual did not have the skills necessary to control rewards (see Radloff, in press, for more details).

It is reasonable to assume that the more frequent and widespread this learning of non-contingency has been, the stronger and more general the helpless beliefs would become. This is a researchable question. Here, we will simply propose a continuum of strength and generality for the expectancy that actions will have no effect on outcomes. It should be possible to measure this expectancy directly, independent of the remaining measures of depression.

If this helpless cognition is a factor in reactive susceptibility to depression, then it would not lead to other symptoms of depression unless appropriate precipitating factors were present. The degree of susceptibility would determine the effect of the important precipitating factors. If one factor in susceptibility is the expectation that behavior cannot control outcomes or that problems cannot be solved, then the corresponding precipitating factor would be a desired outcome or a problem to be solved (a reward to be gained or punishment to be avoided). In the face of such a precipitating factor, the susceptibility would become a self-fulfilling prophecy; i.e., if you believed that nothing you can do will gain the desired outcome, you probably would do nothing. This inaction is seen in the *behavioral* deficit of depression. In the real world, this inactivity would leave you with few rewards and an excess of punishments which would result in a lack of enjoyment and an excess of sadness, the *affective* experience of depression. The link with the *somatic* symptoms is less clear, but there is some evidence (as well as speculation) that strong negative affect can produce somatic and biochemical changes similar to that found in depression (e.g., Arnold, 1970; Brenner, 1979; Izard, 1972; Weiss, Glazer and Pohorecky, 1976).

This depressive sequence is also likely to be a vicious cycle: the symptoms intensify the disorder (see Figure 3). For example, biochemical changes would intensify sleep and appetite disturbances, fatigue, and negative affect; the sleep and appetite disturbances would produce fatigue which would exacerbate the behavioral inactivity; the affective disturbance would interfere with social interactions which might otherwise be rewarding. This implies that an episode of depression could *start* with any one of the four components of the syndrome. Regardless of the original source, these symptoms are probably logically related so that they tend to cause and intensify each other, such that the full syndrome is likely to develop. However, a strong and pervasive helpless cognition is unlikely to develop in the course of a single time-limited experience with the other symptoms unless there is a pre-existing tendency toward such cognititions. If such a theory had validity, therapeutic consequences could follow. For example, treatment of a single episode might be effective if it interrupted the vicious cycle at any point, and set a "benign cycle" in motion. Antidepressant medication, behavior therapy, and cognitive therapy have all been found to be effective treatments, alone as well as in combination. Treatment failures might be explained by failure to affect a crucial component. For example, if intervention at the behavioral level does not lead to full recovery, it may be because an underlying biochemical imbalance has not been adequately corrected; in this case, direct intervention with antidepressants would be indicated. If antidepressants do not lead to full recovery, it may be because helpless cognitions have not been adequately corrected; in this case, cognitive therapy would be indicated.

However, our model suggests that for *primary prevention* of future episodes, reduction of reactive susceptibility—namely, the cognitive dimension—may be most practical and effective. It should reduce the probability of the development of the full depressive syndrome, even if some other symptoms were to recur. The assumption that helpless cognitions are learned implies that they can be changed. Other factors in depression may be much harder to change or prevent. We do not know how to prevent biochemical imbalance; we cannot and should not prevent all sad affect (e.g., normal grief); we cannot always prevent reduced activity (e.g., due to illness) or reduced rates of rewards (e.g., due to loss of a loved one). However, we can change the probability that the individual will interpret these factors as evidence of permanent helplessness. Similarly, we cannot prevent all precipitating factors. According to our model, precipitating factors are problems to be solved, including rewards to be gained as well as punishments to be avoided. In the absence of the relevant susceptibility factor (helpless cognitions), such problems should not lead to depression if they realistically can be solved. However, reduction in the number of precipitating factors, especially of the aversive kind, may be necessary in some cases. Some people may have so many problems to handle that their current situation is, in fact, uncontrollable. In

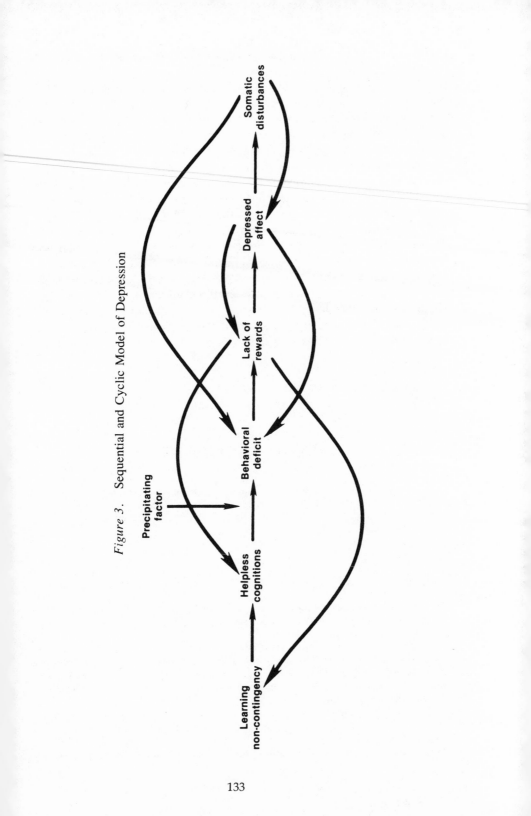

Figure 3. Sequential and Cyclic Model of Depression

133

this case, a helpless belief would be realistic, and trying to change it would be dishonest as well as futile.

In summary, the theory presented here posits that a pre-existing tendency toward helpless cognitions is a reactive susceptibility factor which, when combined with the appropriate precipitating factor, will lead to the whole syndrome of depression. It is *not* suggested that every case of depression must *start* in this way. In other words, it is proposed that the combination of cognitive susceptibility *and* a precipitating factor is a sufficient but not necessary condition for the initiation of depression.

In conclusion, both men and women are exposed to life problems which are difficult to solve. The theory of depression presented here suggests the types of interventions which might be effective to reduce susceptibility or relevant precipitating factors. Ideally, to prevent depression, both social interventions (to reduce life problems to a manageable level) and educational interventions (to reduce susceptibility) should be attempted. The optimistic aspect of our theory is that if susceptibility to depression is learned, then it can be unlearned. Prevention of susceptibility to depression might be seen as training to actualize St. Francis' prayer:

> Give me the strength to change what I can change,
> The humility to accept what I cannot change,
> And the wisdom to tell the difference.

ACKNOWLEDGMENTS

The authors wish to acknowledge the helpful comments on early drafts of this paper from colleagues, with special thanks to Ms. Rochelle Albin and Ms. Anne Rosenfeld. Requests for reprints should be sent to Ms. Lenore Sawyer Radloff, Center for Epidemiologic Studies, National Institute of Mental Health, 5600 Fishers Lane, Rockville, Maryland 20857.

NOTES

1. See the conclusion for further discussion of this issue.

2. Maccoby and Jacklin (1974) do not report sex differences of this type in socialization, although they do not deal specifically with the issue.

3. This issue is discussed in more detail in the conclusion.

4. Field work was conducted by the Epidemiolgogic Field Station, Greater Kansas City Mental Health Foundation, Kansas City, Missouri; and Johns Hopkins Training Center for Public Health Research, Johns Hopkins University, Hagerstown, Maryland; under contract from Center for Epidemiologic Studies, NIMH.

5. For the level of participating in household activities, the intercepts were significantly different, but the observed means at the zero level were not. Examination of Figure 1 suggests that this is due to a higher-than-expected observed mean for males at the zero level of x. If we assume that this is a sampling error, we would accept the results of the test of intercepts. If we believe it is a meaningful

value (e.g., a tendency toward a U-shaped regression), we would accept the t-test result. Since there was no significant deviation from linearity for this variable, the authors lean slightly toward the former interpretation.

REFERENCES

Abramson, L. Y., Seligman, M. E. P., and Teasdale, J. D. (1978), "Learned helplessness in humans: Critique and reformulation." *Journal of Abnormal Psychology* 87:49.

Akiskal, H. S., and McKinney, W. T., Jr. (1975), "Overview of recent research in depression." *Archives of General Psychiatry* 32:285.

Alkire, A. A. et al. (1968), "Information exchange and accuracy of verbal communication under social power conditions." *Journal of Personality and Social Psychology* 9:301.

Altemeyer, R. A., and Jones, K. (1974), "Sexual identity, physical attractiveness and seating position as determinants of influence in discussion groups." *Canadian Journal of Behavioral Science* 6:357.

Arnold, M. B. (1970), "Perennial problems in the field of emotion." Pp. 169–203 in M. B. Arnold (ed.), *Feelings & Emotions,* New York: Academic Press.

Bart, P. B. (1975) Unalienating abortion, demystifying depression and restoring rape victims. Presented at American Psychiatric Association Meetings, Anaheim, California.

Beck, A. T. (1967), *Depression.* New York: Harper & Row.

_____ (1976), *Cognitive Therapy and the Emotional Disorders.* New York: International Universities Press, Inc.

Benefari, R. C., Beiser, M., Leighton, H., and Mertens, C. (1972), "Some dimensions of psychoneurotic behavior in an urban sample." *Journal of Nervous and Mental Diseases* 155:77.

Berkman, P. L. (1971), "Measurement of mental health in a general population survey." *American Journal of Epidemiology* 94:105.

Block, J. H. (1975), Another look at sex differentiation in the socialization behaviors of mothers and fathers. Presented at conference *New Directions for Research on Women,* Madison, Wisconsin, May.

Brenner, B. (1979), "Depressed affect as a cause of associated somatic problems." *Psychological Medicine* 9:737–746.

Bronfenbrenner, U. (1961), "Some familial antecedents of responsibility and leadership in adolescents." Pp. 239–271 in L. Petrullo and B. Bass (eds.), *Leadership and Interpersonal Behavior,* New York: Holt, Rinehart and Winston, Inc.

Brown, G. W., and Harris, T. (1978), *Social Origins of Depression.* New York: The Free Press.

Costrich, N., Feinstein, J., Kidder, L., Marecek, J., and Pascale, L. (1975), "When stereotypes hurt: Three studies of penalties for sex-role reversals." *Journal of Experimental Social Psychology* 11:520.

Dweck, C. S., Davidson, W., and Nelson, S. (1978), "Sex differences in learned helplessness: (II) The contingencies of evaluating feedback in the classroom (III) An experimental analysis." *Developmental Psychology* 14:268.

Feather, N. T., and Simon, J. G. (1975), "Reactions to male and female success and failure in sex-linked occupations: Impressions of personality, causal attributions, and perceived likelihood of different consequences." *Journal of Personality and Social Psychology* 31:20.

Hillman, J. S. (1974), "An analysis of male and female roles in two periods of children's literature." *Journal of Educational Research* 68:84.

Izard, C. E. (1972), *Patterns of Emotion.* New York: Academic press.

Kessler, R. C. (1979), "A strategy for studying differential vulnerability to the psychological consequences of stress." *Journal of Health and Social Behavior* 20:100.

Kessler, R. C. (1978), Sex and Psychological distress: Re-examining the differential exposure hypothesis. Unpublished manuscript. (Available from Ronald C. Kessler at the University of Wisconsin, Madison, Wisconsin).

Langner, T. S., and Michael, S. T. (1963), *Life Stress and Mental Health*. New York: The Free Press of Glenco.

Lewinsohn, P. M. (1975), "The behavioral study and treatment of depression." Pp. 19–64 in M. Hersen, R. M. Eisler and P. M. Miller (eds.), *Progress in Behavior Modification*, Vol. 1. New York: Academic Press.

Maccoby, E. E., and Jacklin, C. N. (1974), *The Psychology of Sex Differences*. Stanford: Stanford University Press.

McLean, P. (1976), "Therapeutic decision-making in behavioral treatment of depression." Chapter 5, pp. 54–83 in P. O. Davidson (ed.), *The Behavioral Management of Anxiety, Depression and Pain*. New York: Brunner/Mazel.

Radloff, L. S. (1975), "Sex differences in depression: The effects of occupation and marital status." *Sex Roles*, 1:249.

Radloff, L. S. (1977), "The CES-D Scale: A self-report depression scale for research in the general population." *Journal of Applied Psychological Measurement*, 1:385.

Radloff, L. S. (in press), "Risk factors for depression: What do we learn from them?", in *Mental Health of Women: Fact and Fiction*. New York: Academic Press.

Radloff, L. S., and Monroe, M. M. (1978). "Sex differences in helplessness: With implications for depression." Chapter 12, pp. 199–221 in L. S. Hanson and R. S. Rapoza (eds.), *Career Development and Counseling of Women*. Springfield, Illinois: Charles Thomas.

Radloff, L. S., and Rae, D. S. (1979), "Susceptibility and precipitating factors in depression: Sex differences and similarities." *Journal of Abnormal Psychology*, 88:174.

Rubin, J. Z., Provenzano, F. J., and Luria, Z. (1974), "The eye of the beholder: Parents' views on sex of newborns." *American Journal of Orthopsychiatry*, 44:512.

Seligman, M. E. P. (1975), *Helplessness: On Depression, Development, and Death*. San Francisco: W. H. Freeman & Co.

Serbin, L. A., O'Leary, K. D., Kent, R. N., and Tonick, I. J. (1973), "A comparison of teacher response to the pre-academic and problem behavior of boys and girls." *Child Development* 44:796.

Silverman, C. (1968), *The Epidemiology of Depression*. Baltimore: The Johns Hopkins Press.

Spitzer, R. L., Endicott, J., and Robins, E. (1978), "Diagnostic Criteria: Rationale and Reliability." *Archives of General Psychiatry* 35:773–782.

Sternglanz, S. H., and Serbin, L. A. (1974), "Sex role stereotyping in children's television programs." *Developmental Psychology* 10:710.

Unger, R. K. (1976), "Male is greater than female: The socialization of status inequality." *The Counseling Psychologist* 6:2.

Wahrman, R., and Pugh, M. D. (1974), "Sex, non-conformity and influence." *Sociometry*, 37:137.

Weiss, J. M., Glazer, H. I., and Pohorecky, L. A. (1976), "Coping behavior and neurochemical changes: An alternative explanation for the original "Learned helplessness" experiments." Pp. 141–173 in G. Serban and A. Kling (eds.), *Animal Models in Human Psychobiology*. New York: Plenum Press.

Weissman, M. M., and Klerman, G. (1977), "Sex differences and the epidemiology of depression." *Archives of General Psychiatry* 34:98.

Weissman, M. M., Sholomskas, D., Pottenger, M., Prusoff, B. A., and Locke, B. Z. (1977), "Assessing depressive symptoms in five psychiatric populations: A validation study." *American Journal of Epidemiology* 106:203.

Winsborough, H. H., and Dickinson, P. (1971), "Components of Negro-white income differences." Proceedings of the American Statistical Association, Social Statistics Section, 6.

Wolman, C., and Frank, H. (1975), "The solo woman in a professional peer group." *American Journal of Orthopsychiatry* 45:164.

APPENDIX
CENTER FOR EPIDEMIOLOGICAL STUDIES
DEPRESSION SCALE (CES-D)

Instructions for questions on the CES-D: Below is a list of the ways you might have felt or behaved. Please tell me how often you have felt this way during the past week. Hand Card A.

Rarely or none of the time (less than 1 day)
Some or a little of the time (1–2 days)
Occasionally or a moderate amount of time (3–4 days)
Most or all of the time (5–7 days)

During the Past Week	*Rarely*	*A little*	*Moderate*	*Most*
1. I was bothered by things that usually don't bother me	0	1	2	3
2. I did not feel like eating; my appetite was poor	0	1	2	3
3. I felt that I could not shake off the blues even with help from my family or friends	0	1	2	3
4. I felt that I was just as good as other people	3	2	1	0
5. I had trouble keeping my mind on what I was doing	0	1	2	3
6. I felt depressed	0	1	2	3
7. I felt that everything I did was an effort	0	1	2	3
8. I felt hopeful about the future	3	2	1	0
9. I thought my life had been a failure	0	1	2	3
10. I felt fearful	0	1	2	3
11. My sleep was restless	0	1	2	3
12. I was happy	3	2	1	0
13. I talked less than usual	0	1	2	3
14. I felt lonely	0	1	2	3
15. People were unfriendly	0	1	2	3
16. I enjoyed life	3	2	1	0
17. I had crying spells	0	1	2	3
18. I felt sad	0	1	2	3
19. I felt that people disliked me	0	1	2	3
20. I could not get going	0	1	2	3

PERSPECTIVES ON SUICIDE IN ADOLESCENCE

Paul C. Holinger and Daniel Offer

INTRODUCTION

This report explores various etiological perspectives on suicide among high-school-aged adolescents, attempts to explain fluctuations in the suicide rates, and suggests further directions of investigation. To accomplish this, mortality data on adolescent suicide and accompanying methodological problems will be examined, followed by a literature review; the current state of knowledge will then be assessed and new research areas offered. This presentation will be restricted to suicide by adolescents (as defined by the years 15–19, essentially high school rather than college age) in the United States. Childhood and early adolescence (10 to 14 years) and late adolescence and early adulthood (20 to 24) will not be considered in this paper. Only successful suicides will be discussed, although, in individual cases, it may be chance alone which stops an attempted suicide from being completed. Literature dealing with adolescent age groups other than 15 to 19 years, with countries other than the United States, and with attempted rather

Research in Community and Mental Health, Volume 2, pages 139–157
Copyright © 1981 by JAI Press, Inc.
All rights of reproduction in any form reserved.
ISBN: 0-89232-152-0

than completed suicides are beyond the scope of this paper but will be the subject of future communications.

Suicide is the third leading cause of death in adolescence in the United States and is similarly ranked in many western countries. (National Center for Health Statistics, 1975; WHO Chronicle, 1975; Holinger, 1978) Only accidents and homicides are responsible for more deaths in that age group in the United States (National Center for Health Statistics, 1975) and many accidents and homicides may also reflect self-destructive tendencies (Wolfgang, 1959; Holinger, 1979; Seiden, 1969). Suicide in adolescence is a major cause of concern for many: for the distressed adolescent, for the parents, and for those in the health care system who try to understand and influence it. If one uses the number of publications on a topic as indicative of the attention paid to it by the scientific community, there would appear to be a recent upsurge of interest in adolescent suicide. Bakwin (1957) noted that his literature review on suicide in children and adolescents yielded only five recent articles of importance, and that by contrast a large number of extensive studies appeared in the last century and during the early years of this century. Seiden (1969) listed a bibliography of more than 200 articles and books on youthful suicides in his review of the literature from 1900–1967; most of his references were published after 1957. Two separate computerized literature searches indicated that a total of about 275 articles had been published from 1967–1977 on suicidal children, adolescents, and young adults.

However, this large number of publications should not belie the fact that significant methodological problems exist in researching and writing about suicide, and, perhaps, about adolescent suicide in particular. In attempting to assess the literature, difficulties are created by the multiple definitions of suicide used; e.g., completed suicide, attempted suicide, partial suicide, suicidal behavior, and theoretical suicide. Also, as described by Seiden (1969), literature evaluation is further complicated by wide differences in study design, generalizability, and validity. Seiden noted that nearly all the studies were retrospective. Tuckman and Connon (1962), elaborating on this retrospective nature of suicide studies, stated that reconstruction on any person's life experiences is a difficult undertaking and particularly so with a suicide, both because the person who committed suicide is dead and inaccessible, and also because of the defensiveness of survivors due to the stigma and guilt surrounding the suicide. Finally, Haim (1974), discussing adolescent suicide specifically, also noted the tactical problems involved but stressed the difficulty in writing about the subject due to the nature of the subject itself and the resistance which develops in attempting to study adolescent suicide. Consideration of the investigator's response as well as the other methodological issues involved perhaps makes understandable the scarcity of detailed case studies (Balser and Masterson, 1959) and presuicidal data (Holinger, 1977; Blanchard and Blanchard, 1976; Finch and Poznanski, 1971) throughout the literature on adolescent suicide.

MORTALITY TRENDS

Methodological Problems

Two major methodological problems occur when using national mortality data to study suicide: (1) underreporting; and (2) data classification. Underreporting may cause reported suicide data to be at least two or three times less than the real figures (Seiden, 1969; Kramer et al., 1972; Toolan, 1962, 1975). The underreporting may be intentional or unintentional. In intentional underreporting, the doctor, family, friends, etc., may contribute to covering up a suicide for various reasons: guilt, social stigma, insurance or pension benefits, malpractice, and so on. Unintentional underreporting refers to deaths labeled "accidents"; e.g., single car crashes, some poisonings, etc., which were actually suicides but were unverifiable as such due to the absence of a note or other evidence. Two types of data classification problems exist. One involves classification at the national level and the changes in this classification over time (Klebba and Dolman, 1975). The second concerns classification at the local level; e.g., the legal issue in which some localities may require a suicide note as evidence of suicide, thereby both decreasing numbers and biasing results so that only the literate could be listed as having committed suicide.

Studies of suicide in the young involve additional methodological problems. There may be greater social stigma and guilt surrounding suicide in childhood and adolescence because of the intense involvement of the parents at that age and the issue of parents failing and being "bad parents." In addition, it may be much easier to cover up suicide in the younger age groups. Poisonings and other methods of suicide are more easily conceived of as accidents in those age groups than in older age groups.

Suicide Rates

A brief overview of suicide rates from 1900 to 1975 is necessary to give perspective to adolescent suicide. Male rates are consistently higher than female, by a ratio of 2–3:1. There were increased suicide rates in years of economic depression and decreased rates during World Wars I and II, with male rates accounting for most of these shifts. For males, there is a striking, almost invariable, age distribution in which the suicide rate increases as age increases. For females, the highest suicide rates occur in the middle age intervals (35–64 years) and the lowest rates in the younger (5–24 years) and older (65–84 years) age groups. The suicide rates for whites are consistently higher than for nonwhites, with a few recent exceptions in the younger age groups. The suicide rates over the past fifteen years demonstrate a decrease in the difference between the younger and older age groups, with older age groups declining while the rates for younger age groups rise gradually (Vital Statistics, 1956; Vital and Health Statistics, 1967; Vital Statistics of the United States, 1961–1973, 1974 and 1975).

The suicide rates for 15–19 year olds are less than for older age groups, and the rates shift less markedly during economic depression and war. The rates for males are higher than for females, and rates for whites higher than nonwhites (see Figure 1). The suicide rates for 15–19 year olds have more than tripled over the past twenty years and are now higher than they ever have been (U.S. Vital Statistics, 1956, 1967, 1974–1975, in press) (see Table 1). The increase is more dramatic for males than for females. While the methods of suicide used by 15 to 19 year olds have been discussed in detail elsewhere (Holinger, 1978), it should be noted that the commonest methods are firearms and explosives, followed by hanging, poisoning by liquids and solids, and poisoning by gas.

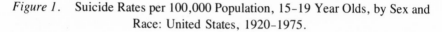

Figure 1.   Suicide Rates per 100,000 Population, 15–19 Year Olds, by Sex and Race: United States, 1920–1975.

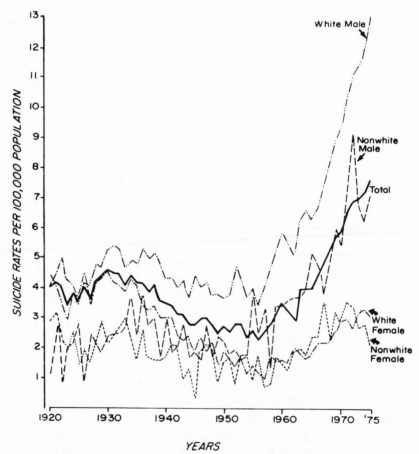

Source: 1920–1929: Number of deaths from *Mortality Statistics,* 1920–1929, Washington, D.C., U.S. Government Printing Office; population (in Death Registration States) for rate derivation from National Center for Health Statistics (unpublished data). 1930–1975: Mortality rates per 100,000 population from National Center for Health Statistics (unpublished data).

Perspectives on Suicide In Adolescence   143

Table 1.   Suicide Rates per 100,000 for 15–19 Year Olds, by Sex and Race:
United States, 1956–1975

Year	Total*	Male*	Female*	White*	White Male*	White Female*	Nonwhite*	Nonwhite Male*	Nonwhite Female*
1975	7.6	12.2	2.9	8.1	13.0	3.1	4.6	7.0	2.1
1974	7.2	11.0	3.2	7.6	11.9	3.3	4.5	6.2	2.8
1973	7.0	10.7	3.1	7.4	11.4	3.2	4.7	6.8	2.7
1972	6.9	10.9	2.8	7.0	11.1	2.7	6.5	9.5	3.4
1971	6.5	9.9	3.1	6.7	10.3	3.0	5.2	6.8	3.6
1970	5.9	8.8	2.9	6.2	9.4	2.9	4.2	5.4	2.9
1969	5.7	8.6	2.7	5.9	9.0	2.6	4.5	5.8	3.2
1968	5.1	7.8	2.2	5.3	8.3	2.2	3.5	4.7	2.2
1967	4.7	7.0	2.4	4.9	7.5	2.2	3.7	3.8	3.5
1966	4.3	6.5	2.1	4.4	6.7	2.1	3.6	4.8	2.4
1965	4.0	6.1	1.9	4.1	6.3	1.8	3.8	5.2	2.4
1964	4.0	6.3	1.7	4.2	6.6	1.7	2.9	4.0	1.8
1963	4.0	6.0	1.9	4.2	6.3	1.9	2.9	3.7	2.0
1962	3.7	5.5	2.0	3.9	5.8	2.0	2.8	3.7	1.9
1961	3.4	5.3	1.5	3.5	5.5	1.6	2.5	3.6	1.3
1960	3.6	5.6	1.6	3.8	5.9	1.6	2.4	3.4	1.5
1959	3.4	5.1	1.6	3.5	5.4	1.6	2.5	3.4	1.7
1958	3.0	4.3	1.7	3.2	4.7	1.8	1.1	1.4	0.8
1957	2.5	4.0	1.0	2.6	4.1	1.0	1.9	3.3	0.7
1956	2.3	3.3	1.3	2.3	3.5	1.2	2.1	2.5	1.8
Pearson correlation between year and suicide rate	.98	.98	.95	.98	.98	.95	.90	.87	.76
% change, 1956–1975	+230	+270	+123	+252	+271	158	+109	+180	+17

< .001, Pearson product correlations between year and suicide rate. Pearson product correlations were done between year
and suicide rate among 15–19 year olds in all categories: total, male, female, white, white male, white female, nonwhite,
nonwhite male, nonwhite female. Correlations between year and suicide rates were significant at p < .001 for each category,
with results showing that rates linearly and almost invariably increased between the years 1956 to 1975.

Sources: Vital Statistics of the United States, 1956–1973, Volume II-Mortality, Washington, D.C., U.S. Government Printing
Office; and Vital Statistics of United States, 1974–1975, Volume II-Mortality, to be published.

LITERATURE REVIEW

Biological

There are few biologically-oriented hypotheses or studies which address the
issue of suicide specifically in adolescents. The exceptions, psychoanalytic
studies which attempt to take the onset of puberty and the accompanying
psychiological changes into account (Zilboorg, 1937), are discussed later. Three
areas of biological research relate to suicide in general: hereditary, biochemical,
and nosological studies. Biologically-oriented nosological research refers to
studies of suicide in mental illnesses which appear to have a biological compo-

nent; e.g., manic-depressive illness and schizophrenia, and these studies are also discussed later.

Studies relating heredity to suicide assume two forms: anecdotal reports of suicide within families and twin studies. Many reports on suicide within families, sometimes through several generations, exist in the literature (Holinger, 1977; Medical Record NY, 1901; Shapiro, 1935; Swanson 1960; Patel, 1974). They provide little evidence that the tendency to suicidal acts is inherited biologically rather than occuring; e.g., on the basis of family and individual psychodynamics or conditioning. The second method of investigation of the heredity of suicide is twin studies (Kallman and Anastasio, 1947; Kallman et al., 1949; Kallman, 1953). Kallman (1947) found only six references to twin suicide cases in the literature, and felt that only two of them could be considered absolutely authentic. Regarding his own data, Kallman stated that if hereditary factors play a decisive role, a concordant tendency to suicide should be more frequent in one-egg than in two-egg pairs, regardless of ordinary differences in environment. He found that in his series of 39 suicidal twin index pairs (18 one-egg and 21 two-egg sets, only a few of which were adolescents), all but one (a monozygotic pair) had remained discordant (1953). He concluded that suicide was one of the few phenomena unlikely to occur in both twins, whether monozygotic of dizygotic, even under similar conditions of maladjustment and privation.

Biochemical studies of affective disorders have increased our knowledge about depression, but this area has produced little direct work on suicide in adolescence specifically. This topic has recently been reviewed in general by Akiskal and McKinney (1975) and, with specific reference to adolescent suicide, by Petzel and Cline (1978). Akiskal and McKinney noted that, despite the many methodological problems associated with biochemical studies, some consensus is gathering on the possible role of lowered serotonin levels in both depression and mania and elevation of catecholamines in the switch process from depression to mania. They felt that the best synthesis of the current data was represented by the permissive amine hypothesis of Prange et al. (1974) which states that central serotonergic deficiency may represent the vulnerability to affective illness, lowered catecholamines correlating with depression and increased catecholamines with mania. Akiskal and McKinney (1975) also noted that although the focus has been on behavioral alterations occurring secondary to changes in biogenic amines, another perspective is possible; i.e., alterations in biogenic amines can occur secondary to developmental and interpersonal events. For example, Bliss et al. (1966) and Weiss et al. (1970) reported evidence from animal models to support the hypothesis that, under stress, changes in certain neurotransmitters in the brain are determined mainly by psychological factors. Petzel and Cline (1978) described the controversial nature and paucity of biochemical investigations related to adolescent suicide (e.g., steroids, neurotransmitters, menstruation, pregnancy), but they did note that a higher risk of adolescent suicide might be associated with evidence of structural neuropathology (e.g., electroencephalographic changes and epilepsy).

Psychoanalytic

Many psychoanalytic theories of suicide in general exist (Litman, 1967; Warren, 1967; Freud, 1917; Jones, 1957; Menninger, 1933; Klein, 1932; Draper, 1976; Zilboorg, 1936) and have been reviewed recently by Warren (1967), but less familiar are the works of several authors who have discussed completed suicide in adolescence from an analytic perspective (Haim, 1974; Zilboorg, 1936, 1937; Gould, 1965; Anthony, 1970; Sabbath, 1969; Rosenbaum and Richman, 1970; Schneer and Kay, 1961; Freud, 1910; Lourie, 1967; Freidman, 1967). Zilboorg (1937) stated that the suicidal drive appeared to be a real elemental psychic force, universal in nature and apparently confined not only to human beings, and he urged that suicide be considered a form of instinctual expression. Zilboorg, noting data that showed marked discrepancy between low suicide rates in children and high rates in adolescents, contended that the age of puberty seems to be the crucial period as far as the development of active self-destructive drives are concerned. He thought that at puberty the task of the ego is to assert itself as quickly and as fully as possible by means of asserting the instinctual drives with which it must make or is inclined to make an unconditional alliance. Should the ego fail in this task the suicidal outcome would offer itself as its paradoxical substitute. Zilboorg also noted that only those individuals who appear to have identified themselves with a dead person and in whom the process of identification took place during childhood or adolescence, at a time when the incorporated person was already actually dead, were most probably the truly suicidal individuals.

Gould (1965) maintained that the psychodynamics of suicide must be differentiated between children, adolescents, and adults, with physical, intellectual, and physiologic levels of development being of particular importance in understanding the psychodynamics of suicide in children and adolescents. Gould suggested that although the conscious reason for the suicide attempt seems to be that it is an escape from a situation too difficult to face, the common theme underlying the precipitating events is rejection and deprivation, which results in loss of love and support. This may even be felt by the child or adolescent as a threat to his survival, and Gould felt that the core factor in the formation of a "suicidal personality" in adolescents was the felt loss of love.

Anthony (1970) described two types of adolescent depression. In type one, the psychopathology would be mainly preoedipal and based on a marked symbiotic tie with the omnipotent, need-satisfying mother. In this type, the discrepancies between the ego and ego ideal, with resulting changes in self-esteem, are of primary focus. The type two depression, as discussed by Anthony, is more oedipal in nature with a great deal of guilt and moral masochism associated with a punitive superego.

Andre Haim (1974) noted from his clinical data that adolescents usually can perform the work of mourning that results from narcissistic wounds, damage to the ego ideal, and object losses. However, the inadequacy of two defense mechanisms seemed to be one of the most constant features in all suicidal adolescents: mobility of investments and the projective mechanism. Regarding the mobility of investments, Haim asserted that in all suicidal adolescents, there is an inability to disinvest the disappointing or lost object. Despite that pain, they maintain their investments, repeat their behavior, and brood on their disappointment. In terms of the projective mechanism, Haim noted that when the adolescent is confronted by the gap between his ideal aspirations and reality, he reacts by making a projective defense; the adolescent constructs projects and theoretical systems with the ultimate intention of bringing reality into line with his own ideal image of it, or he reacts by attempting at once to alter reality. Haim suggested that in the case of the suicidal adolescent, this mechanism is either disturbed, inadequate, or absent altogether.

The role of hostility from significant others has been studied less in suicidal adolescents than the patients' hostility turned inward. Sabbath (1969) proposed the expendable child concept, which presumed a parental wish, conscious or unconscious, interpreted by the child as a desire to be rid of him. Rosenbaum and Richman (1970) found more extreme hostility and less support in families of suicidal patients than nonsuicidal patients.

Sociocultural

An increasingly large literature exists on the sociocultural perspective of attempted suicide among adolescents, but remarkably little literature addresses completed suicide in adolescence. Various aspects of the sociocultural viewpoint on adolescent suicide will be considered: familial, socioeconomic, epidemiologic, epidemics, sibling position, and pregnancy. It is of interest that there is a relative lack of literature on the sociological, student subculture from this point of view (Sanborn et al., 1973) or on religious aspects of completed suicide among high-school-aged adolescents.

Familial. Family interaction and adolescent suicide have been excellently reviewed recently by Williams and Lyons (1976) and also dealt with uniquely by Cain (1972). The classic sociological theory of suicide is Durkheim's (1951). According to Durkheim, suicide rates are likely to be high at one extreme if persons are isolated interpersonally ("egoistic suicide"), and at the other extreme if individuals are so tightly integrated into a group that they devalue their own individuality ("altruistic suicide"). Suicide rates are also likely to be high in situations where the norms and standards are unclear ("anomic suicide"). As Gibbs (1971) notes, the main tenet of Durkheim's theory is that suicide rates vary inversely with the degree of social integration. This theorem would lead one to predict that youth from broken families would have a high suicide rate and there is some evidence in support of this assertion.

However, attempts to understand the relationship between "broken homes" and suicide in adolescence have proven controversial. One difficulty relates to the various descriptions and definitions of broken homes; e.g., broken through divorce, separation, or death of one or both parents at various stages of the adolescent's life. Another problem concerns the paucity of controlled studies in this area. Finally, with few exceptions, (e.g., Cain, 1972) nearly all the studies examined attempted rather than completed suicide.

The relationship between broken homes and psychiatric disorder, depression, and suicide is methodologically complex. Dennehy (1966) and Gregory (1966) emphasized the need to control for the year of birth of the patient, the patient's parents, and social class. Crook and Raskin (1975) noted that the reported association of parental loss with attempted suicide may be due to a primary association between parental loss and severe depression. Depression could be an intervening variable, since it is a variable related to both attempted suicide and parental loss. Crook and Raskin suggested that future studies should establish whether there is an equivalence between those who attempt suicide and control groups on severity of depression.

Major methodological problems in retrospective case-control investigations which utilize interviews should be noted; i.e., observation bias and a lack of blindness.

Socioeconomic Factors. Many studies have investigated the relationships between socioeconomic factors and suicide, but few discuss adolescent suicide specifically. These investigations may be descriptive; i.e., in the course of describing the characteristics of a group of suicidal adolescents, the socioeconomic status (SES) is examined; or they may focus more specifically on socioeconomic factors and their possible etiologic role in suicide. Some researchers have suggested that the distribution of suicide is very democratic and represented proportionately at all levels of society (Farberow and Schneidman, 1961). Other investigators have probed the possible etiologic role of socioeconomic factors in suicide (Bakwin, 1957; Waldron and Eyer, 1975). Epidemiologic data indicate that the highest rates of suicide occurred during the economic depression of the 1930s (Holinger, 1978). However, the rates for the younger age groups were affected less than the older groups by the Depression.

Epidemiologic. Epidemiologic data from the United States as well as from other countries contribute to the sociocultural perspective of adolescent suicide. Within the United States, epidemiologic study of adolescent suicide rates indicates that there are differences by age, sex, and race (white and nonwhite) as described above and elsewhere (Holinger, 1978). Married teenagers have higher suicide rates than single teenagers, i.e., the reverse of what is found among other age groups; divorced teenagers have higher suicide rates than those married or single (Seiden, 1969; Petzel and Clina, 1978; Dublin, 1963). Unfortunately, with the exception of studies of young blacks (Seiden, 1972; Weiss, 1976; Bush, 1976; Hendin, 1969; Morris et al., 1974) and American Indians (Dizmang et al., 1974; Ogden et al., 1970; Shore, 1972, 1975; Westermeyer and Brantner, 1972;

Resnick and Dizmang, 1971), there is little systematic mortality data which addresses the issue of adolescent suicide rates among the various ethnic subcultures within the United States. There has been much recent attention to the rise in suicide among young blacks, as noted above. However, national mortality data indicate that while the white and nonwhite rates among 20- to 24-year-old males are currently about equal, the rates for 15- to 19-year-old white males have increased more over the past 20 years and are almost twice as high as the rates for 15- to 19-year-old non-white males (Holinger, 1978) (see Table 1).

Although the focus of this paper is on adolescent suicide in the United States, it is useful to briefly examine adolescent suicide in crosscultural perspective in order to get a sense of the varying rates. Important methodologic problems arise when comparing suicide rates of various countries and cultures (WHO Chronicle, 1975; Brooke, 1974). However, data do exist which suggest that the adolescent suicide rates vary from country to country and that these differences are real, at least in part, rather than artifact (WHO Chronicle, 1975; Holinger, 1978; Brooke, 1974). Statistical data on adolescent suicide rates for various countries can be found in specific articles (e.g., WHO Chronicle, 1975), as well as in international compilations of such data (e.g., World Health Statistics Annual, 1972; Demographic Yearbook, 1974). Japan, Czechoslovakia, and Hungary have had some of the highest recent suicide rates among adolescents, and Ireland, Mexico, and Greece some of the lowest (WHO Chronicle, 1975; World Health Statistics Annual, 1972). The suicide rates for adolescents in the United States are approximately midway between the highest and lowest of these rates (Holinger, 1978).

Epidemics.   There have been many reports of epidemics of suicide and attempted suicide in young people of various cultures. Such phenomena would appear to lend support to the notion that sociocultural factors may in certain situations be a powerful contributor to adolescent suicide. For example, perhaps the best known suicide epidemics among the young have been associated with Goethe's *The Sorrows of Young Werther.* Youthful suicides were frequently attributed to this book, particularly during the 18th Century following its publication. Popow (1957) described a suicide epidemic among school children in Moscow, in which 70 children took their lives with 18 months. Popow suggested a variety of motives: poor grades, bad examination scores, conflicts with school administrators, adverse home situations, love affairs, and physical illness. The author considered imitation an important factor. Zilboorg (1936) described several suicide epidemics, gleaned from ethnological data as well as from newspaper accounts, involving both adults and young people. Bakwin (1957) and Murphy (1959) have summarized other suicide epidemics among adolescents.

Sibling Position.   Some investigators have suggested that sibling position may be related to adolescent suicide. Kallman et al. (1949) noted that the suicide rate of only children did not differ significantly from that of the general population or from that of twins in his mostly adult sample. In a review of the available data on sibling position and suicide, Lester (1966) concluded that the oldest and perhaps the youngest children are over-represented in adolescent suicide. Among adult suicides, Lester stated the available data showed no relationship to birth order. He felt this might be due to birth order losing some of its significance in later years as compared to childhood and adolescence.

Pregnancy and Suicidal Adolescents. Much literature exists on adolescent pregnancy and attempted suicide, but little on completed suicide. Bengtsson (1965) summarized various surveys of female suicides, and a range of pregnancy from 3 to 20 percent was found. Marek et al. (1976) presented data from Europe which suggested that undesired pregnancy was an important factor in adolescent suicide from 1881–1939, but was not so important in more recent suicidal behavior among adolescents. Many explanations exist to account for the relationship between adolescent suicide and pregnancy; e.g., the biological effect of the pregnancy, the psychological stresses involved, and the underlying psychopathology which accounts for both the pregnancy and the suicide, but little data exist. Lester (1970), studying the relationships between adolescent suicide and the attitudes toward premarital sexual behavior, hypothesized that adolescent suicide would occur more where premarital sexual expression was severely punished. The data failed to support this hypothesis.

Nosology

One important line of inquiry involved in adolescent suicide research concerns the presence of absence of mental illness among suicidal adolescents. At least two major issues can be discerned in the literature: the presence or absence of mental illness, and the type of disorder. Unfortunately, literature on clinical diagnosis of completed adolescent suicides is scarce. Two other problems impair the attempt to uncover the relationship between mental illness and adolescent suicide. First, some studies assign a clinical diagnosis to every subject. Superficially it might appear that all suffered "mental illness," but one must look at the specific diagnosis to reach more useful conclusions. Second, increasing attention is being given to "depressive equivalents"; i.e., boredom, apathy, and acting out behaviors may be evidence of serious depression in adolescence although they may not be so diagnosed (Glaser, 1967).

The evidence tends to suggest that serious mental illness is an important factor in many adolescent suicides. In a large series of suicidal adolescents in which clinical psychiatric diagnoses were made, psychoses and depression represented a proportion of those diagnosed (Stearns, 1953; Otto, 1972). Stearns (1953) noted that 20 of 97 adolescent suicides were "frankly insane," but that 25 apparently normal males hung themselves in unusual circumstances. Other authors incorporated delinquency and antisocial behavior into their diagnosis of adolescents who killed themselves (Dizmang et al., 1974). However, some suggest that mental illness is not a major component of suicide among adolescents. Seiden (1969) wrote that ''there are no modern writers who contend that mental disorder is either a necessary or sufficient cause of suicide.'' Yet, research has rarely shown evidence that suicidal adolescents are normal, healthy individuals. The notion that adolescents who killed themselves were normal and healthy may be due to the denial of the presence of psychiatric symptoms and an inability to recognize such symptoms.

DISCUSSION

The phenomenon of suicide is as old as the history of recorded time. Suicide among the young may be no different from suicide among other groups, if one considers the basic underlying psychological principle of self-destruction. It has always been perplexing for philosophers, theologians, and psychologists to understand why under similarly hellish conditions some people elect to destroy themselves, while others hold on with lingering hope to the future. Similarly, it has been a mystery why other people commit suicide under what seems to the ordinary observer rather hopeful conditions. What is it in man which forces some to resort to self-destruction? Is suicide, as some philosophers and theologians would suggest, the last available option of a free man? Or, closer to psychic determinism, is man subject to varying degrees of self-preservative and self-destructive drives?

It has been suggested that the self-destructive impulse is a manifestation of what Freud called the death instinct—''the task of which is to lead organic life back into the inanimate state'' (1924). While Freud and other analysts (e.g., Benedek, 1973; Klein, 1975) have supported the notion of the death instinct, probably the majority of analysts have rejected it. The universality of self-destructiveness is important. Self-destructiveness, in the form of thoughts of suicide to overt suicide, appears in every culture and individual. It is perhaps useful to conceive of a continuum of self-destructiveness, ranging from the briefest consideration of suicide, to the things one does daily that sabotage one's best efforts and well-being, to a variety of forms of self-mutilation without attempting suicide, to overt attempts to end one's life.

The data presented in this paper indicate that the suicide rates among 15- to 19-year-olds have increased significantly over the past 20 years. Statistically significant increases have been found among white males, white females, nonwhite males, and nonwhite females in the 15 to 19 age group. The increased suicide rate may represent real change, may be partially an artifact that selectively effects younger age groups (e.g., greater acceptance of existence of youthful suicides and better diagnosis), or both (Holinger, 1978). It is unlikely that the increase is an artifact due to changes in federal classification (Holinger, 1978; Klebba and Dolman, 1975).

Why has there been such an increase in the suicide rate among 15- to 19-year-olds in the past 20 years? It is easy to speculate, or to suggest better or more accurate reporting, but in reality little data exists to help answer the question. Perhaps the best tactic is to study subgroups of 15- to 19-year-olds: why do white adolescent males have higher suicide rates, with a greater increase over the past 20 years, than any other subgroup among 15- to 19-year-olds? There is obviously no simple explanation; suicide is a multi-determined phenomenon with a number of variables contributing to the actual event. Yet, it is important to consider the combination of two factors in understanding the high suicide rates among young white males: the action-oriented style of the males, and the pressure for performance on the white male. The male in our society learns to express his feelings in action. Male adolescents who are mentally healthy channel their feelings via action, sports being one of their favorite routes (Offer, 1969). When male adolescents get depressed, it is hard for them to use the verbal channel (as can their female peers). Rather, they turn to the method with which they are most familiar—the action route. The white male appears to have the most pressure for performance: he has the greatest expectations placed on him by others and by himself and hence the greatest potential for self-esteem problems. If, for whatever reason, the white male teenager slips in his school work, does not have good interpersonal relationships, is shy or introspective, the pressure on him is stronger than on other adolescents. This pressure, together with the action-oriented psychological posture of male adolescents in our culture, may begin to explain why the suicide route is relatively higher among white male adolescents.

In addition, interpersonal isolation may enhance the rise in suicide rates, as would be predicted by Durkheim's classic theory of "egoistic" suicide (1951). Longitudinal studies have shown that children and adolescents who do not get along well with peers are less happy and less well adjusted as adults than those who do (Janes et al., in press). There is some, albeit controversial, evidence that suicide is attempted more among youth from broken homes (Crook and Raskin, 1975). Teicher (see Luce, 1971) demonstrated that adolescents who attempted suicide went through progressive isolation from important people in their lives, leading to a chain reaction dissolution of any remaining meaningful social relationships. The vast majority of adolescents do not commit suicide or even attempt it. A tremendously large population of adolescents aged 15 to 19 exists in the United States. This population has increased steadily over the past 20 years from 11,263,000 in 1956 to 20,966,000 in 1975 (Vital Statistics of the U.S., 1956-1974; Health—U.S., 1976-1977), with relatively less fluctuation prior to that span. Paradoxically, this increase may intensify the sense of isolation and tendency to suicide. It may be more difficult for an adolescent to gain a sense of self-worth and find friends in the large impersonal high school of today than in the smaller schools of the past. The lonely, emotionally-depleted, depressed adolescent may look around him and see most of his peers functioning relatively well, sharpening his awareness of his personal problems and increasing his loneliness and isolation. Seeing so many seemingly well-functioning peers may also lower his already low and excessively vulnerable self-esteem, with the consequent sense of hopelessness resulting in a suicide attempt, or, in extreme situations, suicide. This may help explain the continuous increase in suicide among adolescents during the past 20 years. It would also mean that if the number of adolescents decreases (as is predicted for the next decade) and assuming other factors stay the same (e.g., sociocultural factors such as economics, war, etc., and nosological factors such as proportion of adolescents with psychoses), the suicide rate among adolescents may decrease accordingly.

Several directions of research into adolescent suicide appear to have potential for enhancing the understanding, prediction, and prevention of this third leading cause of death in youth. Perhaps most important are epidemiologic studies: it seems essential that better standardized and more reliable epidemiologic data be available at both national and local levels in order to adequately understand the frequency, distribution, and etiology of suicide among the young. National mortality data on adolescent suicides should include more information on their ethnicity and SES, and the data should be compiled and easily accessible by one-year intervals inasmuch as the five-year intervals (e.g., 10-14 years, 15-19 years, 20-24 years, etc.) inappropriately divide up "adolescence." It will probably take many more decades of excellent epidemiologic data to understand the fluctuations in suicide rates, make accurate predictions, and intervene effectively. Thus, it behooves society to take the additional necessary steps now to assure high-quality data over the next several generations. Other epidemiologic work, such as cohort (studies based on exposure; e.g., suicide-risk factors) and case-control (studies based on disease; i.e., attempted or completed adolescent suicide) investigations, would be fruitful. Continued research into the various biological and hereditary components of major mental illnesses, depressions, and suicide is also essential. Future psychoanalytic research might best utilize the developmental perspective and focus upon the jump in adolescent rates over childhood, on the one hand, and the fact that adolescent rates are lower than rates for older age groups, on the other. It is important to understand what intrapsychic as well as sociocultural forces may be protective in childhood as compared with adolescence, and protective in adolescence as compared with adulthood. Finally, while prediction of suicide has received some attention in the literature (Bunney, Fawcett, Davis et al., 1969; Schneidman, 1968; McIntire and Angle, 1975; Farberow and MacKinnon, 1975; Brown and Sheran, 1972; Tuckman and Youngman, 1968; Vecchio, 1969; Davidson, Choquet, and Facy, 1976; Neuringer, 1975; Beck, Resnick, and Lettieri, 1974; Durkheim, 1951.), the predictive concepts need to be applied to intervention studies on individuals and groups in order to optimally enhance effective intervention for those adolescents who have a high risk of suicide.

NOTES

Dr. Holinger is Associate Attending, Institute for Psychosomatic and Psychiatric Research and Training (P&PI), Michael Reese Hospital and Medical Center, Chicago, Illinois. This work was done in part when Dr. Holinger was at the Harvard University School of Public Health, Boston, Massachusetts.

Dr. Offer is Professor and Chairman, Department of Psychiatry, Institute for Psychosomatic and Psychiatric Research and Training (P&PI), Michael Reese Hospital and Medical Center, and Professor of Psychiatry, Pritzker School of Medicine, University of Chicago, Chicago, Illinois.

REFERENCES

Akiskal, H. S., and W. T. McKinney (1975), "Overview of recent research in depression," *Archives of General Psychiatry* 32:285-305.

Anthony, E. J. (1970), "Two contrasting types of adolescent depression and their treatment," *Journal of the American Psychoanalysis Association* 18:841-859.

Bakwin, H. (1957), "Suicide in children and adolescents," *The Journal of Pediatrics* 50:749-769.

Balser, B. H., and J. F. Masterson (1959), "Suicide in adolescents," *American Journal of Psychiatry* 116:400-404.

Beck, A. T., H. L. P. Resnick, and D. J. Lettieri (1974), *The Prediction of Suicide*. Bowie, Maryland: Charter Press.

Benedek, T. (1973), "Death instinct and anxiety," *Psychoanalytic Investigations: Selected Papers*. New York: Quadrangle.

Bengtsson, L. (1965), "Graviditet och sjalvmord," *Svenska Lak.-Tidn.* 28:1469. As cited by Otto, U. (1965), "Suicidal attempts made by pregnant women under 21 years," *Acta Paedopsychiatric* 32:276-288.

Blanchard, J. D., E. L. Blanchard, and S. Roll (1976), "A psychological autopsy of an Indian adolescent suicide with implications for community services," *Suicide and Life-Threatening Behavior* 6:3-10.

Bliss, E., and J. Zwanziger (1966), "Brain amines and emotional stress," *Journal of Psychiatry Res* 4:189-198.

Brooke, E. M. (Ed) (1974), "Suicide and Attempted Suicide," *Public Health Papers* No. 58, Geneva: WHO.

Brown, T. R., and T. J. Sheran (1972), "Suicide prediction: a review," *Life-Threatening Behavior* 2:67-98.

Bunney, W. E., J. A. Fawcett, J. M. Davis et al. (1969), "Further evaluation of urinary 17-hydroxy cortiosteroids in suicidal patients," *Archives of General Psychiatry* 21:138-150.

Bush, J. A. (1976), "Suicide and Blacks: A conceptual framework," *Suicide and Life-Threatening Behavior* 6:216-222.

Cain, A. (Ed) (1972), *Survivors of Suicide*. Springfield, Illinois: Charles C. Thomas.

Crook, T., and A. Raskin (1975), "Association of childhood parental loss with attempted suicide and depression," *Journal of Consulting Clinical Psychology* 43:277.

Davidson, F., M. Choquet, and F. Facy (1976), "The concept of risk in the field of youth suicide," *Rev Epidemiol Sante Publique* 24:283-300.

Demographic Yearbook, 1974 (1975). New York: United Nations.

Dennehy, C. M. (1966), "Childhood bereavement and psychiatric illness," *British Journal of Psychiatry* 112:1049-1069.

Dizmang, L. H., J. Watson, P. A. May et al. (1974), "Adolescent suicide at an Indian reservation," *American Journal of Orthopsychiatry* 44:43-49.

Draper, E. (1976), "A developmental theory of suicide," *Compr Psychiatry* 17:63-80.

Dublin, L. J. (1963), *Suicide: A Sociological and Statistical Study.* New York: Ronald Press.

Durkheim, E. (1951), *Suicide: A Study in Sociology* (trans. by Spaulding and Simpson. New York: The Free Press (Macmillan).

Farberow, N. L., and E. S. Shneidman (Eds) (1961). *The Cry for Help.* New York: McGraw-Hill.

Farborow, N. L., and D. MacKinnon (1975), "Prediction of suicide; a replication study," *Journal Pers Assess* 39:497-501.

Finch, S. M., and E. O. Poznanski (1971), *Adolescent Suicide.* Springfield, Illinois: Charles C. Thomas.

Friedman, P. (Ed) (1967), *On Suicide.* New York: International Universities Press.

Freud, S. (1910), "Contributions to a discussion on suicide," *Standard Edition* (J. Strachey, Ed.), Vol. XI. London: The Hogarth Press.

——— (1917), "Mourning and melancholia," *Standard Edition* (J. Strachey, Ed.), Vol. XIV. London: Hogarth.

——— (1923), "The ego and the id," *Standard Edition* (J. Strachey, Ed.) Vol. XIX, London: Hogarth.

——— (1924), "Economic problem of masochism," *Standard Edition* (J. Strachey, Ed.), Vol. XIX. London: Hogarth.

Gibbs, J. P. (1971), "Suicide," *Contemporary Social Problems* (R. K. Merton and R. Nisbet, Eds.), Third Edition, pp 271-312. New York: Harcourt Brace Jovanovich.

Glaser, K. (1967), "Masked depression in children and adolescents," *American Journal of Psychotherapy* 21:565-574.

Gould, R. (1965), "Suicide problems in children and adolescents," *American Journal of Psychotherapy* 19:228-246.

Gregory, I. (1966), "Retrospective data concerning childhood loss of parents - II. Category of parental loss by decade of birth. Diagnosis and MMPI," *Archives of General Psychiatry* 15:362:367.

Haim, A. (1974), *Adolescent Suicide.* (Translated by A.M.S. Smith). New York: International Universities Press.

Health—United States—1976-1977 (1977), Washington, D.C.: U.S. Government Printing Office.

Hendin, H. (1969a), "Black suicide," *Archives of General Psychiatry* 21:407-422.

Hendin, H. (1969b), *Black Suicide.* New York: Basic Books.

Holinger, P. C. (1977), "Suicide in adolescence," *American Journal of Psychiatry* 134:1433-1434.

——— (1978), "Adolescent suicide: An epidemiological study of recent trends," *American Journal of Psychiatry* 135:754-756.

——— (1979), "Violent deaths among the young: An epidemiological study of recent trends in suicide, homicide, and accidents," in press: *American Journal of Psychiatry.*

Janes, C. L., V. M. Hesselbrock, D. G. Myers et al. (1979), "Problem boys in young adulthood: Teachers' ratings and 12-year follow-up," *Journal Youth Adolescence* 8(4):453-472.

Jones, E. (1957), *The Life and Work of Sigmund Freud,* Vol. 3, p 180. New York: Basic Books.

Kallman, F. J., and M. M. Anastasio (1947), "Twin studies on the psychopathology of suicide," *Journal Nerv Ment Dis* 105:40-55.

Kallman, F. J., J. dePorte, E. dePorte et al. (1949), "Suicide in twins and only children," *American Journal of Human Genetics* 1:113-126.

Kallman, F. J. (1953), *Heredity in Health and Mental Disorder.* New York: Norton.

Klebba, J., and A. B. Dolman (1975), "Comparability of mortality statistics for the seventh and eighth revisions of the International Classification of Diseases," *United States, Vital and Health Statistics,* Series 2, Number 66. Washington, D.C.: U.S. Government Printing Office.

Klein, M. (1932), *Contributions to Psycho-Analysis.* London: Hogarth.

_____ (1975), "On the theory of anxiety and guilt," *Envy and Gratitude & Other Works 1946-1963.* New York: Dell.

_____ (1975), "On the development of mental functioning," *Envy and Gratitude & Other Works 1946-1963.* New York: Dell.

Kramer, M., E. S. Pollack, R. W. Redick, and B. Z. Locke (1972), *Mental Disorders/Suicide.* Cambridge: Harvard University Press.

Lester, D. (1966), "Sibling position and suicidal behavior," *Journal of Individual Psychology* 22:204-207.

_____ (1970), "Adolescent suicide and premarital sexual behavior," Journal of Social Psychology 82:131-132.

Litman, R. E. (1967), "Sigmund Freud on suicide," *Essays in Self-Destruction* (E. Shneidman, Ed.). New York: Science House.

Lourie, R. S. (1967), "Suicide and attempted suicide in children and adolescents," *Texas Medicine* 63(11):58-63.

Luce, G. (1971), "Why adolescents kill themselves" (Teicher, investigator), *The Mental Health of the Child* (J. Segal, Ed.). Rockville, Md.: NIMH.

McIntire, M.S., and C. R. Angle (1975), "Evaluation of suicide risk in adolescents," *Journal of Family Practice* 2:339-341.

Marek, Z., J. Widacki, and W. Zwarysiewica (1976), "Suicides committed by minors," *Forensic Science* 7:103-108.

Medical Record N.Y. (1901), "A family of suicides," 60(17):660-661.

Menninger, K. A. (1933), "Psychoanalytic aspects of suicide," *International Journal of Psychoanalysis* 14:376-390.

Morris, J. B., M. Kovacs, A. I. Beck et al. (1974), "Notes toward an epidemiology of urban suicide, *Comprehensive Psychiatry* 15:537-547.

Murphy, H. B. N. (1959), *The Student and Mental Health.* Cambridge: Harvard University Press.

Neuringer, C. (1975), "Problems in predicting adolescent suicidal behavior," *Psychitric Opinion* 12:27-31.

Offer, D. (1969), *The Psychological World of the Teenager.* New York: Basic Books.

Ogden, M., M. I. Spector, and C. A. Hill (1970), "Suicides and homicides among Indians," *Public Health Reports* 85:75-80.

Otto, U. (1972), "Suicidal acts by children and adolescents," *Acta Psychiatrica Scandinavica Suppl* 233:7-123.

Patel, N. S. (1974), "A study on suicide," *Med Sci Law* 14:129-136.

Petzel, S., and D. W. Cline (1978), "Adolescent suicide: epidemiological and biological aspects," *Adolescent Psychiatry* Vol. VI (S. Feinstein and P. Giovacchini, Eds.). Chicago: University of Chicago Press.

Popow, N. M. (1911), "The present epidemic of school suicides in Russia," *Nevrol Vestnik,* Kazan 18:312,592. As cited by H. Bawkin (1957), "Suicide in children and adolescents," *Journal of Pediatrics* 50:749-769.

Prange, A. I. Wilson, C. W. Lynn et al. (1974), "L-Tryptophan in mania: contribution to a permissive hypothesis on affective disorders," *Archives of General Psychiatry* 30:56-62.

Resnick, H. L., and L. H. Dizmang (1971), "Observations on suicidal behavior among American Indians," *American Journal of Psychiatry* 127:58-63.

Rosenbaum, M., and J. Richman (1970), "Suicide: the role of hostility and death wishes from the family and significant others," *American Journal of Psychiatry* 126:128-131.

Sabbath, J. C. (1969), "The suicidal adolescent—the expendable child," *Journal of the American Acadamy of Child Psychiatry* 8:272-285.

Sanborn, D. E., C. J. Sanborn, and P. Cimbolic (1973), "Two years of suicide: A study of adolescent suicide in New Hampshire," *Child Psychiatry Human Development* 3:234-242.

Schneer, H. I., and P. Kay (1961), "The suicidal adolescent," pp. 180-201. *Adolescents*. (S. Lerand and H. Schneer, Eds.) New York: Paul Hoeber.

Seiden, R. H. (1969), "Suicide among youth: A review of the literature, 1900-1967," *Bull Suicidology* (suppl.)

———— (1972), "Why are suicides among blacks increasing?" *HSMHA Health Reports* 87:3-8.

Shapiro, L. B. (1935), "Suicide: psychology and family tendency," *Journal Nerv Ment Dis* 81:547-553.

Shneidman, E. S. (1968), "Orientation toward cessation: A re-examination of current modes of death," *Journal of Forensic Science* 13:33-45.

Shore, J. H. (1972), "Suicide and suicide attempts among American Indians of the Pacific Northwest," *International Journal of Social Psychiatry* 18:91-96.

———— (1975), "American Indian suicide—fact and fancy," *Psychiatry* 38:86-91.

Stearns, A. W. (1953), "Cases of probable suicide in young persons without obvious motivation," *Journal of Maine Medical Association* 43:16-23.

Swanson, D. W. (1960). "Suicide in identical twins," *American Journal of Psychiatry* 116:934-935.

Toolan, J. M. (1962), "Suicide and suicidal attempts in children and adolescents," *American Journal of Psychiatry* 118:719-724.

———— (1975), "Suicide in children and adolescents," *American Journal of Psychotherapy* 29:339-344.

Tuckman, J., and H. E. Connon (1962), "Attempted suicide in adolescents," *American Journal of Psychiatry* 119:228-236.

Tuckman, J., and W. F. Youngman (1968), "A scale for assessing suicide risk of attempted suicides," *Journal of Clinical Psychology* 24:17-19.

Vecchio, T. J. (1966), "Predictive value of a single diagnostic test in unselected populations," *New England Journal of Medicine* 274:1171-1173.

Vital and Health Statistics (1967), "Suicide in the United States 1950-1964," Series 20, Number 5. Washington, D.C.: U.S. Government Printing Office.

Vital Statistics—Special Reports (1956), "Death rates by age, race, and sex: United States, 1900-1953: Suicide," Volume 43, Number 30. Washington, D.C.: U.S. Government Printing Office.

Vital Statistics of the United States, 1956-1974, Mortality, U.S. Department of Health, Education & Welfare, Public Health Service, National Center for Health Statistics. Washington, D.C.: U.S. Government Printing Office.

Vital Statistics of the United States, 1961-1973, Volume II—Mortality. U.S. Department of Health, Education & Welfare, Public Health Service, National Center for Health Statistics. Washington, D.C.: U.S. Government Printing Office.

Vital Statistics of the United States, 1974 and 1975, Volume II—Mortality, National Center for Health Statistics (in press).

Waldron, I., and J. Eyer (1975), "Socioeconomic causes of the recent rise in death rates for 15-24 year olds," *Soc Sci Med* 9:383-396.

Warren, M. (1967), "On Suicide," *Journal of American Psychoanalysis Association* 24:199-234.

Weiss, M., E. Stone, and N. Harrel (1970), "Coping behavior and brain norepinephrine level in rats," *Journal of Comparative Physiology and Psychology* 72:153-160.

Weiss, N. S. (1976), "Recent trends in violent deaths among young adults in the United States," *American Journal Epidem* 103:416-422.

Westermeyer, J., and J. Brantner (1972), "Violent death and alcohol use," *Minn Med* 55:749-752.

WHO Chronicle (1975), "Suicide statistics: the problem of comparability" 29:188-193. "Suicide and the young" 29:193-198.

Williams, C., and C. M. Lyons (1976), "Family interaction and adolescent suicidal behavior: A preliminary investigation," *Australian New Zealand Journal of Psychiatry* 10:243-252.

Wolfgang, M. E. (1959), "Suicide by means of victim-precipitated homicide," *Clinical Experimental Psychopathology* 20:335-349.

World Health Statistics Annual 1972 (1975), Volume I: Vital Statistics and Causes of Death. Geneva: WHO.

Zilboorg, G. (1936), "Suicide among civilized and primitive races," *American Journal of Psychiatry* 92:1347-1369.

_____ (1936), "Differential diagnostic types of suicide," *Archives of Neurological Psychiatry* 35:270-291.

_____ (1937), "Considerations on suicide, with particular reference to that of the young," *American Journal of Orthopsychiatry* 7:15-31.

Part II

EFFECTS OF A KEY INDEPENDENT VARIABLE UPON MULTIPLE DIMENSIONS OF MENTAL HEALTH

Section A

EFFECTS OF FAMILY EVENTS AND RELATIONSHIPS

MATTERING:

INFERRED SIGNIFICANCE AND MENTAL
HEALTH AMONG ADOLESCENTS

Morris Rosenberg and B. Claire McCullough

The familiar term "significant others," introduced by Harry Stack Sullivan (1947, 1953), succinctly reflects the idea that some people matter to us greatly whereas others do not[1], and that the views attributed to those significant others make more of a difference than the views of those who count little (Hughes, 1962; Denzin, 1966). Research has amply documented the wisdom of this observation (Rosenberg, 1973). What is generally overlooked, however, is the obverse—the degree to which we feel we matter to others. Do we believe that we count in other's lives, loom large in their thoughts, make a difference to them? Are we an object of another's concern, interest, or attention?

So viewed, mattering is the direct reciprocal of significance. Like significance, mattering may rest on different foundations. The conviction that one matters to another person is linked to the feeling that: (a) one is an object of his attention; (b) that one is important to him; and (c) that he is dependent on us.

Research in Community and Mental Health, Volume 2, pages 163–182
Copyright © 1981 by JAI Press, Inc.
ISBN: 0-89232-152-0

Attention

The most elementary form of mattering is the feeling that one commands the interest or notice of another person. The only prospect more bleak than to die unmourned is to die unnoticed. The acts of many assassins or highjackers is frequently understood as the desperate actions of nonentities to impinge, even if briefly or negatively, on the minds of others. In the words of William James (293–4):

> We have an innate propensity to get ourselves noticed . . . by our kind. No more fiendish punishment could be devised, were such a thing physically possible, than that one should be turned loose in society and remain absolutely unnoticed by all the members thereof. If no one turned round when we entered, answered when we spoke, or minded what we did, but if every person we met 'cut us dead,' and acted as if we were non-existing things, a kind of rage and impotent despair would ere long well up in us, from which the cruellest bodily tortures would be a relief; for these would make us feel that, however bad might be our plight, we had not sunk to such a depth as to be unworthy of attention at all.

And Charles Horton Cooley (1912) expresses this idea in the story of Philoctetes, whose greatest woe is not the tribulations he has suffered but the fact that he is no longer of *interest* to others, that he is not an object of their concern (142).

Philoctetes - And know'st thou not, O boy, whom thou dost see?
Neoptolemus - How can I know a man I ne'er beheld?
Philoctetes   - And didst thou never hear my name, nor fame
            Of these my ills, in which I pined away?
Neoptolemus - Know that I nothing know of what thou ask'st
Philoctetes   - O crushed with many woes, and of the Gods
            Hated am I, of whom, is this my woe,
            No rumor travelled homeward, nor went forth
            Through any clime of Hellas.

Importance

Mattering is more strongly expressed in the feeling that we are important to the other person or are objects of his concern. To believe that the other person cares about what we want, think, and do, or is concerned with our fate, is to matter. Whether the adolescent goes on to college or becomes hooked on drugs may deeply concern his parents, whereas they would have no corresponding feelings regarding the fate of the boy or girl down the street. One sure sign of importance is whether we are someone's ego-extension—that we reflect on or constitute a part of him. The adolescent who knows his parents will swell with pride at his achievements feels himself to be their ego-extension; his triumph is their success, his defeat their failure. Mattering, it should be stressed, is independent of approval. That the other person persists in criticizing us does not mean that we do not matter; on the contrary, it may be precisely because we matter so much that makes him so intent on overcoming our imperfections.

Dependence

That our behavior is influenced by our dependence on other people is easily understood, since most of our needs are satisfied by other human beings. What is much more mysterious is why our actions are equally governed by their dependence on us. The mother who rushes to put dinner on the table is impelled by the pressure of the fact that others are dependent on her to appease their hunger. The husband who feels his family is dependent on his earnings is under a tremendous burden of obligation. The executive who feels that his division will go to pot without him is tied to his company not only by his feelings toward it but equally by its (assumed) feelings toward him.

Mattering represents a compelling social obligation and a powerful source of social integration: we are bonded to society not only by virtue of our dependence on others but by their dependence on us. Part of Durkheim's (1951) explanation for the lower rate of suicide among married men and women, especially those with children, rested on this foundation. He pointed out that if suicide were due to stress and the burdens of living, then married people with children should commit suicide more than single people, since the latter were relatively free of obligations. The fact that married people with children had lower suicide rates suggested that it was not simply the individual's dependence on others but also their dependence on him that served as an insulator against suicide.

From the above observations, it is fair to conclude that mattering is a motive; the feeling that others depend on us, are interested in us, are concerned with our fate, or experience us as an ego-extension exercises a powerful influence on our actions. But since mattering is anchored in specific others, different people matter to us for different reasons. The present study deals with adolescents' beliefs that they matter to their parents. These beliefs, incidentally, are not necessarily accurate; but true or false, they have consequences.[2]

RESEARCH STRATEGY

The research strategy employed in this paper is theoretical replication. Theoretical replication involves the use of diverse measures of the same concepts employed in diverse samples. We turn first to a description of these diverse samples and measures.

Four large-scale surveys constitute the data files for this report: (1) a sample of 1678 juniors and seniors in ten high schools in New York State collected in 1960; (2) a sample of 679 adolescents in 13 junior and senior high schools in Baltimore in 1968;[3] (3) a sample of 1998 high school students in two schools in East Chicago in 1966; and (4) a nationwide sample of 2213 tenth-grade boys in 87 high schools in 1966. (Details regarding these samples appear respectively in Rosenberg, 1965; Rosenberg and Simmons, 1972; Dager, 1968; Bachman, 1970; and Bachman et al., 1972).

The four studies differ widely not only in time and space but also in terms of the richness of the parental mattering measures. The items captured diverse expressions of mattering: the feeling that one is an *object of interest* to parents, that one is *important* to parents, that one is an object of concern, that one's opinions count, and that one is *wanted*. Whether the parents were dependent on the child or whether the child was an ego-extension could not be ascertained directly.

The Baltimore parental mattering index was based on three items asking the respondent how often the mother was interested in him, how interested the parents were in what he had to say, and how important a part of the family he was. New York had only a single indicator: how interested parents were in what the child had to say at mealtime conversations. In East Chicago, four items were used: how interested the respondent's father was in him, how interested his mother was in him, whether he had ever felt that he was not wanted by his father, and whether he had ever felt he was not wanted by his mother. Finally, in the nationwide study, subjects were asked whether they felt they had influence in family decisions, how often their parents listened to their side of the argument, how often parents talked over important decisions with them, how often parents ignored them when they did something wrong, and how often their parents acted as if they didn't care. Ignoring the subject or not caring were interpreted as reflections of lack of interest. Wherever possible, items reflecting favorable or unfavorable parental attitudes were excluded, although such attitudes may be implied in some items.

Before presenting the data, a discussion of our research strategy is in order. The rationale for examining common propositions in differing samples using differing measures obviously resides in the principle of replication. La Sorte (1972) has distinguished four types of replication: retest replication, internal replication, independent replication, and theoretical replication. The purpose of retest replication is to repeat the original study with few or no changes in order to provide a reliability check on the original study. Such replication essentially involves duplication. Internal replication tests whether essentially the same results appear among sub-samples of a broader sample; it is reflected in the consistency of the conditional relations (Finifter's, 1975, pseudo-replication is of this type). An important early example of internal replication was Stouffer's (1949: 92–95) "method of matched comparisons." Independent replication is designed to establish empirical generalizations by examining the same proposition among different populations, varying in nature, time, and place. Finally, theoretical replication refers to the question of how diverse data bear on a common theoretical proposition. According to La Sorte (1972: 223): "In order to move toward a theoretical generalization, where empirical variables which have concrete anchoring points are abstracted and conceptualized to a higher theoretical plane, it is necessary to sample a variety of groups using different indicators of the same concepts." The reason is that every concept may be reflected in an infinite universe of indicators, each of which bears on probability relation to the underlying concept. Each indicator—or index—thus reflects both the concept plus some idiosyncratic or other component, characteristically labelled error. This principle is at the root of our present strategy—namely, to examine the same propositions across diverse samples using diverse indicators of the same concepts.

An example may serve to clarify the distinction between a theoretical replication and other types. Assume that we wished to examine the relationship between race and self-esteem and, using the Total Net Positive Score of the Fitts Tennessee Self-Concept Scale, found no racial differences. Since this finding might violate our theoretical expectations, we might wish to replicate it in one or more other studies to insure that the initial result was not the consequence of sampling accident or systematic error. The duplication of these results in other carefully designed studies would increase confidence in the finding. But assume that in various studies we also found no relationship between race and the Butler-Haigh Self-Ideal discrepancy score, Osgood's semantic differential, the Coopersmith Self-Esteem Inventory, the Bills' Index of Adjustment and Values, and the Gough and Heilbrun Adjective Check List. Since these measures differ in various ways, the consistency of the results is almost certainly due to what they have in common; the most plausible interpretation is that this common element is self-esteem. Other things equal, then, the theoretical proposition would appear to rest on a sounder foundation if common results appear when diverse measures are used than if the same measures are repeated.

The use of such diverse indicators, it may be pointed out, represents a more severe empirical test of the theoretical proposition for the following reason: Whereas the identical measure in different studies reflects both the common underlying concept plus some common error, the diverse indicators reflect the common underlying concept plus diverse error. Assuming random error, the likelihood that consistent empirical results across studies will appear is reduced. The severity of this test is exacerbated by the use of samples of diverse populations. In retest replication, the new sample should match the original as closely as possible; if the original study involved a college student sample, the replication should also involve college students. Theoretical replications, on the other hand, may involve samples with diverse populations. Since these populations differ among themselves, even perfect measurement would produce diversity of results. Furthermore, since each sample represents its population imperfectly, sampling error is superimposed on measurement error.

Difficult as it would be to achieve consistent univariate results when using different measures among different samples, it should be all the more difficult to obtain consistent bivariate relationships, because each of the concepts is itself reflected in diverse indicators, *each* of which reflects the underlying concept plus unknown error. Hence, the likelihood of discovering consistent bivariate, or even multivariate, relationships among such concepts is reduced appreciably. Theoretical replication thus constitutes a particularly severe test of a proposition.[4] At the same time, if this test is passed, it deserves respect, for it has overcome powerful forces working toward randomization.

RESULTS

Mattering and Mental Health

Does mattering matter? We suggested earlier that mattering may affect behavior in diverse ways. But if it is true that people have a *need* to matter—that they want to feel that they make a difference in others' lives—then mattering should be associated with diverse aspects of mental health. We shall first consider the dimension of global self-esteem and then turn to other indicators of mental health.

Self-esteem

Self-esteem is defined here as the individual's global positive or negative attitude toward himself as an object. The mental health relevance of this dimension has been amply documented in prior research (Wylie, 1961; Kaplan, 1975; Turner and Vanderlippe, 1958). All four studies contained global self-esteem measures; these measures overlapped but were not identical. The New York State study employed the ten-item Rosenberg Self-Esteem Scale based on a Guttman scoring procedure (Rosenberg, 1965; Wylie, 1974); the East Chicago study used the same items, but scored them according to the Likert procedure; and the nationwide study combined six of these items with four drawn from other sources, scoring them according to the Likert procedure. The Baltimore study used a separate six-item measure of self-esteem (Rosenberg and Simmons, 1972).

Are these diverse measures of parental mattering related to these diverse measures of self-esteem in these four different studies? In turns out that all four studies show clear positive relationships between the adolescent's feeling that his parents are interested in and care about him and his global feeling of self-worth (Table 1). In Baltimore, gamma = .2094; in New York, .2798; in East Chicago, .2754; and in nationwide, .2960. All four relationships are significant at the .001 level.

But is this relationship due to the fact that the adolescent's parents *care* about him or that they *think well* of him? The distinction is crucial. To feel that we matter to others is conceptually distinct from feeling that they think well of us. There is, of course, ample evidence to indicate that our views of how others evaluate us (described as the "perceived self" by Miyamoto and Dornbusch, 1956, and as "subjective public esteem" by Sherwood 1965, 1967, and others) is closely related to our self-esteem (Reeder, Donohue, and Biblarz, 1960; Sherwood, 1965, 1967; Rosenberg and Simmons, 1972). But if mattering per se

Table 1. Self-Esteem and Parental Mattering: Zero-Order Relationship and Relationship Controlled on Perceived Self

	Gamma	Chi-squared P	Partial gamma, controlled on perceived self	N
Baltimore	.2069	.001	.2017	(657)
Nationwide	.2960	.001	—†	(2065)
East Chicago	.2754	.001	.2990	(1855)
New York	.2798	.001	.3211	(1112)

†No perceived self index available.

makes a difference for the adolescent's self-esteem, then it should make a difference whether the youngster's parents think well of him or not. It should, in other words, be independent of the perceived self.

In general, the data on parental perceived selves—whether the child believes his parents hold favorable or unfavorable attitudes toward him—are skimpy in these studies so that a completely adequate test of the issue is not at hand. Nevertheless, the evidence appears highly suggestive.

The Baltimore perceived self items are the most satisfactory and direct. The subjects were asked: "Would you say that your mother thinks you are a wonderful person, a pretty nice person, a little bit of a nice person, or not such a nice person?" The same question was asked for the father, and the two items were combined into a parental perceived self index.

It will be recalled that, in Baltimore, the zero-order gamma of mattering to global self-esteem is .2069. Table 1 shows that, when we control on parental perceived self, the first-order partial gamma is .2017—a trivial difference. To believe that others consider you important, are interested in you, and pay attention to you is related to global self-esteem virtually independently of whether their attitudes are positive or negative.

Both in New York and in East Chicago, the only perceived self items were whether the subject felt he was his mother's favorite child and whether he was his father's favorite child. This index has several limitations: first, most respondents said there was no favorite child; second, although being a favorite child suggests that your parents think well of you, not being a favorite child does not necessarily mean they do not. Despite these limitations, the results are suggestive. In East Chicago, the zero-order relationship of parental mattering and self-esteem is gamma = .2754; the partial gamma (controlling on favorite child) is .2990. In New York, the corresponding figures are .2798 and .3211 (Table 1). Plainly, the original relationship between parental mattering and self-esteem is not attributable to the child's feeling that he is the parental favorite.

In this discussion we have been relating weak measures of mattering to questionable measures of self-esteem controlling on dubious measures of the perceived self. Despite the variety of measures, however, the results across studies—not only the zero-order relationships but the first-order partials—are impressively consistent. They suggest that parental mattering is related to global self-esteem and that this relationship is not attributable to the child's belief that his parents hold positive or negative attitudes toward him.

Parental Mattering and Other Mental Health Measures

The data thus suggest that mattering is important to youngsters, at least as far as self-esteem is concerned. But does it have further mental health implications as well? Again, the measures of mental health across the studies are diverse and vary considerably in quality, ranging from excellent in the nationwide study, fair in the Baltimore study, and poor in the East Chicago and New York studies. Such diversity, of course, militates against cross-study consistency, thus representing a formidable test of the theoretical proposition at issue.

The Baltimore study included a six-item Guttman scale of "depressive affect," asking respondents how happy they were, whether they got a lot of fun out of life, whether they were usually cheerful, etc.; a measure of somatic disturbance (how healthy the adolescent felt, how often he was tired, and how often he felt sick in the stomach); and a measure of "worries" (worrying about doing well in school, about being laughed at, about what others think of you, etc.).

In the nationwide study, depression was measured by a six-item score dealing with the respondent's feeling that the future was bright, that things seemed hopeless, that he was bored, that he was often down in the dumps, etc. Anxiety-tension was measured by a five-item index dealing with feeling jittery, tense, relaxed, worried, and nervous. The nationwide study of somatic symptoms is an 18-item checklist of physical complaints which are frequently interpreted as psychophysiological indicators of anxiety (Stouffer et al., 1950; Srole, 1962; Gurin et al., 1960). This measure includes such symptoms as nervousness, headaches, loss of appetite, shortness of breath, dizziness, and trembling hands. Finally, "negative affective states" is a composite score of six closely related scales (irritability, general anxiety, anxiety and tension, depression, anomia, and resentment) based on a total of 40 items.

Unfortunately, neither the East Chicago nor New York State studies contained direct, adequate measures of mental health. Each, however, contained a small number of items which expressed certain feelings of depression. In New York, subjects were asked whether or not they were usually in good spirits and whether they had generally been happy or unhappy earlier in life. The East Chicago items had a stronger flavor of anomia (Srole, 1956) or fatalism combined with depression: one item dealt with the respondent's view that planning was futile since plans never worked out anyway, that these days one didn't know who one could count on, and that the subject was less happy than he used to be.

Table 2 shows that, with the exception of the worry measure in Baltimore, the feeling that one matters to parents is clearly related to various measures of

Table 2. Mattering and Mental Health Measures: Zero-Order Relationships and Relationships Controlled on Global Self-Esteem

	Zero-order Gamma	Chi-squared P	Partial gamma, controlled on self-esteem	N
Baltimore				
Depression	.3042	.001	.2685	(659)
Worries	.0142	.331	.0525	(680)
Somatic	.1276	.022	.1662	(662)
Nationwide				
Depression	.3360	.001	.2483	(2053)
Worries	.1875	.001	.1514	(2052)
Anxiety-tension	.2176	.001	.1557	(2061)
Somatic	.3577	.001	.2786	(2053)
Negative affective	.3725	.001	.2960	(2047)
East Chicago				
Anomia-Depression	.2070	.001	.1895	(1866)
New York				
Depression	.4209	.001	.3813	(1310)

emotional disturbance in all of the studies; the nine other relationships vary between gamma = .12 and .42, and all are significant at the .001 level.

The adolescent who feels he matters little to his parents is thus strikingly more likely to be depressed, anxious, and otherwise disturbed, however measured. But is this because his self-esteem is inordinately low? The data in Table 2 suggest that this is the explanation in part, but only in part. Leaving aside the Baltimore worries measure (essentially a null relationship), the various other relationships decline somewhat when self-esteem is controlled, but still remain strong. The feeling that one matters to one's parents is thus associated with a number of fundamental dimensions of mental health *independent of the adolescent's global self-esteem.*

Mattering and Social Adjustment

Delinquency. There is thus a clear connection between the adolescent's feeling that he matters to his parents and diverse dimensions of mental health, variously measured. The question is: are these effects solely in the mind of the adolescent or do they connect with socially significant behavior? One type of behavior that is particularly relevant during adolescence is delinquency. When we speak of delinquency, we shall not be referring primarily to serious crime but chiefly to minor infractions, acts which are not uncommon among adolescents. Since delinquency is primarily a male phenomenon at this age, we shall confine our analysis in this section to the boys in the samples.

The Baltimore study contained a somewhat vague "trouble" index asking youngsters how often they got into trouble at home, in school, with friends, and with the police. As Table 3 shows, youngsters who scored low on the mattering index were more likely to get into trouble with others, although the relationship was not strong or significant (gamma = .1097).

Unlike the Baltimore measure, which spoke vaguely of "trouble," the nationwide delinquency measures were very concrete. Five measures of delinquency are available. Delinquent behavior in school is a seven-item index based on such experiences as getting into school fights, being suspended or expelled from school, cutting classes, damaging school property, hitting a teacher, etc. Frequency of delinquent behavior is a nine-item measure assessing how often the youth has stolen from stores, run away from home, trespassed, injured someone in a fight, etc. The seriousness of delinquency index is a ten-item score (overlapping with frequency) measuring whether the infraction was minor (stealing hubcaps, pilfering, etc.) or major (committing armed robbery, arson, etc.). Theft and vandalism is a nine-item index referring to pilfering, damaging school property, car stealing, etc. Finally, total delinquency is a 26-item scale based on the other four measures. There is, then, overlap among the five delinquency measures.

The conceptualization of delinquency as a continuum avoids the labeling fallacy which views delinquency as an absolute property of the individual. Few youths have committed most of these infractions, but few have committed none at all. Table 3 shows that school delinquency, frequency of delinquency, seriousness of delinquency, theft and vandalism, and total delinquency are all related to parental mattering at the .001 level; the gammas range between .22 and .38.

The East Chicago data were quite flimsy, but there are two items which reflect rather minor deviance, nonconformity, or social difficulty: the first dealt with how often the boy smoked; the second with how often he skipped school. The

Table 3. Mattering and Delinquency Among Boys

	Gamma	Chi-squared P	N
Baltimore			
Trouble	.1097	.248	(324)
Nationwide			
School delinquency	.2538	.001	(2013)
Frequency delinquency	.2604	.001	(2015)
Seriousness delinquency	.3785	.001	(2013)
Theft/Vandalism	.2230	.001	(2014)
Total delinquency	.2887	.001	(2014)
East Chicago	.2662	.001	(918)

two items were combined to form a "rule violation" score. The relationship of this score to parental mattering was gamma = .2662 (p < .001).

Why the adolescent who believes his parents have little interest in him or care little for him should turn to delinquency is a question that merits speculation. William James tells us that we have an "innate propensity" to get ourselves noticed and that the failure to command the attention of other people is painful. But if the need to feel that one makes a difference is so powerful, then may not the recourse to delinquency sometimes be a device designed to make an impression, attract attention, command notice, or have an impact, even if these are all negative? The delinquent may then be deplored, but he cannot be ignored. The angry reaction of his teachers, his parents, and the police are all vivid testimony to the fact that he makes a difference, that he counts; and this sense of significance is intensified by the support of his delinquent peers who value his contribution to the group's collective purposes. Furthermore, what incentive does he have for remaining nondelinquent? Many a youth who does as he is told is rewarded by remaining unnoticed, and is treated as a cipher and a nonentity. Thus, one reason for delinquency may be that it makes unimportant people feel important.

SIGNIFICANCE AND MATTERING

We suggested earlier that mattering may be viewed conceptually as the reciprocal or inverse counterpart of interpersonal significance. A significant other is one who matters to us; mattering refers to how much we matter to them. That the two concepts need not necessarily be empirically linked is recognized in the age-long theme of unrequited love: the beloved matters to us but we don't matter to him or her.

The question is, then, whether mattering and significance are empirically related. Like the other measures, the measures of parental significance vary across the studies. The Baltimore index of parental significance was straightforward: subjects were asked whether they cared very much, somewhat, a little, or not at all about what their mothers thought of them, and the same question was asked about fathers. Table 4 shows a strong empirical association between parental significance and parental mattering. Those whose parents are significant to them are considerably more likely to believe they are important to their parents (gamma = .3691, p < .001).

In the East Chicago study, the indicators of parental significance were more abundant though less straightforward. Respondents were instructed as follows:

"Some of the people below are very CLOSE TO YOU—you care about them very much. There are others that you may not care about at all—you don't feel close to them at all. Would you say that the following people are very close to you, close, a little close, or not at all close to you?" A number of individuals were mentioned including "my father" and "my mother."

"Now think for a second about how much each of the following people

Table 4. Parental Mattering and Parental Significance

		Chi-squared	
	Gamma	*P*	*N*
Baltimore	.3691	.001	(640)
Nationwide	.4337	.001	(1913)
East Chicago	.6564	.001	(1853)
New York†	—	—	—

†No indicators of parental significance available.

INFLUENCE YOU. Think about their influence in ALL AREAS of your life. Would you say that the following people influence you very much, some, a little, or not at all?'' Again, mother and father were included on the list.

These four items were combined to form a parental ''significant others'' index. The gamma = .6564 (p < .001) shown in Table 4 indicates that parental significance is very closely tied to parental mattering in East Chicago.

In the nationwide study, respondents were asked whether they felt extremely, quite, fairly, or not close to their fathers, and the same question was asked about mothers. On the assumption that the youngster who feels close to his parents considers them more important to him that one who does not, these two items were combined to form a parental significance index. The association between this index and the measure of parental mattering in this study was gamma = .4337 (p < .001).

Since the New York State study lacked any indicators of parental significance, the hypothesis could not be tested in this sample. Nevertheless, the strong relationships in the other three samples, as well as the absence of evident confounding factors, offers persuasive evidence that there is a tendency toward reciprocity between mattering and significance: we tend to care about those who, we believe, care about us.

SOCIAL AND CULTURAL INFLUENCES

That the adolescent wants to matter to his parents is evident. The question is: why do youngsters differ in this respect? To some extent, idiosyncratic factors in the family are decisive. Many years ago, Horney (1950) observed that, although the childhood circumstances that may be associated with neurotic personality development are almost infinitely varied, they have one element in common, namely, parental egocentricity. Speaking of such adverse circumstances, she held that ''when summarized, they all boil down to the fact that the people in the environment are too wrapped up in their own neuroses to be able to love the child, or even to conceive of him as the particular individual he is; their attitudes toward him are determined by their own neurotic needs and responses'' (Horney,

1950: 19). We interpret this to suggest that the neurotic parent is not genuinely interested in the child for what he is, and that the child can sense whether or not he matters to his parents.

Idiosyncratic factors aside, however, are there any factors rooted in the structure of society or the norms of cultures or sub-cultures that would contribute to the child's view that he does or does not matter to his parents? An obvious problem involved in attempting to answer this question by means of the theoretical replication method is that one or another study may lack the requisite data, making it impossible to assess trans-study consistency. Thus, the nationwide study lacks information on gender (the sample is male), Baltimore and East Chicago lack data on rural-urban residence, and New York, Baltimore and East Chicago lack regional variation data. Hence, the effect of certain structural factors could not be examined because information was not uniformly available. We shall, however, consider three factors: socioeconomic status, sibling structure, and religious affiliation.

Socioeconomic Status

Do adolescents in different social classes vary in the tendency to believe that they matter to their parents? Once more, we are faced with a diversity of measures. The Baltimore and East Chicago studies both used the Hollingshead Two-Factor Index of Social Position; the nationwide study used a composite socioeconomic level measure based on father's occupational status, father's education, mother's education, possessions in the home, number of books in the home, and number of rooms per person in the home; and New York used a weighted index based on father's occupation, education, and primary source of income.

Although it is not easy to summarize the results crisply, the data suggest a rather weak ordinal association between SES and mattering. In all four studies, the highest class ranked higher on mattering than the middle class and in three of the four the middle class ranked higher than the lowest class (in the fourth study they were tied). The linear effect is generally weak, chiefly because the difference between the middle and lowest class is rather small (4–7 percent). The most conspicuous difference, then, is between adolescents in the highest classes and those in the other classes. (Since the SES measures varied across studies, "highest class" does not have an identical meaning in all studies; it refers simply to those who ranked in the first or second categories in each study.) In Baltimore, 47 percent of the highest class ranked high in mattering compared with 39 percent of the others (gamma = .2177); in nationwide, the corresponding figures are 49 percent and 35 percent (gamma = .2240); in East Chicago, 41 percent and 37 percent (gamma = .2235); and in New York, 43 percent and 31 percent (gamma = .2532) (Table 5). The relationships are similar in strength, and all are significant at the .10 level.

The adolescents in the highest class are thus consistently, though not con-

Table 5. Mattering by Highest Socioeconomic Status

| | | Chi-squared | |
	Gamma	P	N
Baltimore	.2177	.083	(657)
Nationwide	.2240	.001	(2030)
East Chicago	.2235	.011	(1370)
New York	.2532	.066	(1031)

spicuously, more likely than others to feel that they matter greatly to their parents. Our data do not enable us to ascertain why these class differences appear, but it is possible to speculate on this issue. In his investigations in the area of social class and child-rearing values, Kohn (1959, 1969) has found that middle class and working class parents differ strikingly in the qualities they value in their children; these differences, Kohn holds, can be traced to the concrete content of adult work activity. The working class is primarily concerned with those qualities in the child that are overt, visible, and behavioral; these parents are particularly concerned that the child is obedient, that he is neat and clean, and that he is honest. The higher classes—and, in particular, the highest class—tend to be concerned with inner psychological and emotional states; these parents place primary stress on whether the child is happy, is curious to learn new things and, to a lesser extent, can exercise self-control (Kohn, 1969: 29–30).

We suggest that the child whose parents are concerned with, and interested in, his inner thoughts, feelings, and wishes is more likely to feel that they are really interested in him as a person than the one whose parents are concerned primarily with his external appearance and overt behavior. Unfortunately, the data to test this interpretation are unavailable. Whether or not it is correct, it does appear that the adolescent's location in the social structure influences his sense of parental mattering and, by extension, his mental health and social adjustment.

Sibling Structure

In his classic discussion of the role of numbers in social life, Simmel (1950) pointed out that as the group increased in size, each member (other things being equal) came to count for less. This observation suggests the possibility that children from larger families would be less likely to feel that they mattered greatly to their parents than children from smaller families. A second possibility is that birth order would make a difference—those coming earlier mattering more than later arrivals.

An examination of these two aspects of family structure to parental mattering showed no clear or consistent results across the four studies. One aspect of sibling structure, however, did appear to make a difference: being an only child. Despite the differences in the mattering indices used in the four studies, in each case there is a tendency for only children to rank higher on the mattering indices

* *Table 6.* Mattering and Only Child: Zero-Order Relationship and Relationship
Controlled on Race, Socioeconomic Status, and Both

			Partial gammas			
	Zero-order gamma	Chi-squared P	Controlled on race	Controlled on SES	Controlled on both	N
Baltimore	.2346	.211	.2661	.2554	.2338	(679)
Nationwide	.1109	.008	.1001	.0917	.0892	(1992)
East Chicago	.2439	.036	.2354	.1952	.2036	(1325)
New York	.2946	.002	.2902	.3051	.3115	(930)

than children with siblings (Table 6). In Baltimore, 48 percent of the only children ranked high compared with 40 percent of the others (gamma = .2346, p < .211); in New York, the corresponding figures were 46 percent and 29 percent (gamma = .2946, p < .002); in East Chicago, 50 percent and 34 percent (gamma = .2439, p < .036); and in nationwide, 27 percent and 18 percent (gamma = .1109, p < .008).

The data are thus consistent in suggesting that this aspect of family structure has some bearing on the child's feeling that he is an object of concern and importance to his parents, although one of the relationships does not meet the conventional significance levels. Although this conclusion is plausible, it is not inescapable since it could conceivably be the product of certain extraneous variables. Two possible confounding factors would be race and class. Black families tend to be larger than white and hence to have a smaller proportion of only children, and the same is true of lower and working class families. The data in Table 6, however, show that controlling on race or class separately or simultaneously has virtually no effect on the relationships. It thus seems plausible to think that the structural fact of being an only child increases the likelihood that one will feel significant in the life of one's parents.

Religion

Anthropological investigations have suggested that certain cultures or subcultures are "child-centered"; that is, children represent the focal objects of parental interest. To be sure, it is easy to exaggerate such differences if one confuses overt behavior with underlying attitudes, but the possibility of cultural differences in parental mattering is still worth considering.

The only cultural difference that we have been able to discern—and even here the results are modest and not always statistically reliable—is religion; Jewish children tend to score somewhat higher on parental mattering indices than non-Jewish children. One problem, however, is that since Jews constitute only about 3 percent of the population, the number of Jewish respondents likely to appear in samples of the general population is small. Hence, the data must be treated with caution since they may be consequences of statistical chance.

Keeping these caveats in mind, what do the data show? In Baltimore 57 percent of the Jewish children but 41 percent of the non-Jewish children score high on the mattering index (gamma = .2616, p < .129); in New York, the corresponding figures are 41 percent and 32 percent (gamma = .2187, p < .046); in East Chicago, the figures are 46 percent and 35 percent (gamma = .3341, p < .235); and in nationwide, the figures are 21 percent and 19 percent (gamma = .0512, p. < .9598) (Table 7).

There thus appears to be some tendency for Jewish children to score somewhat higher than others on these mattering indices, although only one of the four studies reaches an acceptable level of statistical significance, and the nationwide study shows virtually no association. One can thus place little confidence in any of the individual studies in this respect; however, the consistency of the findings across three studies suggests the possibility that the observed association may be real.

But even if the findings were statistically reliable, the results might still not be due to religious differences in child-centeredness but to associated factors. For one thing, Jewish respondents tend to be above average in socioeconomic status; for another, they tend to come from smaller families and hence may be more likely to be only children. Hence, Table 7 examines the association of religious background and mattering controlling on each of these factors independently and jointly. The partial gammas show that socioeconomic status is indeed partly responsible for the original relationships, but that being an only child is not. Controlling on SES reduces the Baltimore relationship from .2616 to .1202; the New York relationship from .2187 to .1778; the East Chicago relationship from .3341 to .2158; and the nationwide relationship from .0516 to .0157. Independent of socioeconomic status, then, the religion-parental mattering relationship is moderate in two studies, modest in one, and non-existent in the fourth. Samples with larger numbers of Jewish respondents would be required before we can place great confidence in such findings.

Table 7. Mattering and Jewish Affiliation: Zero-Order Relationship and Relationship Controlled on Socioeconomic Status, Only Child, and Both

			Partial gammas			
	Zero-order gamma	Chi-squared P	Controlled on SES	Controlled on only child	Controlled on both	N
Baltimore	.2616	.129	.1202	.2973	.2227	(616)
Nationwide	.0516	.960	.0157	.0444	−.0245	(1828)
East Chicago	.3341	.235	.2158	.3783	.2716	(1327)
New York	.2187	.046	.1778	.1866	.1559	(918)

SUMMARY AND DISCUSSION

This paper has attempted to shed light on certain psychological consequences and social causes of the important though neglected interpersonal attitude of inferred significance; that is, the individual's feeling that he matters in other people's lives. By mattering, we refer to the person's sense that, as far as other people are concerned, he is an object of interest and importance, that he is wanted or serves as an ego-extension, or that others depend on him. In this paper, we have limited our discussion to adolescents and have restricted our analysis to *parental* mattering. In principle, mattering is anchored in specific individuals so that generalizations based on parental mattering are not necessarily transferable to sibling, teacher, or classmate mattering.

The data suggest that mattering is important both for the individual and for society. As far as the individual is concerned, the adolescent who feels he matters little to his parents has lower self-esteem, is more depressed and unhappy, is more anxious and experiences other negative affective states, and is more likely to be delinquent. However, since these conclusions are based on correlational data, we cannot at this point be certain that mattering is responsible for psychological disturbance. In the absence of panel data, the assumption that mattering is a causal influence remains at the level of plausibility.

At first glance, these results would appear to be explained by learning theory. Mattering is associated with many of our major life gratifications, since more good things come to us from those who care about us than those who do not. But if this is so, how can one explain the fact that parental punishment is associated with *more favorable* self-attitudes than parental indifference; there is certainly no reward associated with being punished or criticized (Rosenberg, 1963). A second possible explanation for the relationship of mattering to mental health is that mattering serves the self-esteem motive which, according to James (1890), is irreducible. And it is true that the adolescent's feeling that he matters to his parents is strongly related to his global self-esteem. But that explanation also does not suffice because, self-esteem aside, mattering continues to be strongly related to emotional disturbance.

The finding that the adolescent who infers that he is significant is happier is doubly interesting because mattering is usually a burden, an obligation, and a restriction on freedom. When others depend on us, worry about us, expect things of us, we are constrained and inhibited by these expectations. The key figure on the team may give more of himself than the inessential one in part because his teammates depend on him. Furthermore, the person who infers that he is significant may consciously experience this situation as a burden and a constraint; but the unhappy person is the one who is free of the burden.

It has been suggested that one problem of retirement is that one no longer matters; others no longer depend upon us. "What we owe the old is reverence but all they ask for is consideration, attention, not to be discarded, forgotten" (Herschel, 1971). The reward of retirement, involving a surcease from labor, can be the punishment of not mattering. Existence loses its point and savor when one no longer makes a difference.

The wish to make a difference is thus not easily reduced to other motives. Whether or not James is correct in referring to it as an "innate propensity," it is plain that the feeling that one is an irrelevance touches the profoundest depths of self and relates to depression, anxiety, and delinquency. From the viewpoint of the adolescent, mattering matters profoundly.

But mattering also is important for society, for it is a significant source of social cohesion. It is frequently held that one of the main forces binding people to society is their dependence on others. Humans cannot survive, or even be truly human, without other people. But perhaps equally important is others' dependence on us. Discussions of freedom frequently overlook the fact that people assume burdens happily and accept restraints freely if it gives them a feeling of significance, a feeling that they matter to others, that they make a difference. Not all people, we hasten to add, do embrace these obligations happily. Some raise to the pinnacle of their value systems the state of independence, a state in which they care nothing for others and others care nothing for them. Perhaps such people alone can be free. But, in losing their attachment to society, they come to constitute prime candidates for Durkheim's (1951) egoistic suicide; and in losing their feelings of significance for others, they become vulnerable targets for depression and associated emotional states.

Finally, we suggest that mattering may be relatively high among children and adults, low among adolescents and old people. The young child feels that he matters because the world revolves about him, because he is the center of the universe. The adult matters because he runs the world.

The adolescent, on the other hand, is something of a sociological superfluity, an irrelevance. In less advanced societies, mattering presumably would be high because the adolescent would already have established his or her own family. In America half a century ago, the adolescent's family would have depended on his earnings or his work on the farm. Today, the family is less dependent on the adolescent for his material contribution. It may be that one reason why the adolescent clings so tenaciously to his peers is that to them, at least, he matters. If it is true that the feeling of being socially irrelevant is widespread among adolescents, this fact may underly some of the problems of contemporary youth.

ACKNOWLEDGMENTS

Paper presented at the annual meeting of the American Sociological Association, Boston, Massachusetts, August 27, 1979. The research reported in this article was funded by a grant from the National Institute of Mental Health (MH27747). The data and tabulations were made available (in part) by the Institute for Social Research Social Science Archive (originally collected under the supervision of Jerold G. Bachman, Survey Research Center) and by Edward Z. Dager, who permitted us to examine his East Chicago High School Study data. Neither investigator bears responsibility for the analyses or interpretations presented here. The authors are also grateful to Mary Collins for her excellent computer assistance.

NOTES

1. Although the term "significant other" is usually treated rather loosely to refer to any way in which the other is important to us, recent research has shown that there are different types of significance (e.g., valuation, credibility, personalism: Rosenberg, 1973; Gergen, 1971) and that others are differentially significant to specific aspects of the self (e.g., role-specific or orientational others: Denzin, 1966; Quarantelli and Cooper, 1966).

2. The work of Hess and Goldblatt (1957) makes clear that adolescents have rather mistaken perceptions of adults' views of them. Specifically, adolescents believe that adults hold more derogatory attitudes toward adolescents than adults in fact do. This finding is especially noteworthy in light of the well-documented tendency for individuals and groups to believe that other people hold them in higher regard than these others actually do (Reeder, Donohue, and Biblarz, 1960; Wylie, 1979). It is possible that adolescents err equally in their assumption of how much they matter to others.

3. The original study consisted of 1988 school children from grades 3–12 in Baltimore City public schools. The present analysis is confined to those subjects in the seventh grade or above.

4. Ruth Wylie's (1979) review of the literature dealing with the relationship of academic achievement and self-esteem leads to a similar conclusion. She notes: "It is obvious that the 19 reports discussed above involved a wide range of types of subjects, self-regard measures, achievement measures, ability measures, and means of trying to control for ability while looking at the relationship between over-all self-regard and achievement. In one way, this variety is a weakness, since direct replications are not at hand, and systematic comparisons between and among studies are not possible. In another way, however, such variety may strengthen one's confidence in the more usual . . . trends for higher over-all self-regard to be associated with higher achievement levels" (pp. 392–393).

REFERENCES

Bachman, J. G. (1970), *Youth in Transition,* Volume II: *The Impact of Family Background and Intelligence on Tenth-Grade Boys*. Ann Arbor, Michigan: Survey Research Center, Institute for Social Research.

Bachman, J. G., R. L. Kahn, M. T. Mednick, T. N. Davidson, and L. D. Johnston (1972), *Youth in Transition,* Volume I: *Blueprint for a Longitudinal Study of Adolescent Boys*. Ann Arbor, Michigan: Institute for Social Research.

Cooley, C. H. (1912), *Human Nature and the Social Order*. New York: Scribners.

Dager, E. Z. (1968), *A Study of Social Interactions Which Lead to Decisions to Drop Out of School*. U.S. Department of Health, Education and Welfare, Office of Education, Bureau of Research, Project No. 7-E-082.

Denzin, N. K. (1966), "The significant others of a college population." *Sociological Quarterly* 7:298–310.

Durkheim, E. (1951), *Suicide*. New York: The Free Press.

Finifter, B. (1975), "The generation of confidence: evaluating research findings by random subsample replication." Pp. 112–175 in H. Costner (ed.), *Sociological Methodology 1972*. San Francisco: Jossey-Bass.

Gergen, K. (1971), *The Concept of Self*. New York: Holt, Rinehart, and Winston.

Gurin, G., J. Veroff, and S. Feld (1960), *Americans View Their Mental Health*. New York: Basic Books.

Herschel, A. (1971), *To Grow in Wisdom*. Private publication by Synagogue Council of America, New York.

Hess, R., and I. Goldblatt (1957), "The status of adolescents in American society." *Child Development* XXVIII:459–468.

Horney, K. (1950), *Neurosis and Human Growth*. New York: Norton.

Hughes, E. C. (1962), "What other?" Pp. 119–127 in A. M. Rose (ed.), *Human Behavior and Social Processes*. Boston: Houghton-Mifflin.

James, W. (1890), *The Principles of Psychology*. New York: Henry Holt and Company.

Kaplan, H. B. (1975), *Self-Attitudes and Deviant Behavior*. Pacific Palisades, California: Goodyear Publishing.

Kohn, M. L. (1959), "Social class and parental values." *American Journal of Sociology* 64:337–351.

——— (1969), *Class and Conformity: A Study in Values*. Homewood, Illinois: Dorsey Press.

LaSorte, M. A. (1972), "Replication as a verification technique in survey research: a paradigm." *Sociological Quarterly* 13(2):218–227.

Miyamoto, S. F., and S. Dornbusch (1956), "A test of the symbolic interactionist hypothesis of self-conception." *American Journal of Sociology* 61:399–403.

Quarantelli, E. L., and J. Cooper (1966), "Self-conceptions and others: a further test of Meadian hypotheses." *Sociological Quarterly* 7:281–297.

Reeder, L. G., G. A. Donohue, and A. Biblarz (1960), "Conceptions of self and others." *American Journal of Sociology* 66:153–159.

Rosenberg, M. (1963), "Parental interest and children's self-conceptions." *Sociometry* 26:35–49.

——— (1965), *Society and the Adolescent Self-Image*. Princeton: Princeton University Press.

——— (1973), "Which significant others?" *American Behavioral Scientist* 16:829–860.

Rosenberg, M., and R. G. Simmons (1972), *Black and White Self-Esteem: The Urban School Child*. Rose Monograph Series. Washington, D.C.: American Sociological Association.

Sherwood, J. J. (1965), "Self identity and referent others." *Sociometry* 28:66–81.

——— (1967), "Increased self-evaluation as a function of ambiguous evaluations by referent others." *Sociometry* 30:404–409.

Simmel, G. (1950), "The stranger." Pp. 402–408 in K. Wolff (ed.), *The Sociology of Georg Simmel*. New York: The Free Press.

Srole, L. (1956), "Social integration and certain corollaries: an exploratory study." *American Sociological Review* 21:709–716.

———, T. S. Langner, S. T. Michael, M. K. Opler, and T. A. C. Rennie (1962), *Mental Health in the Metropolis: The Midtown Manhattan Study*. New York: McGraw-Hill.

Stouffer, S. A. et al. (1949), *The American Soldier*. Volume I. *Adjustment During Army Life*. Princeton, New Jersey: Princeton University Press: 92–95.

Stouffer, S. A., L. Guttman, E. A. Suchman, P. F. Lazarsfeld, S. A. Star, and J. A. Clausen (1950), *Measurement and Prediction*. Princeton, New Jersey: Princeton University Press.

Sullivan, H. S. (1947), *Conceptions of Modern Psychiatry: The First William Alanson White Memorial Lectures*. Washington, D.C.: The William Alanson White Psychiatric Foundation.

——— (1953), *The Interpersonal Theory of Psychiatry*. New York: Norton.

Turner, R. H., and R. Vanderlippe (1958), "Self-ideal congruence as an index of adjustment." *Journal of Abnormal and Social Psychology* 57:202–206.

Wylie, R. (1961), *The Self-Concept: A Critical Survey of Pertinent Research Literature*. Lincoln, Nebraska: University of Nebraska Press.

——— (1974), *The Self-Concept: Revised Edition*. Volume 1. *A Review of Methodological Considerations and Measuring Instruments*. Lincoln, Nebraska: University of Nebraska Press.

——— (1979), *The Self-Concept: Revised Edition*. Volume 2. *Theory and Research on Selected Topics*. Lincoln, Nebraska: University of Nebraska Press.

A LONGITUDINAL STUDY OF TEENAGE MOTHERHOOD AND SYMPTOMS OF DISTRESS:

THE WOODLAWN COMMUNITY EPIDEMIOLOGICAL PROJECT

Hendricks Brown, Rebecca G. Adams, and Sheppard G. Kellam

INTRODUCTION

In recent years, many people have become concerned with the consequences of teenage motherhood. This interest seems to have become more widespread as the birth rate has increased among very young (ages 15 to 17) and unmarried teenage women (Baldwin, 1980; Sklar and Berkov, 1974). The public concern seems to be based on a belief, increasingly supported by evidence, that women who begin

Research in Community and Mental Health, Volume 2, pages 183–213
Copyright © 1981 by JAI Press, Inc.
All rights of reproduction in any form reserved.
ISBN: 0-89232-152-0

childbearing early in life are at a disadvantage and that this disadvantage makes it difficult for them to rear their children effectively.

The transition to motherhood requires women to take on many complex and demanding roles and to modify or abandon others (Bacon, 1974). The adoption of a new role is often accompanied by stress (Turner, 1978). Potentially, the transition to motherhood is more stressful than other role transitions as the change occurs abruptly and is irreversible (Rossi, 1968). There is supporting evidence from relatively recent research that becoming a mother early in life is associated with a variety of negative sociological and psychological consequences (Chilman, 1979; Hofferth and Moore, 1979; Mindick, 1979). Becoming a mother as a teenager might thus be even more stressful than adopting the role as an adult.

The general hypothesis underlying our work and the work of others is that teenage mothers are a high risk group (Baizerman, 1974). In other words, exposure to motherhood at an early age is hypothesized to be related to a variety of negative characteristics—both psychological and social structural—that prevent the woman from adequately performing in this role. A related research question is whether or not teenage mothers continue to be adversely affected long after the birth of their first child.

Although this paper will be concerned with the mother's own psychological well-being, her moods may have direct impact on her children (Kellam et al., 1979c; Fleck, 1966). Blumenthal and Dielman (1975) found that depressive symptomatology among 160 married couples was associated with a decline in satisfaction and functioning in work, social, and marital life. The most marked decline in function observed was in the area of child rearing. Weissman and Paykel (1974) state similar conclusions more strongly:

> . . . acute symptoms of depression conflict with the demands of being a mother and produce a widespread negative impact on the children (p. 121).

Many researchers have suggested a link between depressive symptoms in women and various aspects of the child rearing cycle. The most commonly studied periods are the early postpartum (Butts, 1969; Brown and Shereshefsky, 1972) and "empty nest" stages (Deykin et al., 1966), the former marking the entry into the social role of motherhood and the latter marking the departure of the children from the home and a drastic modification of the role of mother. Both periods are characterized by increased reports of depression in women.

In this paper, we will report on the psychological consequences of women giving birth at various ages and points in their child rearing cycle. We will specifically focus on the consequences for the teenage mother. Underlying this research is our concern with the life cycle and its relationships to social structural conditions. We measured the mother's feelings of distress while she was raising a first-grade child and when that same child was a teenager. For some mothers, this child was the firstborn, for others it was later-born.

We will focus on two symptoms: self-reports of sadness and tension. Sadness is a central characteristic of the depressive mood (Weissman and Paykel, 1974) and tension, or anxiety, often accompanies depression. Tension may also occur by itself with enough intensity to disorder women's lives.

Two characteristics of these measures are of considerable interest. First, these symptoms are self-reports of distress, not clinical diagnoses; they express the way an individual feels. Weissman et al. (1979), however, have found self-reports of psychiatric symptoms predictive of clinical depression in longitudinal studies.

Second, we are studying a general epidemiological population, not a clinical one. This distinction is important, because the course of symptoms in a clinic population may be different from the course of sadness or tension among unhappy people not under psychiatric treatment. In comparing clinical and non-clinical populations of women, Weissman et al. (1975) found that depression in the latter group is less likely to be characterized by somatic complaints and somatic anxiety, but that both clincial and non-clinical depressives imporved over a four-month period. They also concluded that more research is needed on the frequency, patterns and course of symptoms of depression found in non-clinical populations.

The data reported in this paper are part of a community-wide study of Woodlawn, which is an urban, poor, black neighborhood on the South Side of Chicago. Each mother was interviewed in 1966, when one of her children was in first grade, and again in 1975, when this same child was a teenager. Although the data was collected prospectively, we will use some retrospective data to give a fuller picture of the mothers' child rearing histories.

PRIOR STUDIES OF TEENAGE MOTHERHOOD

Psychological Correlates

Although the social structural correlates of teenage motherhood have been studied widely, the psychological correlates have received very little attention. As far as we know, there have been no studies focused on the relationship between being a teenage mother and the course of psychiatric symptoms.

Numerous studies have investigated how psychological motivations or responses relate to the biological state of pregnancy during adolescence. These studies have tended to concentrate on two topics. First, there have been many studies of the psychological factors that predispose women to become pregnant or to fail to use contraceptives effectively (Wilson, 1979; Hatcher, 1973; Wolf, 1973; Lefheldt, 1971; Cobliner, 1974; Zelnick and Kantner, 1979). As Mindick (1979) has observed, such studies often have inadequate sample designs, often lack control populations, and are based on retrospective data. Despite these problems, there is evidence that unwanted teenage pregnancies are sometimes the result of psychiatric dysfunction.

A second set of studies has focused on psychological reactions to abortion. The results suggest that severe reactions are rare (Blumberg and Golbus, 1975). Reactions also seem to be less negative when the teenager's parents or partner have not forced her to have an abortion (Barglow and Weinstein, 1973; Evans et al., 1976) or when they offer her emotional support (Bracken et al., 1974). As Chilman (1978) has observed, there is a lack of long-term studies in this area. Often, reactions are measured in the hospital or clinic immediately after the abortion.

Social Structural Deficits and the Teenage Mother's Psychological Well-being

Many of the social structural findings from studies to be cited below suggest that teenage mothers have difficulty in providing the child with an adequate environment for growth and development. The results discussed in this section imply that teenage mothers may also suffer from psychological deficits, as well as from social structural ones. For example, the social conditions surrounding adolescent parenthood decrease the mother's chances of maintaining collaborative and intimate relationships with others, including the father of her children. This disconnectedness may contribute to distressed feelings on the part of mothers, or it may result in part from earlier psychological deficiencies. In either case, the accompanying psychological disturbances would seem likely to affect the children as well as the mothers.

In a recent article about the evolution of the family structures of the Woodlawn mothers studied in this paper, we found a very strong tendency for teenage mothers, especially those with two children, to be the only adult in the household (Kellam et al., 1979a). At approximately six years postpartum, a higher proportion of teenage mothers than older mothers lived alone (42 percent compared to 30 percent) and a lower proportion lived with the study child's father (roughly 25 percent compared to 50 percent). By 16 years postpartum, a much greater proportion of mothers lived alone than at six years postpartum. This shift towards mother-aloneness was much more noticeable among teenage mothers than among older mothers. About 65 percent of the former teenage mothers lived alone at this second point in time, whereas 41 percent of the other mothers lived alone. In addition, we found that mothers of all ages who lived alone were less likely than others to receive any help with child rearing, less likely to belong to social and political organizations, and less likely to attend religious services.

Furstenberg and Crawford (1978) have described the residential careers of the teenage mothers in their black, poor, East Baltimore clinic sample through five years postpartum. The most common arrangement was for the teenage mother to be living with one or both of her parents or with another family member throughout the five years. Few of these teenage mothers lived alone from the start, but the proportion increased over time. By the end of the five-year study, 26 percent of the mothers lived in households in which they were the only adult.

Other studies have reported the instability of teenage marriages (Johnson,

1974; Hardy et al., 1978). Osofsky et al. (1973) reported that when adolescent pregnancy is accompanied by marriage, divorce has been three to four times more frequent than among couples married later in life. Glick and Mills (1974), reporting on 1960 and 1970 census data, found that early marriages (before the age of 20 for males and before 18 for females) are more likely to end in divorce for both whites and blacks.

Another indication of the teenager's difficulty in providing an adequate environment for her child is the tendency for these mothers to live in poverty or to depend on welfare (Trussell, 1976; Moore and Caldwell, 1977; Chilman, 1979). Ensminger (1979) has recently reported that welfare dependency and poor psychological well-being are closely connected over an extended period of time for the same population of Woodlawn women studied in this paper. In a recent article, Hofferth and Moore (1979) reported that teenage mothers tend to have low economic well-being later in life because of their tendency to have more children, less education, and less work experience. This finding is particularly important since teenage mothers tend to be the only adult in the family (Kellam et al., 1979a).

Most of the information thus far about the long-term consequences of teenage motherhood concerns such effects as those on the family, on education, on work, and on income. In these social structural areas, the effects or correlates appear long-lasting and often become worse over time. The psychological consequences of teenage motherhood, which may be partially related to social structural deficits, need not follow a course similar to that of social structural consequences. In this paper, we will examine the occurrence and course of psychological symptoms over time for teenage and older mothers, considering both child rearing cycles and life cycles of the mothers as background for the analyses and in the interpretation of the results.

METHOD

Population: The Woodlawn Longitudinal Epidemiological Studies and Teenage Motherhood

The Woodlawn community is an urban, poor community on the South Side of Chicago. Between 1955 and 1966 (at which time the first of two interviews of Woodlawn mothers took place), the community underwent a change from 40 percent black to almost totally black. There was substantial overcrowding and high unemployment. Economically, Woodlawn ranked among the four most impoverished Chicago neighborhoods in 1966. While the median income was low, there was and still is social and economic heterogeneity.

With the support of Woodlawn community leaders and service agencies, the Social Psychiatry Study Center, between 1963 and 1968, assessed the mental health of first-grade children and gathered information on the families through interviews with the mothers. These assessments were coupled with service and evaluation programs (Kellam et al., 1975).

One cohort, the 1966–67 first-grade class, along with the children's mothers (or, if the mother was not present, the primary child-rearing adult), were reassessed in 1975–76. About 80 percent of these adults were still locatable in the Chicago area at the time of second interview, although more than two-thirds had moved away from the Woodlawn community (Agrawal et al., 1978). Of the 1242 families of first-grade children completing the 1966–67 school year in Woodlawn, we reinterviewed 939 (75 percent) of the mothers. The difference between percent located and percent reinterviewed reflects a small percentage (5.9) of mothers who refused to participate in the second interview.

We compared the early information on the mothers that we reinterviewed with the mothers we did not. We found no differences between the population which was reassessed and that which was not, in the areas of the mother's or child's 1966–67 psychological well-being, the child's adaptation to school, the family's early income, welfare status, or combination of adults at home. The differences we did find were in early family mobility before the child's first-grade year, age of mother at time of interview (younger mothers refused more often), and child's enrollment in a parochial school in first grade. At that time, the parochial schools lacked a centralized, computerized student record system like that maintained by the public schools. We used these school records in an effort to locate families for reinterview, and students enrolled in parochial schools were harder to trace. The population under study in this paper includes all biological mothers of the 1966–67 first-graders of Woodlawn who were living with the study child. Approximately seven percent of the children were not living at home with their natural mothers at time of first interview, when the study child was in first grade. Hereafter this point is referred to as time 1. The study population at time 1 consists of 1145 biological mothers while the reinterviewed population (at time 2) consisted of the 828 biological mothers who were found and were willing to be interviewed.

The Woodlawn data, which is community-wide, longitudinal, and includes much retrospective data, offers a good opportunity to study further the consequences of teenage motherhood. The data extends to a minimum of 16 years after the birth of the mother's first child. Although most of the data was collected prospectively, rich retrospective data gives us a full picture of the mother's childbearing history.

Community-wide studies such as this one are important complements of broader studies such as those on national probability samples. Relationships among variables may vary considerably according to community (Kellam et al., 1975) thereby limiting the utility of broader based samples.

Many studies have included only teenage mothers at early stages of their child rearing cycles (Osofsky et al., 1973; Jekel et al., 1973; Furstenberg, 1976). In order to identify the consequences of early childbearing or the importance of the mother's stage of child rearing one should use an epidemiological study involving mothers of all ages and at all stages of child rearing. The population studied in this article is community-based and satisfies the requirements above. However, this study contains only women with at least one child, so that we are unable to compare young mothers to non-mothers of the same age.

It is important to view the interviews as occurring at different points in the child rearing portion of the mother's life cycle. For some of the mothers, the study child was firstborn; for others, the study child was preceded by other children. Because all of the study children were born close to the year 1960, this latter group of mothers began childbearing prior to that time. Differences in mothers' life courses and child rearing histories which have bearing on feelings of distress are examined in these analyses. Childbearing typically follows a pattern closely associated with age of mother; and by examining feelings of distress in women who have somewhat atypical childbearing patterns—in this instance, women who began childbearing in their teenage years—we can hope to distinguish the effects of child rearing itself on psychological well-being. Besides mother's age at the beginning of childbearing, we also use other factors: her age at the birth of the study child, the birth order of the study child, and total number of children being raised by the mother.

By considering both the mother's age at the birth of her *first* child and her age at birth of *study*-child (the latter of which is directly related to her age at time of interview), we can partially describe the duration of the effects of early childbearing on later psychological well-being. (Other complementary analyses also explore this issue.) If mothers who start childbearing early generally have poorer psychological well-being only during their teenage years and early twenties, we should find an improvement among teenage mothers as they grow older. Without an epidemiological, total population, we might miss finding such a relationship.[1]

The longitudinal character of the data further helps us to chart the evolution of psychological well-being with regard to child rearing and other relevant events or conditions within the family. Our analyses include a partial description of the course of symptoms of distress in teenage and older mothers over a period that extends to at least 16 years postpartum. Many important studies of teenage motherhood extend to fewer than five years postpartum (Stone and Rowley, 1966; Jekel et al., 1973; Lorenzi et al., 1977). This longer-term data makes it possible to describe further the duration of the consequences.

Measures: Validity of Sadness and Tension Measures

Mothers were asked to rate their own feelings of sadness and tension at both time periods on a single global sadness and a single global tension scale. Assessment of distress is made on the basis of these measures. Distributions are given in Appendix I. Feelings of tension at the moderate or severe levels on the global items were roughly twice as frequent as feelings of sadness at similar levels.

The mothers' follow-up interview in 1975–76 also included 15 more specific self-assessment questions relating to recent psychiatric symptoms, but these questions were not asked at time 1. The 15 items were divided into *a priori* categories of anxiety (three items), depression (four items), bizarreness (four items), and self-esteem (four items). The questions and their distributions on a six-point scale are given in Appendix I. We have used these time 2 measures both individually and as constructs to assess the validity of our time 1 and time 2 global measures of sadness and tension. (In this paper, we do not utilize them in their own right as dependent variables, but concentrate on the variables for which we have measures at both time 1 and time 2.)

The correlation structure within and between constructs indicates that the 15 items do fit reasonably well within their own clusters. Measures of anxiety and depression are positively correlated; their correlations range from 0.2 to 0.4, and the two constructs obtained by summing scores on the relevant items have a correlation of 0.5. The within-construct correlations among items are larger than correlations between items of the two constructs. Additionally, self-esteem items are all negatively correlated with anxiety, depression, and bizarreness items. Bizarrenness is positively correlated with both anxiety and depression and is more common in depressed mothers as compared with anxious mothers. Reliability coefficients for the constructs of anxiety, depression, bizarreness, and self-esteem, as measured by Cronbach's Alpha (Cronbach, 1951), are all between 0.65 and 0.75.

We now describe the relationships that the global sadness and global tension scales, measured at time 1 and time 2, have with the 15 individual items and the four constructs measured at time 2. The most important relationships we expect to find, if indeed the measures of sadness and tension are meaningful, are:

1. Global sadness and global tension should each be similarly related to all items within a construct, and this relationship should be similar for both the time 1 and time 2 global measures of sadness and tension.
2. At either point in time, global sadness should be more closely related to the four depression items than to the three anxiety items.
3. At either point in time, global sadness should have a smaller correlation with items within the anxiety construct than global tension has.

The last two relationships can be used to show that anxiety and depression, as we have measured them, are in fact somewhat separate feelings.

Sadness and tension both at time 1 and time 2 are positively correlated with anxiety, depression, and bizarreness and negatively correlated with self-esteem. These relationships conform to the structure of within and between construct correlations among the 15 psychiatric symptom measures at time 2.

In regression of the 15 time 2 symptom items on sadness and tension at time 1, sadness was significantly related to all depression items, all three anxiety items, and three of the four bizarreness items. Tension at time 1 was significantly related to two of the three anxiety items, but none of the depression items. The multivariate regressions also showed that sadness was significantly related to depression and bizarre items ($p < .001$), and tension was related primarily to anxiety ($p < .0001$). The explained variance for each first canonical variable was about 6 percent, but because the measurements were made ten years apart, we should not expect this value to be very large.

These analyses were repeated with the time 2 measures of sadness and tension. As expected, these two variables measured at time 2 were more closely related to all of the time 2 symptom measures than were the time 1 global measures of sadness and tension. Only two regression coefficients were not significant, and these were related to one bizarreness item and one self-esteem item.

Multivariate regressions of the four time 2 constructs on global sadness and global tension showed that mothers with high and low sadness at either time point differed most on their depression scores and much less on the three other construct scores. Similarly, almost all of the difference in symptom construct scores between mothers with low and high levels of tension appeared in the anxiety construct. These multivariate results were highly significant, in a large measure because the analyses are based on more than 800 women. Nevertheless, 13.4 percent of the first canonical variable was explained by sadness and 45.9 percent of the first canonical variable was explained by tension.

As one last validation test, we compared the relative sizes of global sadness and global tension correlations with anxiety and depression items. Of the 14 possible comparisons (using time 1 and time 2 measures), all but two supported our hypothesis that sadness would relate more strongly to depression items than tension and less strongly to anxiety items. In the two cases where the order of correlation coefficients was reversed, the differences between the correlations were insignificant.

While our measures of sadness and tension are not especially focused on precisely defined concepts, they do appear to be useful measures of general levels of depressed and anxious feelings. The measures of sadness and tension show reproducible and increasingly strong relationships over time to our 15 self-reports of psychiatric symptoms, specifically to depression and anxiety respectively.

In another analysis of this data on Woodlawn children (Kellam et al., 1979), we found that these same mothers' ratings of daughters' symptoms during first grade—especially sad and worried feelings, trouble with feelings, and muscular tension—were moderately related to the daughter's own symptom reports ten years later. This mother/daughter concordance over a ten-year period also suggests that the symptom reports are valid measures of psychological well-being.

RESULTS

The general hypothesis guiding the following analyses is that mothers who begin childbearing during their adolescence are at a higher risk of distress than mothers who begin later. A major research question concerns the prevalence and course of the distressed feelings experienced by mothers.

In testing this hypothesis, we have compared and contrasted two models of teenage motherhood. In one model, the distress is viewed as transitory and a result of the young mother's immaturity and inexperience. The other model suggests that teenage motherhood is a more permanent position, one that a woman may continue to occupy despite aging, experience with child rearing, and maturation.

The analyses that we present, using prospective and retrospective data, examine the risk of distress in teenage mothers throughout a large portion of their child rearing years. If the effects of teenage motherhood start as far back as the birth of the mother's first child and continue to influence her later in life, we should observe a higher level of distress not only in teenage mothers whose first child had just entered first grade at time of interview, but also in women who had given birth as a teenager but were considerably older by time of interview. Age of mother at first birth would then show an effect on distress regardless of mother's current age. If the effects of teenage motherhood are more transitory, we should find that a past history of early childbearing is not relevant once we control for the current age of mother.

A further indication of the continuing or discontinuing nature of distressed feelings can be seen in the longitudinal analyses we report. The presence of distressed feelings at both times suggests a continuing or recurrent state, even though measurement error may be somewhat large since interviews were conducted at just two time points.

Two other analyses are presented to examine further child rearing effects on mothers' symptoms. A transitory effect of early childbearing would lead us to predict that raising a first child, especially for teenage mothers, would produce more distress than the demands of later-born children. We will thus examine the influence of the stage of child rearing on mothers' distress. A second issue relates to the number of children raised by the mother; more children are generally associated with more demands and stressful situations. For these reasons, mothers with many children may have a high risk of distress. If this is correct, teenage mothers, who generally have more children than other mothers, would be exposed to a long-term risk of distress.

In reporting and discussing the following analyses we will refer to women who first gave birth at 19 years or younger as "teenage" mothers. All other mothers, regardless of their age at interview or at the birth of the study child, will be referred to as "non-teenage" mothers.

Cross-Sectional Analyses of Psychological Effects of Childbearing

At time 1 (1966–67), mothers who began childbearing before 18 years of age had the highest rate of symptoms. Over 23 percent of these "early teenage" mothers—those beginning childbearing before 18—reported frequent feelings of sadness compared to a low of 13.7 percent for mothers who began childbearing between 20 and 24. For tension, the percentages were higher, with 44.7 percent of the early teenage mothers and less than 30 percent of the mothers who began childbearing between 20 and 24 reporting frequent feelings of tension. As can be seen from Figure 1, tension almost invariably accompanied feelings of sadness. Mothers who began childbearing before 18 were also more likely to report frequent feelings of both sadness and tension, and almost half of these early teenage mothers felt either sad or tense. The lowest levels of distress (sadness, tension, or both) were felt by mothers who began childbearing between 20 and 24, and feelings of distress followed a clear curvilinear relationship with age of mother at beginning of childbearing; the fewest symptoms were in the 18–24 age category.

We then included in the analysis a second variable, that of age of mother at birth of study child, as contrasted with her age at birth of her first child. We could then examine whether the effects of early childbearing continue for an extended time in the mother's child rearing career or relate only to a more limited period involving the rearing of her first child.

Results of log-linear analyses with these two age variables are given in Table 1 of Appendix III. The chi-square statistics in the first row of that table may be used to test for independence between feelings of distress and the age variables (feelings of distress (FD) appears alone in the model specification) against the model that describes the table exactly (fully saturated model). For all three measures, sadness and tension separately and "sadness or tension," the p-values are very small, indicating that important age dependencies do exist. (In effect, a model which acts as if there were no age dependencies is significantly different from the actual data in the observed table.) The other three rows of this table decompose these age relationships in different ways. The second row tests for a partial association between age at first birth and feelings of distress but does not use age at study child's birth as a predictor of distress. For tension and "sad or tense" feelings, this model fits reasonably well, as shown by relatively large p-values, but it does not fit as well to the table of sadness. (A larger "p" value means, in effect, that this model is not significantly different from the actual data). Not only does age at first birth show a strong relationship to distress, with mothers who began childbearing before 18 reporting the higher frequency of distress feelings,[2] but the tests involving tension and "sad or tense" feelings suggest that age of mother at study child's birth has minimal effect given age at first birth. Row 3 of Table 1 tests the adequacy of age at study child's birth in predicting feelings of distress, while discounting any effect from age at first birth on feelings of distress. Although it works moderately well for sadness, we see from the small p-values that it inadequately explains the associations of mother's age variables with tension or "sad or tense" feelings. The models which do it the actual data reasonably well, as measured by large p-values and a high number of degrees of freedom, have been marked by an asterisk.

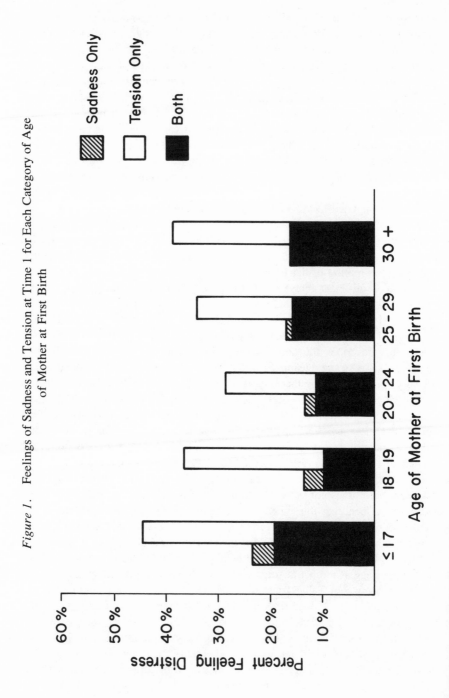

Figure 1. Feelings of Sadness and Tension at Time 1 for Each Category of Age of Mother at First Birth

The last row in Table 1 tests for a joint effect of age at first birth and age at study child's birth on feelings of distress. Under such a model, one would expect that mothers in high risk states of both age at first birth and age at study child's birth should experience the most distress. The small p-values indicate that some actual observed cell counts deviate significantly from this more general model. An examination of residuals reveals that women who had at least two children born while they were teenagers—the first before 18 and the second, the study child, born while the mother was 18 or 19—reported the highest level of distress on all three measures. For example, 76 percent of these 21 mothers had frequent sad or tense feelings. The fairly small number of mothers in this category carries with it sizeable uncertainty about the deviation of this group from the other mothers; nevertheless, even if we disregard this cell, the level of distress— particularly in regard to tension and sad or tense feelings—still appears to be high in mothers who began childbearing as early teenagers regardless of their age at study child's birth.

More details about log-linear models are contained in a footnote to Table 1 of Appendix III. Basic references on log-linear and logit analyses are given in Goodman (1972), Goodman (1969), and Haberman (1978).

This last finding is related to the major research question in this paper: given that we have found a teenage mother to be more prone to distressed feelings than a non-teenage mother, does this difference continue throughout her child rearing years? The indication from this last analysis is that tension and sad or tense feelings continued to be common in mothers who began childbearing before 18, but by 1966–67 were raising later-born children. Even for sadness, the highest percentages of high distressed mothers were recorded for mothers who began childbearing as teenagers.

For the sake of comparison, we have repeated these same analyses on the time 2 (1975–76) reports of distressed feelings. Significant age relations to distress at this later time point might indicate a latency period in some mothers, a continuing risk of distress into the child's teenage years, or a changing nature of psychiatric symptoms between the two points in time. There are differences in these analyses from those of time 1. By time 2, both feelings of sadness and tension were less prevalent than they were at time 1 for all ages. Compared to 42 percent of the mothers experiencing frequent feelings of sadness or tension at time 1, only 25 percent of the mothers experienced frequent sad or tense feelings ten years later.

In Table 2 in Appendix III, the model in row 1 fits the observed data; this is the model in which age of first birth and age of study-child are both independent of distress at time 2. That is, this model is not significantly different[3] from the observed data, especially in the cases of "tenseness" or "sad or tense." Since it is customary to accept the most parsimonious model, this model, as described in row 1, is the one that should be accepted. In effect, then, this analysis indicates that the relationship between age of mother at first birth and distress is no longer significant at time 2. Nevertheless we should note that in all measures of distress, the teenage mothers did report slightly higher levels of distress than other mothers (e.g., 28 percent versus 23 percent for "sad or tense"), and the mothers who waited until after 30 to begin having children reported the least occurrence of distress (21 percent). In summary, then, the fact that we must accept the model in row 1, means that neither age at first birth, nor age at study child's birth, can be considered to relate *significantly* to levels of distress at time 2, although there is some indication that younger first-time mothers are more likely to feel distress even at time 2. (See table 2 of Appendix III.)

The weaker age dependencies, coupled with lower prevalence of frequent distressed feelings at time 2, indicate a limiting effect of early childbearing on distressed feelings. This finding does not necessarily imply that the condition of early motherhood loses its impact by 15 years postpartum. For this question, we need to explore symptoms from a developmental viewpoint.

A Longitudinal Study of Psychological Effects of Early Childbearing

In the previous section we have seen that teenage mothers were at higher risk of distress at time 1 than non-teenage mothers and that by time 2 the prevalence of distressed feelings had decreased for all age groups of mothers. This section describes two aspects of symptom evolution by age of mother at time of first birth.

In this analysis, we further examine the transience or longevity of symptoms in teenage mothers. We have found that distress is more often found in these mothers at time 1 compared to non-teenage mothers. Consequently, the proportion of teenage mothers who report symptoms at both times, plus the proportion who improve from time 1 to time 2, must be larger than that of non-teenage mothers. It may be that age differences appear primarily in one of these two groups, those reporting distress at both times or those improving between interviews. If teenage mothers differ mostly from non-teenage mothers by reporting symptoms at both time periods, this would suggest that internal conditions or negative consequences continue to affect teenage mothers long after first birth. Alternatively, the observed age differences at time 1 may be associated with acute feelings of distress that disappear over time. From Figures 2a and 2b, we see that differences in distress by age of mother appear to be stronger for continued or recurrent feelings of sadness and tension (Figure 2a) than for shorter-term distress (Figure 2b). By chi-square tests, age differences are significant at the 0.05 level for the data presented in Figure 2a on long-term distress and non-significant for the data on shorter-term distress in Figure 2b.

This supports the view that teenage mothers have a higher risk of long-term distress. For example, 18 percent of the teenage mothers felt sad or tense at both times, whereas from five to 12 percent of the mothers who waited until age 20 to begin childbearing reported distress at both times (see Figure 2a). Mothers who waited until 25 to have children were considerably less likely to show continued distress than teenage mothers.

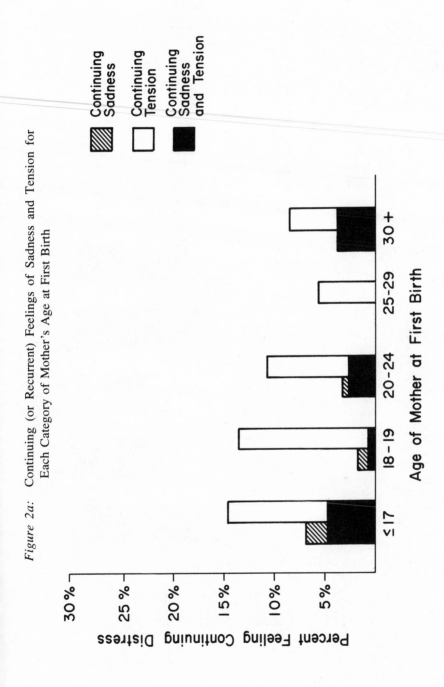

Figure 2a: Continuing (or Recurrent) Feelings of Sadness and Tension for Each Category of Mother's Age at First Birth

197

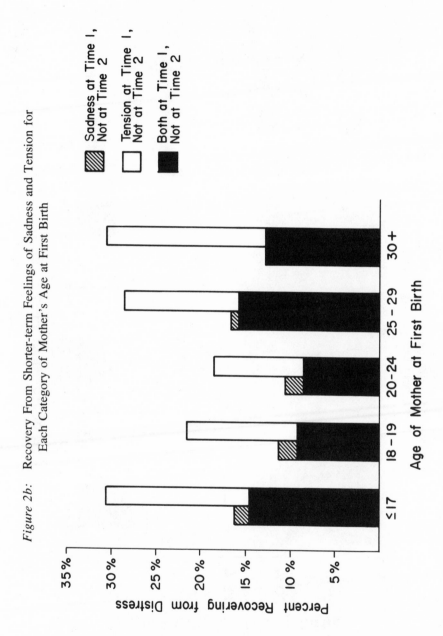

Figure 2b: Recovery From Shorter-term Feelings of Sadness and Tension for Each Category of Mother's Age at First Birth

Sadness at Time I,
Not at Time 2

Tension at Time I,
Not at Time 2

Both at Time I,
Not at Time 2

Percent Recovering from Distress

35%
30%
25%
20%
15%
10%
5%

≤17   18 - 19   20-24   25 - 29   30+

Age of Mother at First Birth

The additional risk of continuing distressed feeling in teenage mothers (which is shown in Figure 2a) may be due to two factors. We have established a higher incidence rate of distressed feelings among teenage mothers at time 1 and a lower rate for mothers between 20 and 24. If the course of distress, once established at time 1, is independent of age, teenage mothers would naturally continue to be at higher risk by time 2; feelings of distress at the two points in time are not independent, as we have seen in the section on validity. However, if after conditioning on the early state of distressed feelings, we still find that teenage mothers are more likely to remain in a distressed state, then they would suffer twice, once from an increased risk of initial distress and secondly from an additional age-related risk of continuing distress. The analyses (in Table 3 of Appendix III: Compare row 4 and 5) show, however, that conditional on the levels of distress at time 1, the chance of a teenage mother remaining distressed is statistically similar to that of a non-teenage mother. Likewise, the chance of entering a distressed state at time 2 from a state of low distress at time 1 is not significantly related to age of mother at first birth.[4]

Stage of Child Rearing and Its Relation to Distress

There may be specific child rearing stages that entail a greater risk of distressed feelings to all mothers and particulrly to teenage mothers. The role transition to motherhood brought about by the birth and growth of the first child is often considered particularly stressful to the mother. Raising the first child, as opposed to a later-born child, may result in more frequent distressed feelings for the mothers, particularly those who were adolescents at time of first-birth.

The analyses we report in this section are based on the time 1 measurement of distress. We found no evidence that teenage mothers, or mothers in general, fared poorly when their first child was entering first grade but then improved with later born children. The differences in sad or tense feelings that we found regarding age at beginning of childbearing and birth order of the study child may be explained by teenage mothers having more distress regardless of whether the study child was firstborn, middle-born, or last-born (at time of first interview) (see row 2 in Table 4 of Appendix III). The predicted order that would place teenage mothers of firstborn children in the most severe category is unsupported in this analysis; although birth order could be interpreted as having an effect on sad or tense feelings (row 3), raising later-born children seemed to be associated with greater risk than a firstborn child. Teenage motherhood entails a risk of distress beginning as far back as the firstborn child, and this risk does not diminish in succeeding child rearing stages.

Number of Children at Time 1 and Its Relation to Distress

As we have seen, there is no evidence to suggest that teenage mothers or any mothers in this cohort who were raising their first child felt more feelings of distress than mothers who were raising later-born children. While it seems the "newness" of the tasks of motherhood does not affect feelings of distress, it is possible that the quantity of these tasks does. The number of children raised by the mother would thus be a more important influence on her feelings of distress than whether or not she was raising her first child. We would predict that a teenage mother with a given number of children would feel more distress than an older mother with a comparable number of children.

A plot of percent of mothers who felt sad or tense within categories of age at first birth and total number of children being raised by the mother would show a pronounced trend towards higher symptoms as the initial childbearing age decreases and as the number of children increases to more than two. (Only in the category of 25- to 29-year-old mothers did this relationship appear to be unsupported.) Analysis of these proportions suggests that each of these trends are moderately significant. (See rows 2 and 3 in Table 5 of Appendix III; neither of these models differs significantly from the actual data). As statistically plausible explanations of the reports of distress, one could choose either an effect stemming from age at first birth or from total number of children raised by the mother at time of interview. The number of children appears to influence the distress of mothers who began childbearing between 18 and 19 years of age more than other mothers, and the early teenage mothers have the highest risk irrespective of number of children. It is not surprising that we should have difficulty distinguishing between these two models considering that teenage mothers have more children and tend to space them closer together (Kellam et al., 1979a; Trussell and Menken, 1978).

DISCUSSION

In this paper, we have presented results suggesting that beginning child rearing during adolescence adversely influences the mother's psychological well-being for a period that extends well beyond her teenage years. At the time her first child enters school, a teenage mothers show a strong tendency to feel distress. The risk of frequent feelings of distress does not subside with additional children who are born after the mother's teenage years. Early childbearing also involves a higher risk of continued distress both initially and ten years beyond the time when the study child was in first grade. We discuss below the evidence for these conclusions and their implications for the mother, her children, and treatment or intervention programs.

Two alternative models have been presented in explaining the relationship between early childbearing and feelings of distress. One model views the psychological effects of teenage motherhood as transient, and specific to adolescence and early adulthood, while the other presumes that the effects are likely to continue through later stages of life. Both the cross-sectional and longitudinal analyses presented in this chapter support the latter model.

In our cross-sectional analyses using both mother's age at study-child's birth, as representative of her current stage of life, and her age at first birth, we found that the timing of the mother's first birth had a stronger effect on both sad and tense feelings than did her age at birth of the then-current first grader. At time of first interview, the women who first gave birth as teenagers ranged in age from 20 to 40 years. For some, the birth of their first child was quite remote, yet their chances of feeling distress were still relatively high. This suggests that the psychological consequences of teenage motherhood are of long duration.

Further support for this conclusion was found by comparing the frequency of distressed feelings among mothers at different stages of child rearing. Teenage mothers of later-born study children showed no less tendency to report feelings of distress than teenage mothers of firstborn study children. The consequences are not transient; they do not diminish as the mother gains experience in her role.

The longitudinal analyses implied that teenage mothers in this population had a higher risk of feeling distress at both time periods than did other mothers. Women who waited until 25 or 30 to have children also seemed to have a fairly high rate of distress by time 1, but were unlikely to feel distress at both times. Feelings of distress at both time points may imply a more serious and continuing condition of poor psychological well-being.

The more children raised by a mother, the more adverse is the effect on her feelings of distress. This is especially important for teenage mothers, who tend to raise more children. Again, this indicates that the effects of teenage motherhood, either direct or indirect, are not limited to the early period of child rearing.

We have seen that adolescent child rearing seems to effect mothers adversely by increasing their risk of distressed feelings at least until the study child reaches first grade, which is well beyond the mother's teenage years. The origins of this distress may stem from a combination of social structural, social adaptational (Kellam et al., 1975) and psychological factors that predate the mother's first pregnancy. Young women who live in stressful environments amid poverty and discrimination may feel helplessness toward their own futures. This in turn may give rise to perceptions of a low internal locus of control. Such a belief has been found in teenage mothers (Cobliner, 1979) and probably also relates to the occurrence of unplanned or unwanted pregnancies. Premarital sex and pregnancy may also be the result of a compensation on the part of the woman for a lack of intimacy or poor social adaptation in the home or school (Cobliner, 1974). Such predating factors may become important contributors to distress for women who undergo the marked change in life course brought about by young motherhood.

Additionally, or alternatively, teenage motherhood may bring about this distress as a result of unfinished adolescent development or the social consequences that accompany early childbearing. By assuming childrearing tasks at an early age, the young mother is often forced to disrupt social ties and educational plans thus differentiating her life course from those of her peers. The teenage mother may be unwilling to assume care-taking responsibilities and may experience distress as a result. The added risks of separation or divorce in families of teenage mothers can lead to distress later in life. We have observed that teenage mothers, later in life, are more likely to be raising their children without the support of another adult (Kellam et al., 1980). Without the necessary time to develop working skills of her own, the mother is often forced to depend on welfare assistance or support from others which would be unnecessary without a child. Having a child during adolescence therefore leads to long-term changes in social structural position which may well increase the mother's distress.

Although we have not established the reason, our data indicate that early mothers are vulnerable to feelings of self-reported distress. In fact, although the measures of symptoms we have used are self-reports, not clinical diagnoses, they may possibly be predictive of more serious psychological problems. Weissman et al. (1979) have found self-reports of depressive symptoms similar to sadness to be predictive of later diagnosable depression. Of particular interest here is the finding by Weissman et al that women who reported high levels of symptoms at both times of measurement (1967 and 1969) were at higher risk of subsequent diagnosable depression than those who reported symptoms only at time 1. The teenage mothers in our sample were more likely than mothers who started childbearing later in life to report feelings of distress that continued or occurred at both times of measurement.

Although we have been concerned with the mother's own psychological well-being in this chapter, her moods and feelings of potency may have a direct impact on her children. In a recent paper on this same population of women, for example, we found that the mother's own symptoms at both interview times were predictive of her daughter's symptoms as teenagers (Kellam et al., 1979c). Other researchers have also reported that the mother's psychological well-being can have a direct impact on her children (Weissman and Paykel, 1974; Fleck, 1966; Blumenthal and Dielman, 1975). The results reported in this paper show that this distress endures long enough to have an important impact on the children of teenage mothers born during the mother's adolescence *and* on those children born later.

The inference that teenage mothers follow a life course with risk of distress still allows for the influence of subsequent events or decisions by the mother. For example, we have reported that the more children a mother has, the more likely she is to report feelings of distress. If teenage mothers, by conscious decision or otherwise, do not have additional children, they are less likely to experience distress than their multiparous counterparts.

The question that remains is how to help effectively the teenage mother counteract the effects of early childbearing. Others have criticized past intervention programs oriented toward teenage mothers. It seems that most of these programs have had a crisis orientation and have been designed to help the mother and her child only during the prenatal and early postpartum periods (Furstenberg, 1976; Schinke, 1978). The data in this paper describe the distress experienced by teenage mothers as frequently long-lasting and not simply an acute reaction to a stressful situation. In fact, this maternal distress lasts long enough to have an impact on the children born after the mother's adolescence (Kellam et al, 1979c). As Furstenberg (1976) and Schinke (1978) have concluded, if services are to be successful, they must be available on a continuing and long-term basis.

In addition to being long-lasting, the adverse consequences or correlates of early childbearing seem to be broad in scope. We have reported elsewhere that, in addition to being at a high risk of distress, teenage mothers tend to live alone, be isolated from formal organizations, and lack help with the tasks involved in rearing a child (Kellam et al., 1979a). Other researchers have discussed the adverse effects of teenage motherhood on educational attainment (Moore and Waite, 1977), welfare dependency (Trussell, 1976), income (Hofferth and Moore, 1979), and marital stability (Jekel et al., 1973).

In combination, the evidence presented here and elsewhere suggests the need for comprehensive programs designed to deal simultaneously with the social and psychological aspects of teenage motherhood. Other researchers have discussed this need and the inadequacy of programs in the 60s and 70s that dealt with only one aspect of teenage motherhood at a time (Furstenberg, 1976; Schinke and Gilchrist, 1977). Providing the mother only with such social resources as welfare assistance or access to day care centers may only cause her more distress by decreasing her sense of self-sufficiency. In a recent study on this same population of women, for example, it was found that welfare dependency was associated with poor psychological well-being (Ensminger, 1979). On the other hand, programs that offer the mother the opportunity to acquire the social skills she lacks, through vocational training, returning to high school, or instruction in child care, may be unsuccessful if the mother lacks the social and economic support to remain in the program, or if she is not psychologically prepared to accept the opportunity. We found that acceptance of an offer to participate in a free, broad, psychiatric treatment program in Woodlawn was not related to high psychiatric symptoms, at least among the teenage offspring of the mothers studied in this paper (Kellam et al., 1979b). In order to design and more accurately predict the effectiveness and utilization of comprehensive programs, more research is needed on the interrelationships—both concurrently and longitudinally—among the social and psychological aspects of teenage motherhood.

This paper has used prospective, epidemiological data on the occurrence and course of distress in mothers in the Woodlawn community to examine psychological consequences of teenage motherhood. The origins of distress, which may predate pregnancy or be initiated in sociological or psychological conditions related to early child rearing, have important policy implications. While the origins of this distress have not been fully addressed in this report, we have chartered the evolution of distressed feelings as related to the child rearing cycles of the mothers over a period that extends well beyond the mother's first birth. Establishing the existence of long-term consequences and describing their characteristics on the community level are necessary first steps in the design of treatment or itnervention programs. Without the merging of research results relating to consequences and their distinguishable origins, the possible effectiveness of these programs will be unknown.

ACKNOWLEDGMENTS

The authors wish to acknowledge the crucial contributions of the Woodlawn community, its families and children, and the community board members who over the last 18 years have provided support and guidance for this research and service enterprise. Particular thanks are due Mrs. Rose Bates who continues to instruct us regarding community issues. The faculty and staffs of the Woodlawn public and Catholic elementary schools and those of the Chicago Public High Schools made crucial contributions. Over the years, Dr. Curtis Melnick, former Associate Superintendent of the Chicago Board of Education, was very important to this project.

Jeannette Branch, the former Director of the Woodlawn Mental Health Center and later, during the follow-up, the South Side Youth Program, has been involved in all aspects of the research. We are grateful for the assistance of our other colleagues, past and present, at the Social Psychiatry Study Center in many aspects of the study, especially Margaret Ensminger, Ph.D., for work in the early analyses and design of the long-term follow-up and its field supervision. Early analyses by Grant Blank were very helpful. Professor George Bohrnstedt provided comment on early drafts of the paper. Wendy Baldwin, Ph.D., and Virginia Cain provided important clarification regarding national demographic trends. We are indebted to Shelby Haberman for discussions relating to the log-linear analyses in this chapter.

These studies have been supported by the following grants: State of Illinois Department of Mental Health Grant Numbers 17–224 and 17–322; P.H.S. Grant Number MH–15760 and Research Scientist Development Award (Kellam) Grant Number 1–K01–MH–47596; the Maurice Falk Medical Fund; and National Institute on Drug Abuse Grant Number DA–00787. This study of teenage motherhood was supported by National Institute on Child Health and Human Development Contract Number N01–HD–72821.

NOTES

1. We are only able to separate out partially the effects of "growing older" from changing characteristics of teenage mothers over time which may be attributable to environmental or exogenous factors. See Maddox and Wiley (1976) for a discussion of the identification problems involved in the study of aging.

2. These data indicating the direction of findings are not presented in Table 1 (see Figure 1).

3. Using a $p = .050$ cut-off.

4. Table 3, row 1 tests the hypothesis that feelings of distress, cross-classified by their time 1 and time 2 measures, are independent from age at first birth. The significance level ($p = .011$) indicates that this model is significantly different from the actual data; that is, age at first birth is not independent of feelings of distress. These two distress measures appear to be related to age in the following manner: while time 1 distress is clearly age-related (Appendix III, Table 1), we find no additional age relationship to distress at time 2 once we have conditioned on the initial level of distress (row 4). If we subtract the chi-square and degrees of freedom in line 5 from those of line 4, we can make a more specific test of the partial association between age at first birth and feelings of distress at time 2 taking into account feelings of distress at time 1; the result of this test also confirms that this partial association is insignificant. That is, row 5 considers all possible 2-variable relationships to be meaningful, while row 4 implies no partial association between age at first birth and feelings of distress at time 2. This model does not significantly reduce the fit to the observed data. Row 4 does just as well, as it considers the relationship between age at first birth and time 1 distress plus the relationship between feelings of distress at time 1 and time 2.

REFERENCES

Agrawal, K. C., S. G. Kellam, Z. E. Klein, and R. J. Turner (1978), "The Woodlawn mental health studies: tracking children and families for long-term follow-up," *American Journal of Public Health* 68(2):139–42.

Bacon, L. (1974), "Early motherhood, accelerated role transition, and social pathologies," *Social Forces* 52(March):333–341.

Baizerman, M. C., D. L. Ellison, and E. R. Schlesinger (1974), "Critique of the research literature concerning pregnant adolescents, 1960–1970," *Journal of Youth & Adolescence* 3(1):61–75.

Baldwin, W. H. (1980), "Adolescent pregnancy and childbearing—growing concerns for Americans." Washington, D.C.: Population Reference Bureau, Inc. [mimeo addendum to Baldwin 1976, same title, *Population Bulletin* 31(2):3–33.

Barglow, P., and S. Weinstein (1973), "Therapeutic abortion during adolescence: psychiatric observations," *Journal of Youth & Adolescence* 2(4, Dec.):331–342.

Blumenthal, M. D., and T. E. Dielman (1975), "Depressive symptomatology and role function in a general population," *Archives of General Psychiatry* 32(Aug.):985–991.

Blumberg, M., and M. Golbus (1975), "Psychological sequelae of elective abortion," *Western Journal of Medicine* 123(3, Sept.):188–193.

Bracken, M. B., M. Hachamovitch, and G. Grossman (1974), "The decision to abort and psychological sequelae," *The Journal of Nervous & Mental Disease* 158(2):154–162.

Brown, W. A., and P. Shereshefsky (1972), "Seven women: a prospective study of postpartum psychiatric disorders," *Psychiatry* 35(May):139–159.

Butts, H. E. (1969), "Post-partum psychiatric problems: a review of the literature dealing with etiological theories," *Journal of the National Medical Association* 61(2, March):136–139, 204.

Chilman, C. S. (1978), *Adolescent Sexuality in a Changing American Society: Social and Psychological Perspectives,* U.S. Department of HEW, Public Health Service, NIH, DHEW Publication No. (NIH) 79-1426.

_____, (1979), "Teenage pregnancy: a research review," *Social Work* 24(6, Nov.):492–498.

Cobliner, W. G. (1974), "Teenage out-of-wedlock pregnancy, a phenomenon of many dimensions," *Bulletin of the New York Academy of Medicine* 46:438–447.

Cronbach, L. J. (1951), "Coefficient alpha and the internal structure of tests," *Psychometrika* 16:297–334.

Deykin, E. Y., S. Jacobson, G. L. Klerman, and M. Solomon (1966), "The empty nest: psychosocial aspects of conflict between depressed women and their grown children," *American Journal of Psychiatry* 122(2):1422–1426.

Ensminger, M. E. (1979), "Welfare Status and Feelings of Psychological Distress." Paper presented at the American Sociological Association, August 28, 1979, Boston, Mass.

Evans, J., G. Selstad, and W. Welcher (1976), "Teenagers: fertility control behavior and attitudes before and after abortion, childbearing or negative pregnancy test," *Family Planning Perspectives* 8(4, July/August):192–200.

Fleck, S. (1966), "An approach to family pathology," *Comprehensive Psychiatry* 7(5 Oct.):307–320.

Furstenberg, F. F. Jr. (1976), *Unplanned Parenthood.* New York: The Free Press.

_____, and A. G. Crawford (1978), "Family support: helping teenage mothers to cope," *Family Planning Perspectives* 10(6):322–333.

Glick, P., and K. Mills (1974), "Black Families: Marriage Patterns and Living Arrangements." Paper presented at the W.E.B. DuBois Conference on American Blacks, October 3-5, 1974, at Atlanta, Georgia, as quoted in Chilman (1978).

Goodman, L. A. (1968), "The analysis of cross-classified data: independence, quasi-independence, and interaction in contingency tables with or without missing entries," *Journal American Statistical Association* 63:1091–1131.

Goodman, L. A. (1969), "On Partitioning X^2 and Detecting Partial Association in Three-Way Contingency Tables," *Journal of the Royal S-atistical Society*, Series B 31:486-498.

Goodman, L. A. (1972), "A General Model for the Analysis of Surveys," *American Journal of Sociology* 77:1035-1086.

Haberman, S. J. (1978), *Analysis of Qualitative Data*, Volume 1. New York: Academic Press.

Hardy, J. B., D. W. Welcher, J. Stanley, and J. R. Dallas (1978), "Long-range outcome of adolescent pregnancy," *Clinical Obstetrics & Gynecology* 21(3, Dec.):1215-1232.

Hatcher, S. L. M. (1973), "The adolescent experience of pregnancy and abortion: a developmental analysis," *Journal of Youth & Adolescence* 2(1):53-102.

Hofferth, S. L., and K. A. Moore (1979), "Early childbearing and later economic well-being," *American Sociological Review* 44(Oct):784-815.

Jekel, J. F., L. V. Klerman, and D. R. E. Bancroft (1973), "Factors associated with rapid subsequent pregnancies among school-age mothers," *American Journal of Public Health* 63(9, Sept.):769-773.

Johnson, C. (1974). "Adolescent pregnancy: intervention into the poverty cycle," *Adolescence* 9(35):391-406.

Kellam, S. G., R. G. Adams, C. H. Brown, and M. E. Ensminger (1979a), "The long-term evolution of the family structure of teenage and older mothers." Paper presented at the annual meeting of the Society for the Study of Social Problems, August 29, 1979, Boston, Mass.

Kellam, S. G., J. D. Branch, K. C. Agrawal, and M. E. Ensminger (1975), *Mental Health and Going to School: The Woodlawn Program of Assessment, Early Intervention and Evaluation*. Chicago: University of Chicago Press.

Kellam, S. G., J. D. Branch, C. H. Brown, and G. Russell (1979b), "Why Teenagers Come for Treatment: A Ten-Year Prospective Study of Woodlawn." Accepted for publication in the *Journal of the American Academy of Child Psychiatry*.

Kellam, S. G., M. B. Simon, and M. E. Ensminger (1979c), "Antecedents in the First Grade of Teenage Drug Use and Psychological Well-Being: A Ten-Year Community-Wide Prospective Study." To be published in *Origins of Psychopathology: Research and Public Policy*, eds. D. Ricks and B. Dohrenwend. Cambridge: Cambridge University Press. Also in *Prevention of Drug Abuse: Hearings Before the Select Committee on Narcotics Abuse and Control, House of Representatives, Ninety-Fifth Congress, Second Session, April 18, 20, 25, May 16, 25, 1978*. Washington, U.S. Printing Office: SCNAC-95-2-4.

Lehfeldt, H. (1971), "Psychology of contraceptive failure," *Medical Aspects of Human Sexuality* 5:68-77.

Lorenzi, M. E., L. V. Klerman, and J. F. Jekel (1977), "School-age parents: how permanent a relationship?" *Adolescence* 12(45, Spring):13-22.

Maddox, G. L., and J. Wiley (1976), "Scope, concepts and methods in the study of aging," pp. 3-34 in R. H. Binstock and E. Shanas (Eds.), *Handbook of Aging and the Social Sciences*. New York: Van Nostrand Reinhold Company.

Mindick, B. (1979), "Teenage pregnancies: psychiatric or educational problem?" *Psychiatric Opinion* 16(5):32-36.

Moore, K., and S. Caldwell (1977), *Out of Wedlock Childbearing*. Washington, D.C.: The Urban Institute.

Moore, K., and L. J. Waite (1977), "Early childbearing and educational attainment," *Family Planning Perspectives* 9(5, Sept./Oct.):220-225.

Osofsky, H., J. D. Osofsky, N. Kendall, and R. Rajan (1973), "Adolescents as mothers: an interdisciplinary approach to a complex problem," *Journal of Youth & Adolescence* 2(3):233-249.

Rossi, A. S. (1968), "Transition to parenthood," *Journal of Marriage & the Family* 30:26-39.

Schinke, S. P. (1978), "Teenage pregnancy: the need for multiple casework services," *Social Casework* (July):406-410.

_____, and L. D. Gilchrist (1977), "Adolescent pregnancy: an interpersonal skill training approach to prevention," *Social Work in Health Care* 3(2):159–167.

Sklar, J., and B. Berkov (1974), "Teenage family formation in postwar America," *Family Planning Perspectives* 6(2 Spring):80–90.

Stone, F. B., and V. N. Rowley (1966), "Children's behavior problems and mother's age," *Journal of Psychology* 63:229–233.

Trussell, T. J. (1976), "Economic consequences of teenage childbearing," *Family Planning Perspectives* 8(4, July/August):184–190.

_____, and J. Menken (1978), "Early childbearing and subsequent fertility," *Family Planning Perspectives* 10(4, July/August):209–218.

Turner, R. H. (1978), "The role and the person," *American Journal of Sociology* 84(1):1–23.

Weissman, M., J. K. Meyers, W. D. Thompson, and A. Belanger (1979), "Depressive symptoms as a risk factor for a subsequent first episode of an affective disorder." Paper presented at the Society for Life History Research in Psychopathology Conference, "Society for the Study of Social Biology." Statler Hilton Hotel, New York, New York, November 9, 1979.

Weissman, M., and E. Paykel (1974), *The Depressed Woman: A Study of Social Relationships.* Chicago: University of Chicago Press.

Weissman, M., B. Prusoff, C. Pincus (1975), "Symptom patterns in depressed patients and depressed normals," *Journal of Nervous & Mental Disease* 160(1):15–23.

Wilson, F. (1979) "The antecedents of adolescent pregnancy," Paper presented at the Workshop on Adolescent Pregnancy and Childbearing, January 10–12, 1979 at the Center for Population Research, National Institute of Child Health and Human Development, Bethesda, Maryland.

Wolf, S. R., P. A. Lachenbruch et al. (1973), "Psycho-sexual problems associated with the contraceptive practices of abortion-seeking patients," *Medical Aspects of Human Sexuality* 7:169–182.

Zelnick, M., and J. F. Kantner (1979), "Reasons for nonuse of contraception by sexually active women aged 15–19," *Family Planning Perspectives* 11(5, Sept./Oct.):289–296.

APPENDIX I

Original Scale Distributions of Psychological Well-being Variables (N = 828)

	Percentage in Response Category*				
	Hardly Ever	Occasionally	Fairly Often	Very Often	No Response
Time 1					
How often do you have days when you are nervous, tense, on edge?	15.5	47.0	15.6	21.4	0.5
How often do you have days when you are sad and blue?	38.6	43.1	8.8	8.3	1.2
Time 2					
How often do you have days when you are nervous, tense, on edge?	23.7	53.4	10.5	12.3	0.1
How often do you have days when you are sad and blue?	45.9	43.4	5.6	5.1	0.1

*When the variables were dichotomized, "fairly often" and "very often" were contrasted with the other categories.

APPENDIX I—(Continued)

Original Scale Distribution of Psychological Well-being Variables (N = 828)

	Not at all				Very, very much		No Answer
	1	2	3	4	5	6	Answer
Time 2 (Continued)							
Anxiety							
1. Mother (M) has felt nervous, last few weeks	25.8	20.4	21.8	10.3	11.3	10.2	0.1
2. M has felt tense, last few weeks	25.2	30.9	20.9	8.9	9.4	4.2	0.6
3. M has felt anxious, last few weeks	28.9	20.8	20.4	9.6	14.0	5.6	0.6
Depression							
4. M has felt sad, last few weeks	54.8	22.2	13.2	3.7	3.8	1.9	0.2
5. M has felt hopeless, last few weeks	83.5	7.2	4.4	1.7	2.0	0.7	0.4
6. M has felt ashamed, last few weeks	85.7	9.1	2.9	0.7	0.7	0.5	0.4
7. M has felt "Blame Yourself," last few weeks	59.7	21.7	12.0	2.9	2.0	1.1	0.5
Bizarre							
8. M has felt stony-faced, last few weeks	78.3	10.7	7.4	1.2	1.5	0.7	0.7
9. M has felt in another world, last few weeks	85.1	7.0	4.4	1.9	0.5	0.7	0.4
10. M has felt strange, last few weeks	85.2	9.1	3.2	1.0	1.0	0.0	0.5
11. M has heard voices, sounds, last few weeks	95.7	1.7	1.7	0.2	0.7	0.1	0.5
Self-Esteem							
12. M has felt good person, last few weeks	0.8	2.5	5.5	17.9	45.7	26.9	0.6
13. M has felt capable, last few weeks	2.4	2.6	6.0	16.3	44.2	27.7	0.7
14. M has felt self-confident, last few weeks	4.6	4.2	6.8	18.1	40.2	25.8	0.2
15. M has felt "like yourself," last few weeks	1.4	2.4	3.2	12.2	45.1	35.3	0.2

APPENDIX II

Cross Tabulation of Age of Mother at First Birth by Age of Mother at Birth of Study Child at First and Second Interviews

FIRST INTERVIEW (1966-67)

		Age at First Birth					
		≤17	18–19	20–24	25–29	30+	Total
Age at Birth of Study Child	≤17	89	—	—	—	—	89
	18–19	35	77	—	—	—	112
	20–24	79	109	193	—	—	381
	25–29	58	65	131	42	—	296
	30+	4	23	78	75	87	267
	Total	265	274	402	117	87	1145

SECOND INTERVIEW (1975-76)

		Age at First Birth					
		≤17	18–19	20–24	25–29	30+	Total
Age at Birth of Study Child	≤17	56	—	—	—	—	56
	18–19	21	46	—	—	—	67
	20–24	56	77	140	—	—	273
	25–29	45	50	104	35	—	234
	30+	4	16	59	56	63	198
	Total	182	189	303	91	63	828

APPENDIX III

Log Linear Analyses of Distressed Feelings in Relation to
Childbearing and Child Rearing Variables [a]

Table 1. Effects of Age at First Birth and Age at Birth of Study Child
on Time 1 Feelings of Distress†

		Feelings of Distress at Time 1					
		Sadness		Tension		Sad or Tense	
Model[+]	df	χ^2	p	χ^2	p	χ^2	p
(AFB, ASC)(FD)	9	19.78	.019	20.58	.015	22.06	.009
(AFB, ASC)(AFB, FD)	6	13.31	.038	9.95*	.126	10.93*	.090
(AFB, ASC)(ASC, FD)	6	11.18*	.082	14.18	.028	16.92	.010
(AFB, ASC)(AFB, FD)(ASC, FD)	3	9.20	.027	8.24	.041	10.07	.018

a These analyses are based on the population reassessed at time 2 and excludes mothers who began childbearing after 30. Not only did this eliminate small cells from the table, but it limited the possible retrospective errors in measuring age of mother at first birth. There was no relationship between distress and reassessment status at time 2; however, younger mothers were less likely to be reinterviewed (Kellam et al., 1979a). Reinterview status did not affect the relations between age of mother, child rearing variables and feelings of distress.

†The presence of structural zeros—age at birth of first child was never smaller than age at birth of study child—in these tables required the use of special log-linear procedures discussed and implemented by Goodman (1968).

+AFB = age at first birth, ASC = age at birth of study child, FD = feelings of distress.

The symbols in parentheses indicate the model being tested. For example, the last model in Table 1 specifies two-way partial associations between each pair of variables while the first model specifies a two-variable association between the two measures of mother's age. All models include this term because the interrelationship of the two age variables is a function of experimental design. The first model also implies that feelings of distress are unrelated to either age variable. The second model implies that the distribution of FD depends on the category of AFB. This model is similar to that used in analysis of variance, except that the outcome variable is expressed in terms of the logarithm of the cell total (hence the term log-linear). The other two models imply that FD is related to ASC and to both AFB and ASC. For a description of these same models from the viewpoint of logit analysis, see Haberman, Chapter 3 (1978).

*Statistically, these models fit the observed table reasonably well. They have reasonably large p-values (at least larger than p = .050) and a large number of degrees of freedom indicating that few parameters are needed for specification. More complete interpretations, which are also based on residual analysis, may be found in the text.

APPENDIX III—(Continued)

Table 2. Effects of Age at First Birth and Age at Birth of Study Child on Time 2 Feelings of Distress†

Model[+]	df	Feelings of Distress at Time 2					
		Sadness		Tension		Sad or Tense	
		χ^2	p	χ^2	p	χ^2	p
(AFB, ASC)(FD)	9	16.77*	.052	11.07*	.270	8.33*	>.5
(AFB, ASC)(AFB, FD)	6	8.81	.183	3.97	>.5	1.71	>.5
(AFB, ASC)(ASC, FD)	6	8.03	.235	8.21	.229	6.77	.353
(AFB, ASC) (AFB, FD) (ASC, FD)	3	3.75	.290	2.11	>.5	1.19	>.5

†Structural zeros in these models necessitated special log-linear analyses described earlier.
[+]AFB = age at first birth, ASC = age at birth of study child, FD = feelings of distress. Pairs of variables enclosed in parentheses represent pairwise dependence.
*Statistically, this is a satisfactory model for the observed table.

Table 3. Effects of Age at First Birth and Feelings of Distress at Time 1 on Feelings of Distress at Time 2

Model[+]	df	Sad or Tense	
		χ^2	p
(AFB)(FD$_1$, FD$_2$)	9	21.48	.011
(AFB$_1$, FD$_1$)(FD$_2$)	7	29.56	.000
(AFB, FD$_1$)(AFB, FD$_2$)	4	22.90	.000
(AFB, FD$_1$)(FD$_1$, FD$_2$)	6	10.80*	.095
(AFB, FD$_1$)(AFB, FD$_2$)(FD$_1$, FD$_2$)	3	5.05	.17

[+]AFB = age at first birth, FD$_1$ = feelings of distress at time 1, FD$_2$ = feelings of distress at time 2.
*Statistically, this is a satisfactory model for the observed table.

Table 4.   Effects of Age at First Birth and Study Child's Birth Order on Time 1 Feelings of Distress

| | | Feelings of Distress at Time 2 | | | | | |
| | | Sadness | | Tension | | Sad or Tense | |
Model[+]	df	χ^2	p	χ^2	p	χ^2	p
(AFB, SCB)(FD)	11	11.83*	.38	15.76*	.15	20.26	.042
(AFB, SCB)(AFB, FD)	8	5.37	>.5	4.57	>.5	9.21*	.32
(AFB, SCB)(SCB, FD)	9	9.68	.38	13.00	.16	14.27*	.11
(AFB, SCB)(AFB, FD)(SCB, FD)	6	3.86	>.5	2.55	>.5	4.34	>.5

[+]AFB = age at first birth, SCB = study child's birth order, FD = feelings of distress.
*Statistically, this is a satisfactory model for the observed table.

Table 5.   Effects of Age at First Birth and Total Number of Children on Time 1 Feelings of Distress

| | | Feelings of Distress at Time 2 | | | | | |
| | | Sadness | | Tension | | Sad or Tense | |
Model[+]	df	χ^2	p	χ^2	p	χ^2	p
(AFB, TC)(FD)	11	14.98*	.18	16.86*	.11	19.41*	.054
(AFB, TC)(AFB, FD)	8	8.52	.38	5.67	>.5	8.37*	.40
(AFB, TC)(TC, FD)	9	12.14	.21	11.35	.25	11.95*	.22
(AFB, TC)(AFB, FD)(TC, FD)	6	5.83	.44	1.82	>.5	2.78	>.5

[+]AFB = age at first birth, TC = total children at Time 1, FD = feelings of distress.
*Statistically, this is a satisfactory model for the observed table.

Section B

EFFECTS OF A MAJOR CRISIS OR STRESSOR

A STUDY OF HEALTH AND MENTAL HEALTH STATUS FOLLOWING A MAJOR NATURAL DISASTER

James N. Logue, Mary Evans Melick,
and Elmer L. Struening

INTRODUCTION

Descriptions of major disasters frequently include some discussion of the numbers of dead and severely injured persons and may also include an estimate of the number of missing persons. Journalistic and medical accounts of the disaster often report on the handling of casualties and the health problems experienced by the survivors during the first few days following disaster, particularly if these problems involve epidemics or the threat of communicable diseases. It is less common to read accounts of the health of the post-disaster population once outside medical personnel have left the area. In recent years, a number of investigators have become interested in studying the long-term health consequences of

Research in Community and Mental Health, Volume 2, pages 217–274 many types of disasters. In order to examine and compare these studies, several definitions may be useful.

Disasters are massive stress situations. Barton (1970, p. 38) defines disasters as being part of the larger category of collective stress situations which occur when many members of a social system fail to receive the expected conditions of life from the system. Disasters are usually divided into two categories, natural and man-made, depending on the causative agent. There is fairly good general understanding about the nature of natural disasters, sometimes called acts of God. These disasters, including floods, tornados, earthquakes, tidal waves, and landslides, to name a few, are crisis events which are the result of natural agents and involve little, if any, human causation. Man-made disasters differ in that they are, as their name implies, the creation of man. Such disasters include wars and concentration camps; some might also include famines and chronic economic deprivation and its correlates. Recently, the definition of man-made disasters has been extended to include events which are the result of technological failures or other threats to ecological balance which are the result of technology or its byproducts. Such events may be of a chemical, mechanical, electrical, biological, or nuclear nature, to cite a few possible examples. Recent examples of such events include the Love Canal in Buffalo, New York, involving disposition of chemical wastes over several years, and the Three Mile Island nuclear plant accident in Harrisburg, Pennsylvania. Such events can confidently be assumed to be of increasing importance in the future.

Disasters can be divided into various time periods for purposes of analysis and intervention. Powell and Rayner (1952) suggest the following division: (1) warning, (2) threat, (3) impact, (4) inventory, (5) rescue, (6) remedy, and (7) recovery. Nearly all studies of disaster concentrate on the first six periods, extending from immediately before the disaster to two to four weeks following the impact of the disaster. It seems reasonable to assume that the health consequences of disaster might differ from immediately post-impact, when casualties are being cared for, to the recovery period when stress-related chronic diseases might predominate. For this reason, health consequences of the remedy and recovery periods will be examined separately.

Health and Illness in the Remedy Period

According to Powell and Rayner (1952), the remedy period, which follows immediate rescue activities, is the period during which more deliberate and formal activities are undertaken to relieve the population.

Studies of the health of populations during this time period tend to focus on injured victims and their treatment. Chapman (1962), reporting on illness in the remedy period, noted that a sizeable proportion of survivors experienced insomnia, digestive upsets, nervousness, and other products of emotional tension. These problems tended to subside within several days after the disaster. The immediate response of various groups to disaster is so uniform that a "disaster syndrome'' has been defined by Wallace (1956) and described by others. This syndrome is characterized by an absence of emotion, inhibition of activity, docility, indecisiveness, lack of responsiveness, and automatic behavior, together with the physiological manifestations of autonomic arousal. Kinston and Rosser (1974, p. 442) describe this syndrome as a psychic closing-off from further stimuli.

Short term mental health consequences of disaster have been discussed by Wilson (1962), Parker (1977), Knaus (1975), Greeson and Mintz (1972), and Farberow and Frederick (1978). During the remedy period, these authors reported psychosomatic disorders, depression, and lessened ability to function competently. Their general impression is that the individuals affected should not be considered psychiatric cases since their impairments are usually transient. Wilson (1962), however, indicates that disaster may fix propensities toward physical or behavioral disorders and may in the long run lead to mental illness.

One study, based on observations of patients known to the two psychoanalysts (Greeson and Mintz, 1972), reported regressive phenomena following an earthquake. This report, however, differed from other studies in that the authors concluded that for most patients, the disaster resulted in eventual improvement in the therapeutic experience.

One study of the remedy period had essentially negative results. Spiegal (1957), studying the English flood of 1953, found that little physical or emotional illness occurred despite exposure and tension and despite an influenza epidemic which was in progress when the flood came. However, in the adjustment period people began to get sick. The nature of this illness, the length of time after the flood, and methods of data collection were not discussed in detail. Chapman (1962) also observed that little serious mental illness results from the tension, crisis and deprivation of disaster. He postulated that the emotional mobilization required of survivors may counteract some existing cases of mental illness and prevent some incipient cases from becoming florid.

Recently, Perry and Lindell (1978) reviewed the literature on the psychological consequences of natural disasters in American communities. Based on this review, they presented a conceptual model isolating important variables and suggesting the channels through which disaster might produce positive or negative psychological consequences. Variables associated with initial psychological consequences, those lasting up to one week post-impact, include: (1) community variables, such as level of preparedness, forewarning, disaster subculture, and formation of a therapeutic community; (2) disaster variables such as scope and duration of impact and the resulting property damage and destruction of kin and friendship networks, which may result in grief reactions; and (3) personal variables such as demographic variables and pre-impact psychological stability. Later psychological consequences, those occurring from one week to six months following disaster, are influenced by all of the variables associated with initial consequences, and, in addition, are influenced by institutional rehabilitation.

Health and Illness in the Recovery Period

The recovery period, as described by Powell and Rayner (1952) is the extended period during which the community and the individuals in it either recover their previous stability or achieve adaptation to the changed conditions brought about by the disaster. The length of this period may vary from several months to several years following the disaster, and its termination is more or less subjectively defined.

Examination of the literature concerned with health and illness in the recovery period following natural disaster indicates a lack of general agreement among researchers regarding estimates of physical and/or mental impairment following disaster. These estimates range from Bates et al. (1963), who found no significant impairment four years after disaster, to Lifton and Olson (1976), who found overwhelming evidence that everyone exposed to the Buffalo Creek disaster has experienced some or all of the manifestations of the survivor syndrome. These manifestations include death imprint and anxiety, death guilt, psychic numbing, and impaired human relationships. The decreasing number of impairments over time has been noted by Takuma (1978), who reported that few respondents indicated they had no symptoms at seven weeks following an earthquake (5 percent), but that symptoms became less serious as time passed. Parker's (1977) study following Cyclone Tracy in Darwin, Australia, generally supported Takuma's findings. Parker found that after 10 weeks 41 percent (N=13) of the respondents were characterized as probable psychiatric cases, while after 14 months only 22 percent (N=4) were characterized this way.

The type of symptom or impairment shown has great variability. Specific health problems have been reported, such as increased mortality (Lorraine, 1954); psychiatric symptoms such as anxiety, depression, childhood behavior problems, and nervousness (Okura, 1975; Abrahams, 1976; Penick et al., 1976; Price, 1978; Titchener and Kapp, 1976); hypertension (Titchener and Kapp, 1976); duodenal ulcers (Titchener and Kapp, 1976); and increased alcohol and drug use (Erikson, 1976). Other authors, such as Janney (1977), are less specific about the health problems experienced, noting only that there was a change in health status following the disaster. Finally, Bennet (1970; p. 457) found such diverse symptoms that he concluded, "In all aspects studied the health of those flooded was worse in the 12 months after the flood than the health of those not flooded..."

Most reports of post-disaster health have not used a control or nondisaster comparison group (e.g., Moore and Friedsam, 1959; Bates et al., 1963; Kafrissen, Heffron, and Zusman, 1975; Titchener and Kapp, 1976; Erikson, 1976; Newmann, 1976; Rangell, 1976; Lifton and Olson, 1976; Penick et al., 1976; and Takuma, 1978). Some recent studies have tended to use a comparison group on which data are collected (e.g., Bennet, 1970; Abrahams et al., 1974; Janney, 1977) or make use of comparisons with data collected for other purposes—for example, comparison with a household health survey (Parker, 1977).

The subgroups at greater risk have been reported to be: females—at risk of emotional stress or psychiatric symptoms (Moore and Friedsam, 1959; Bennet, 1970; Abrahams et al., 1974); males—increase in surgery, increase in physical symptoms (Bennet, 1970); the aged (Bennet, 1970; and Poulschock and Cohen, 1975); and community leaders (Bates et al., 1963).

The duration of symptoms is difficult to evaluate because of the cross-sectional nature of the samples selected for examination. The range probably extends from somewhat longer than seven weeks (Takuma, 1978) to 18 months (Erikson, 1976) or several years (Rangell, 1976). On the other hand, several studies have reported that symptoms or impairments no longer existed or were minimal at 14 months (Parker, 1977) or at four years (Bates et al., 1963). The only longitudinal study which was located was Parker's study of the effects of Cyclone Tracy on the population of Darwin, Australia. Based on a small sample (N=68) he concluded that psychological morbidity was increased above an Australian general community population initially and at ten weeks after the disaster, but was not increased at 14 months.

In addition to studies of the effects of natural disasters on health, reports have been published on the long-term effects of man-made disasters, particularly concentration and prison camp internment (e.g., Cohen, 1953; Eitinger, 1971) and atomic warfare (Lifton, 1967). The estimates of impairment include long-term physical (Eitinger, 1971) and emotional (Lumry, 1970) disorders which affect not only the individual exposed, but also the unexposed children of holocaust victims (Segal, 1971; and Klein, 1971). Those victims exposed to the disaster stressors during childhood or adolescence seem particularly vulnerable to the development of psychosomatic diseases (Krystal, 1971).

Numerous symptoms and/or disease states have been cited as resulting from man-made disasters. Many of these are classified as post-concentration camp syndrome (post K-Z syndrome). The symptoms associated with this syndrome have included: weight loss, emotional and autonomic lability, instability, irritability, apathy, decreased self-esteem, depression, difficulty concentrating, startle reaction to ordinary stimuli, anxiety, restlessness, apprehension, and obsessive ruminative states (Lumry, 1970). Hocking (1970a, 1970b, 1971) has added depression, sleep disturbances, traumatic dreams, and headaches to this list. In addition, long-term malnutrition, psychoneuroses, impotence, gastrointestinal disorders, cardiovascular, respiratory and neurological problems have been reported (Cohen and Cooper, 1954; and Eitinger, 1971). The health problems which have followed exposure to radiation have included: leukemia and other cancers, cataracts and other eye problems, and impaired growth and development of children (Lifton, 1967). The psychological consequences have included: interpreting any sign of illness as radiation-related, psychic numbing, and A-Bomb neurosis (Lifton, 1967).

One physician observer (Cohen, 1953) has indicated that during the period of concentration camp internment, many diseases met in routine medical practice were less frequent. Among those diseases less frequently seen were: urticaria, asthma, influenza, gastric and duodenal ulcers, eczema, and hypertension. In addition, few of the usual symptoms of diabetes mellitus were seen.

None of the studies reviewed has made use of a control group. Use of such groups seems especially critical when examining victims 20 to 30 years following the disaster since victims are then generally of the age in which the clinical findings of disease are fairly common.

As with the reporting of long-term effects of natural disaster, it is difficult to assess the duration of symptoms and disease because careful longitudinal studies are lacking. Nor has it been possible to accurately determine the prevalence of health problems since convenience, rather than saturation or random, samples of victims have been examined.

Near-Miss Phenomenon

While the sociological and medical literatures have tended to focus on disaster victims, the psychological literature has also included reports on the effects of the near-miss phenomenon. This is a disaster situation in which an individual has barely escaped being a victim (Lazarus, 1966). The concept evolved out of a study of World War II survivors, both military personnel and civilians. Janis (1971) notes that narrow escapes from danger, loss of persons with whom one identifies, and witnessing maimed bodies appear to shatter psychological defenses which maintain a sense of invulnerability. Lazarus (1966) sums up literature about the near-miss phenomenon by stating that the effects will depend on how the experience is interpreted by the individual. Most of the studies of near-miss have followed traumatic events or disasters by a short period of time and have tended to focus on the present psychological status and the psychological defenses used for coping. No studies have been located which deal primarily with the long-term health consequences of being a near-miss survivor.

Discussion

A number of reports have appeared in the literature concerning the short-term consequences of disaster, particularly natural disaster, on the health and well-being of the post-disaster population. These reports have tended to focus on treatment of victims and on minor stress-induced physical and emotional problems which seem to last for several days following impact. A disaster syndrome, as described by Wallace, is of particular importance because of the validation this finding has received in a number of studies. It has been unusual for investigators to follow this same population over an extended period of time to determine the implications that the disaster experience has for the subsequent health of the population.

Those few studies which have been reported concerning the long-term consequences of natural disaster have been based on general observations or have often suffered from methodological problems, such as the lack of a comparison group.

Most have relied on retrospective techniques and victims' self-report of illness and its treatment or on clinical interviews conducted for the purpose of establishing pathology. Comparison of the findings from these studies has been difficult for many reasons, including the failure, in some cases, to discuss sampling procedure, the variety of instruments and assessment techniques used, and the unique characteristics of the population studied.

In the past decade, a number of reports concerning the health consequences of man-made disasters have appeared in the literature. Most have reported both physical and emotional sequelae existing over an extended time period, often 20 to 30 years. As with natural disasters, however, most, if not all of these reports, have suffered from the absence of a comparison group. In addition, it is difficult to generalize health findings from these studies of man-made disasters to natural disaster populations, since these two types of disasters may differ in ways which are crucial. Such differences often include contact with the oppressors, intent to harm, malnutrition, and the length of time the stressor(s) is experienced.

The overall impression which follows a review of disaster literature, particularly literature on natural disasters, is that this is a field of stress research which has not received much systematic attention. This is particularly true in regard to the long-term health effects of disaster.

THE PRESENT STUDY

The Disaster

Disasters are unique, not only because of the peculiarities of the event itself, but because of differences in the populations affected. For these reasons, it is necessary to have an understanding of the particular disaster situation and community in which the disaster occurred.

The disaster to be reported in this present study was the widespread flooding and destruction which occurred in 1972, as a result of Tropical Storm Agnes. The National Oceanic and Atmospheric Administration (U.S. Department of Commerce, 1972) noted that Agnes was unusual because she caused floods and flash floods over a large area, resulting in the declaration of seven states (New York, Pennsylvania, Virginia, Maryland, West Virginia, Ohio, and Florida) as major disaster areas. The storm, which developed in Yucatan during the evening of June 14, 1972, hit the coast of Florida on June 18 and began moving up the coast of the United States causing wind and water damage until she moved out to sea the evening of June 21 (U.S. Army Corps of Engineers, Undated). Instead of continuing out to sea, following the path of similar storms, Agnes shifted her course inland on the evening of June 22 and established a double center over the Wyoming Valley of Pennsylvania and the Corning-Elmira area of the Southern Tier of New York State. The storm continued to move westward until it disintegrated over Western Pennsylvania on June 24. By the time it was over, Agnes had dumped an estimated 28.1 trillion gallons of water on the eastern seaboard, mostly on the Middle Atlantic States. The final statistics showed that 13,500 miles of streams and rivers had been flooded, and an estimated 116,000 homes, 2,400 farm buildings, and 5,800 businesses were damaged or destroyed. This meant at least a $2.5 million property loss and $700 million lost in damage to highways, bridges, and public buildings (U.S. Army Corps of Engineers, Undated). Considering the tremendous amount of property damage, the loss of life was relatively low, with 118 deaths attributed to the storm (Metropolitan Life Insurance, 1977).

Both the widespread damage and the relatively low number of mortalities—only three flood-related deaths in the study communities—made this disaster unlike other disasters such as Buffalo Creek (Erikson, 1976), where major loss of life and more localized destruction occurred.

It has been generally agreed that Agnes caused the greatest amount of damage in the Susquehanna River Basin. The Susquehanna is the longest river draining into the Atlantic Ocean. It has its origin in Otsego Lake in Central New York and flows in a generally southeastern direction toward the Chesapeake Bay. Although many towns and cities, as well as farms, along the Susquehanna suffered damage, the hardest hit communities were located in the Wyoming Valley of Pennsylvania. This valley which extends from Duryea on the Lackawanna River southwestward to Nanticoke, south of Plymouth on the Susquehanna River, is a part of Luzurne County, the county hardest hit by Agnes. Wilkes-Barre, the county seat, is located about 110 road miles from Harrisburg and 120 road miles from Philadelphia (U.S. Army Corps of Engineers, 1972). Of the 39,000 Pennsylvania homes either destroyed or sustaining major damage, about 25,000 were in the Wyoming Valley.

Floods are not uncommon phenomena in the Wyoming Valley. Major flooding during this century occurred in 1902, 1904, 1936, 1940, 1946, and 1964 (Mussari, 1974; Romanelli and Griffith, 1972). Several local businesses have marked the height of each of these successive floods on their buildings. The worst flood of this century, until 1972, was the 1936 flood when the river crested at 33.7 feet. In response to this and other floods, a 15-mile system of dikes was built in the early 1940s to contain flood waters up to 33 feet. In addition to the construction of dikes, six reservoirs have been built on tributaries of the Susquehanna upstream from the Wyoming Valley in an effort to prevent flooding. Obviously, they have failed to achieve this purpose, since the 1972 flood was the most expensive natural disaster in the history of this country.

Natives of the Wyoming Valley are quick to note that although many of them have experienced flooding before, particularly in 1936, this most recent flood was unlike previous floods. Aside from the extent of the flooding and the magnitude of the property damage, the 1972 flood was a "dirty" flood. One native explained the difference between clean and dirty floods this way:

I live along Solomon's Creek, and I've gotten wet before. I got flooded in 1936, but it was a clean flood. The water came up and went down. We let the walls dry out, scraped the mud off the rug and went back to living. This flood (Agnes, 1972) wasn't like that; it was dirty. The water contained all kinds of mine wastes—acids and things. When it went down, everything stank. The walls, everything was ruined. I had to tear out all the walls, throw everything out, and start over. This is the flood of the century.

Agnes dumped 4.90 inches of water on the Valley causing the Susquehanna to crest at 40.9 feet, 7.9 feet above the level of the dikes. On Friday, June 23, the headquarters of the 109th Field Artillery was notified of activation and alert for flood duty. They were ordered to report for such duty at 5:00 a.m., June 24. Meanwhile, the Luzerne County Civil Defense Director requested that television and radio announcements be made asking Plymouth residents, whose homes had been flooded in the 1940 flood, to go to the homes of friends and relatives in Kingston and Wilkes-Barre. About 5,000 people evacuated Plymouth that evening (Mussari, 1974).

By 1:30 a.m., Saturday morning, the situation was worse than anticipated, and Mercy Hospital in Wilkes-Barre and Nesbitt Hospital in Kingston were told to evacuate their patients. Still, the Civil Defense Director did not issue an announcement to the residents of Kingston and Wilkes-Barre for evacuation, because he was concerned about panic and confusion if such an evacuation occurred in the dark. At 4:20 a.m., the Director made a public announcement that the river was 32.3 feet high and was expected to rise to 40 feet. He requested evacuation of the area, and sandbagging of the dikes was begun at 6:00 a.m. About 10,000 people volunteered to work on the dikes, but their efforts proved fruitless when the dikes broke in six locations. The final evacuation siren sounded at 11:14 a.m., and, by evening the water crested at 40.0 feet.

While the waters were rising, most residents went about their usual activities. One department chairman at a local college located immediately adjacent to the river described his Saturday morning this way:

On Saturday I went to the office like I always do. It's quieter there, and I can get a lot of work done. It was about 8:00 a.m. when I got there, and there were people on the street as usual. When I looked out my office window I could see people sandbagging the dikes. Sometime between 10 and 11 a.m. my wife called and asked if I had looked out the window recently. She had heard that Wilkes-Barre was being evacuated, and she told me to pack up my case right away and come home.

When she hung up I looked out the window. The water was even with the top of the dikes and flowing fast. It was still raining lightly. I thought she's probably right, so I packed up and came home. As I crossed the bridge out of town, they put barriers across the entrance so no one else could get across. I must have been the last person out of town. I really didn't know things were that bad.

Approximately 80,000 people were evacuated, many of them to the homes of friends and relatives elsewhere in the Valley. The remainder were housed in public shelters, established in local schools, including the appropriately named Heights area of Wilkes-Barre. The evacuation period lasted three days for most of the residents.

At the public shelters, the evacuees experienced a number of hardships, including food and water lines, lack of privacy, high noise levels, exposure to large numbers of inadequately supervised children, insufficient hygiene facilities, and lack of necessary supplies such as baby diapers. Most remained relatively calm and patient, believing that they would shortly be allowed to return home.

When the residents did return to their homes, most saw greater destruction than they had anticipated. Many reported crying and stating that everything was lost. Some residents had nothing to come home to but a foundation. Many of these people moved in with friends or relatives until the government provided temporary housing in the form of mobile homes. Fairly typical of the disrupted family life which followed the flood is the case of the W family. Mr. W, his wife and five children, ages 9 to 18, and four children Mrs. W cared for during the day were evacuated from their house when the waters flooded the basement. Eventually, the first floor was flooded also. They went to live for four days with Mr. W's uncle in a neighboring town. When they returned, they gutted the downstairs and began major repair while continuing to live upstairs. They cooked on a hot plate, worked during the day, and repaired their home at night and during weekends. When they completed their repairs, their home was purchased and demolished in preparation for urban renewal. The family had to find a new residence, move, and settle in once again.

Damages due to flooding have been estimated at about $3.4 billion. Nearly 25,000 dwelling units were seriously damaged or destroyed and 2,728 commercial establishments were damaged. All but 20 of the buildings in Kingston—a borough of 18,325 people, across the river from Wilkes-Barre—were flooded. Approximately 150 industrial firms, employing 11,335 people, were affected (Franke, 1974; Krantz, 1973). It has been estimated that the unemployment rate in the Wyoming Valley rose to nearly 20 percent (Department of the Army, 1972).

The Community

Unemployment was not unknown in the Wyoming Valley before the flood. Many of the largely working class towns were just beginning to recover from the effects of a decline in the coal industry. Anthracite coal production reached its zenith in 1918, when 37.7 million tons were mined, while peak employment in this industry occurred in 1926 when 67,207 workers were employed in the mining industry, and tonnage had dropped to 2,719,940 tons (Franke, 1974). There are, however, many reminders of the golden era of mining still to be found in the Valley. Large homes, once owned by wealthy businessmen, line the River Common, and the mountains surrounding the residential areas of the Valley show the scars of strip mining. In addition, there is a sizable population of older persons, especially men, who have evidence of anthracosilicosis or other mining-related disabilities.

The mining industry has left other reminders, too. In the Valley, one finds people from many different ethnic backgrounds who came to find employment in the mines. Persons of foreign birth or parentage still constitute 29.1 percent of the population, while only 1.8 percent of the population is black (Franke, 1974). The largest ethnic groups at present are Polish and Italian, but many waves of immigrants from different countries were attracted to the area for employment in the mines. Many of these persons are now elderly, speak broken English, and maintain social ties with ethnically homogeneous institutions.

Following the gradual closing of the mines, an attempt has been made to attract other industries to the area. At present, one-third of all workers, largely women in low-paying jobs, are employed in apparel manufacturing (Franke, 1974). Other important industries include: food processing, fabricated metals, electrical machinery, tobacco, printing and publishing, and transportation.

The 1970 census showed an area still economically depressed with the median value of real estate set at $9,300, the median gross rent at $62.00, and a median income of $8,047. The population of Wilkes-Barre City (58,865) had shown a decrease of 7.4 percent since the 1960 census, and a 4.2 percent of the work force was unemployed (U.S. Department of Commerce, 1972). Many of those who have remained in the area are elderly so that Wilkes-Barre and the surrounding flooded communities have a population with a median age well above that of the national average. This is especially important since it is generally agreed that the elderly are a high risk group for physical and emotional problems as a result of disasters (Friedsam, 1962; Kinston and Rosser, 1974).

Clearly, the terrible devastation wrought by Agnes in this section of the country created an extremely stressful situation for flood victims whose community was already plagued by numerous social and economic problems. Mussari (1974), a native of the area, described the post-disaster population several years after Agnes as "... older, more exhausted, and more heavily in debt than they ever expected to be" and noted that, "Daily they try desperately to restore the normal pace of their disaster scarred lives, but everyday something reminds them of what they have lost."

This loss is much more than property loss, although nearly all residents can provide a dollar value for their property losses, many of them based on the amount of money which has been borrowed to repair these losses. Most residents, however, will also describe their losses in more personal terms such as loss of the children's baby pictures, family heirlooms, handmade items and other irreplaceable objects with special meanings. Some residents literally lost everything. Even individuals who lived in the same community but who were not generally labeled disaster victims experienced loss. Their loss included loss of kin or friends due to moving from the area, and disruption of businesses. One kosher butcher who did not experience flooding of his home or business in the Heights area put it this way:

> How did the flood affect me? I'll tell you. People couldn't get here (to the butcher shop) because of the flood and because of being too busy repairing things. They started eating non-kosher meats, especially during the evacuation, and they found out they didn't die. Since they didn't die, and since non-kosher meat is cheaper, they kept right on eating it. Things will never be the same for me.

It was this post-flood community which was selected for the study of the influence of disaster on the health and well-being of the residents for the period of time up to five years following the flood.

A Social Stress Model

Social stress theory asserts that certain conditions or changes in the environments of populations might contribute to the development of stress and, subsequently, symptoms of physical or mental disorders, in selected members of these populations. Those conditions or changes in the environment which create *stress* in selected organisms are referred to as *stressors*. If stress as a condition of the organism is experienced over a period of time, with a certain intensity and in a particular social context, the organism might manifest symptoms of physical or mental disorders. Should these conditions continue to prevail at a sufficiently high level of intensity, the symptoms might become chronic and eventually result in organ failure and, in the extreme, death.

There is evidence to indicate that a number of mediating factors, some protective and others destructive, stand between vulnerable organisms and the stressors of their environments.

The stress model diagrammed in Figure 1 indicates a sequence of events and processes, including sets of mediating factors, which occur following a major disruption in the environment. The havoc caused by the Agnes flood is conceived as a major set of stressors experienced by selected subjects of this study and referred to as Objective Effects. The first line of defense, indicated under C, is the person's subjective appraisal of the objective events. Variability in this evaluative process is at least partially a function of a person's individual, economic and social resources, indicated under D, E, and F of the diagram. Beyond influencing the person's appraisal of the stressor's impact, the three types of mediating factors may help to protect the organism from the impact of the stressors and lessen the degree of stress experienced. Such characteristics as the person's demonstrated ability to cope with adversity, the presence of financial resources and the existence of a dedicated and supportive family may be important determinants of whether or not symptoms of mental and physical disorders become manifest.

Even if the organism does experience considerable stress, his or her current

Figure 1. Applications of a Stress Model to a Major Natural Disaster

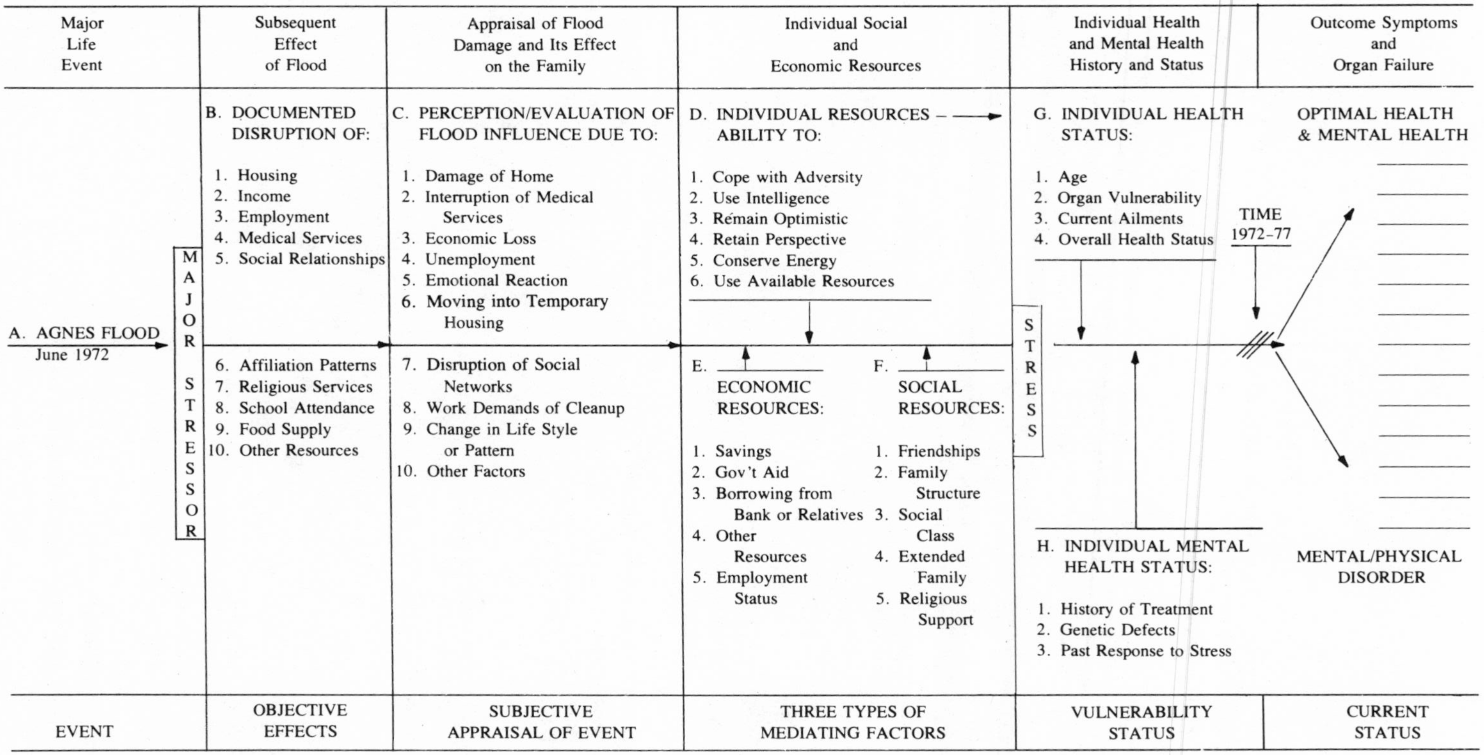

Major Life Event	Subsequent Effect of Flood	Appraisal of Flood Damage and Its Effect on the Family	Individual Social and Economic Resources	Individual Health and Mental Health History and Status	Outcome Symptoms and Organ Failure
A. AGNES FLOOD June 1972	B. DOCUMENTED DISRUPTION OF: 1. Housing 2. Income 3. Employment 4. Medical Services 5. Social Relationships 6. Affiliation Patterns 7. Religious Services 8. School Attendance 9. Food Supply 10. Other Resources	C. PERCEPTION/EVALUATION OF FLOOD INFLUENCE DUE TO: 1. Damage of Home 2. Interruption of Medical Services 3. Economic Loss 4. Unemployment 5. Emotional Reaction 6. Moving into Temporary Housing 7. Disruption of Social Networks 8. Work Demands of Cleanup 9. Change in Life Style or Pattern 10. Other Factors	D. INDIVIDUAL RESOURCES — ABILITY TO: 1. Cope with Adversity 2. Use Intelligence 3. Remain Optimistic 4. Retain Perspective 5. Conserve Energy 6. Use Available Resources	G. INDIVIDUAL HEALTH STATUS: 1. Age 2. Organ Vulnerability 3. Current Ailments 4. Overall Health Status TIME 1972–77	OPTIMAL HEALTH & MENTAL HEALTH
			E. ECONOMIC RESOURCES: 1. Savings 2. Gov't Aid 3. Borrowing from Bank or Relatives 4. Other Resources 5. Employment Status F. SOCIAL RESOURCES: 1. Friendships 2. Family Structure 3. Social Class 4. Extended Family 5. Religious Support	H. INDIVIDUAL MENTAL HEALTH STATUS: 1. History of Treatment 2. Genetic Defects 3. Past Response to Stress	MENTAL/PHYSICAL DISORDER
EVENT	OBJECTIVE EFFECTS	SUBJECTIVE APPRAISAL OF EVENT	THREE TYPES OF MEDIATING FACTORS	VULNERABILITY STATUS	CURRENT STATUS

MAJOR STRESSOR — STRESSORS — STRESS

physical and mental health status may help to prevent the expression of symptoms and organ dysfunction. Characteristics of the individual such as age, the condition of major organs, and the response properties of immune systems would probably play a key role in mediating the effects of stress on the organism. In a similar manner, the mental health status of the individual, indicated by treatment history and reactions to previous crises, will probably predict the emergence of mental symptoms and behavioral deviance as the organism continues to experience stress.

Although the factors listed under C, D, E, and F are presented in a temporal sequence, they quite obviously interact and influence each other, resulting finally in some degree of stress within the organism. The degree of stress experienced by the organism may also create conditions which alter the perceptual/evaluative processes and subsequent coping behaviors. This process, although occurring in a temporal sequence, is conceived as interactive and dynamic in nature and probably fluctuates considerably within individuals until a somewhat stable mode of adaptation has been reached.

In conclusion, social stress theory makes the general assertion that selected characteristics of individuals and of their socio-economic context will mediate, and, therefore, predict the effects of a major stressor on the health and mental health status of those experiencing the stresses.

In this chapter the following very general hypotheses are derived from social stress theory and serve as a guide to more specific hypotheses subsequently tested:

1. The respondent's retrospective evaluation of the effects of the flood, including the degree of disruption of family life, social networks, and economic welfare during the recovery period, will be related to his or her current physical and mental health status and that of his or her family.

2. The coping styles (increased use of alcohol, taking tranquilizers, neglecting medical care, becoming more religious) employed by respondents during the recovery period will be related to their current physical and mental health status.

3. Characteristics of the familial and social context of respondents, both during and after the flood, will be related to their current physical and mental health status.

4. Characteristics of the individual, such as age, education, and socioeconomic status will predict the current physical and mental health status of the individual.

Subsequent parts of this chapter will present more specific hypotheses as they are directly linked to sampling procedures, operational definitions of constructs and data analysis.

METHODS

Melick's Study

The objective of this research, conducted in 1975, was to investigate the relationship between stress and the incidence and prevalence of physical illness and emotional disorder in a sample of working-class men, ages 25–65, during the recovery period of a natural disaster. The study was conducted nearly three years following the flood and focused on three time periods: six months before the flood (January to June, 1972); the period from the impact of the flood to two and one-half years later (June, 1972 to January, 1975); and the most recent six months (January to June, 1975).

This study was designed specifically to compare the life change and illness experience of two groups of men, residents of the same community, who were essentially the same except for their disaster experience. In addition, an attempt was also made to assess the relationship between the social integration of the respondent and his post-disaster illness experience.

Population and Sample

The population consisted of all working-class males, ages 25 to 65, living in Wilkes-Barre and Kingston, Pennsylvania. This study was limited to this population because: (1) it was expected that the vast majority of persons meeting these criteria were employed at the time of the flood and, therefore, had the possibility of life change in terms of alterations in the nature and extent of employment and income; (2) previous research has shown that the lower classes are especially susceptible to the effects of disaster (Wilson, 1962)—lacking resources such as monetary reserve and jobs with high salaries, they may experience a more stressful post-disaster period than persons in Hollingshead's (1957) Classes I to III; and (3) a smaller sample can be used if one does not need to take account of differential rates of illness and differential reporting of illnesses as one would if both sexes and persons across the life span and class structure were to be included in the study population.

The sample was stratified on one type of loss, flooding of the housing unit with damage to possessions and the possibility of loss of the unit itself. The purpose of this stratification was to produce increased homogeneity within strata and to maximize the chances of detecting differences in the dependent variable, number of illnesses, between groups. In addition, a moderate reduction in standard error accompanies sample stratification (Lazerwitz, 1968).

A sample of 120 was drawn from the population using the following procedure:

1. The areas of the community which had been flooded were identified on a block basis from a map prepared at the time of the flood (Dansbury, 1973). All city blocks in Wilkes-Barre and Kingston were identified as flood or non-flood.

2. Four pretest respondents, who had lived in the Wilkes-Barre area at least 20 years, were asked to indicate on a city map the areas in which working men like themselves lived. In addition, two other people who had lived in the community at least 15 years were asked to indicate areas of the city in which working class men, such as factory workers, truck drivers, and warehousemen lived. These people were a college professor whose specialty is labor relations and a dietician and mother of four who had lived in the Wyoming Valley all her life. Finally, a realtor in a large real estate firm was interviewed and asked to identify working

class neighborhoods. The areas identified by all of these people were marked on a map, and the areas of overlap in the neighborhoods selected as the study areas. There was great overlap in the neighborhoods selected by this group, and the boundaries suggested rarely varied more than two or three blocks in any direction.

3. All streets in the study area were listed by blocks as either flood or non-flood. There were 84 flooded streets composed of 3,057 housing units and 140 non-flooded streets with 5,280 housing units.

4. A sample of 120 was desired, 60 flood and 60 non-flood respondents; therefore, dividing 60 into the number of households on target blocks for each condition produced a skip interval for use in selection of respondents.

5. Using the *Greater Wilkes-Barre City Directory* (1974), and following a random start for each condition, every fiftieth respondent in the flood blocks and every eighth respondent in the non-flood blocks was selected for inclusion in the sample.

6. If the target respondent listed in the *Greater Wilkes-Barre City Directory* was female, retired, or a white collar worker, the next head of house was selected for inclusion. If this person was ineligible on the basis of sex or occupation, the next head of house was considered and so on until an appropriate respondent was identified.

Each respondent selected by this method was sent a letter on Wilkes College Institute of Regional Affairs stationery, stating that he had been selected for inclusion in a study of working men in the community, informing him that an interviewer would be calling on him shortly and requesting his cooperation. Wilkes College Institute of Regional Affairs was selected as the auspice because it was believed that respondents were more likely to recognize the Wilkes College name than the name of the university with which the investigator was associated and more likely to cooperate with a local institution. Also, the director of the Regional Institute had been instrumental in working on the Flood Recovery Task Force and was well known to the people of the community.

Instrumentation

Testing of the study hypotheses required the collection of five types of data: demographic information, flood experience, life events, social integration, and health-illness experience over a period of nearly three years. The demographic information included: age, occupation, perceived social class, religious affiliation, education, and income. Flood experience included: whether or not the respondent's home had been flooded, whether he had been evacuated, if he had lost time from work, participation in rescue and recovery operations, losses experienced as a result of the flood, and self-perceived result of the flood for himself and his family and for other people in the Wyoming Valley.

The respondent's life events were determined for three time periods through the administration of the Schedule of Recent Experience (SRE) (Holmes and Rahe, 1967). This is a self-administered questionnaire consisting of two parts: personal history and recent experience sections. The former includes information such as the number of marriages and divorces, age when parents died, number of siblings and number of times the place of residence has been changed within the past five years. The recent event section consists of 42 items requesting information about the time periods when certain events were experienced. Items 13 through 42 of this section inquire about the frequency of events during each of these same time periods. This instrument, developed using a method adapted from psychophysics, provides a measure of the comparative stressfulness of common life events. In addition to the life events on the SRE, respondents were asked about other important life events which occurred during the three time periods under study.

Social integration items obtained information on marital status, family size, religious participation, group memberships and participation, and leisure activities, both before and after the flood. Finally, health-illness information included: the occurrence, duration and treatment of injuries and illnesses for three time periods, self-assessment of present health as compared to pre-flood status, stress-related problems experienced by family members and completion of the Checklist of Twenty Symptom Items (Gurin, Veroff, and Feld, 1960) to indicate the respondent's current psychological symptoms. This checklist, as reported in Gurin, Veroff, and Feld (1960), was developed from 12 items used in the Stirling County Study (MacMillan, 1957) and/or the Midtown Manhattan Study (Rennie, 1953). Four additional items were modifications of those used in these two studies, and four items were prepared specifically for the Gurin, Veroff, and Feld study. Factor analysis indicates that four factors exist—two represent psychological expressions of life dysfunction and two represent somatization of distress. Total scores range from 20 (maximum impairment) through 80 (total absence of symptoms).

Self-reports were selected to obtain the health-illness information not only to acquire factual information, but because it may more accurately reflect the respondent's health-illness experience, a subjective experience, than do medical records. In addition, it is often difficult to gain access to health records, and they have been shown to have difficulties such as the significant difference in the symptoms reported and the diagnosis made by two physicians examining the same patient (Elson et al., 1960; Schor, 1964). Further, a study of octogenarian retirees from the automobile industry, with access to survey interviews and medical record data, showed high levels of congruence between factual information gathered by these two methods (Richardson and Freeman, 1972). Finally, it would have been difficult to rely on hospital and physician records for the pre-flood period because many of these records were destroyed in the flood.

Data Collection

Each respondent was given a personal interview. Interviewers were recruited locally and trained in the administration of the interview schedule.

Interviewers reported that locating the respondents was often time-consuming and frustrating. The flood had significantly altered neighborhoods and considerable time was spent by interviewers and the project director in locating the designated respondents. The following are some of the methods and resources which were helpful in locating respondents: neighbors, calling persons with the same last name listed in the phone book, contacting the last known employer, post office forwarding addresses, utilities company and taxation office files, and the Urban Redevelopment Authority, which helped to locate some non-flood respondents living in an area under development. Use of these methods resulted in location of all but 13 of the 120 respondents. It was anticipated that a relatively high proportion of the sample would be difficult to locate in a community disrupted by disaster and widespread reorganization. In addition to the men who could not be located, two men had died since the *Greater Wilkes-Barre City Directory* (1974) had been published, and 14 men refused to be interviewed. Data analysis was based on 91 cases, 76 percent of the original sample. Of these, 43 were flood respondents and 48 were non-flood respondents. Comparison of available data, last known address and occupation, indicated no important differences between responders and non-responders.

Immediately following data collection, another interviewer was hired to conduct a reliability study. Ten names of respondents were selected at random to be reinterviewed on three items from the interview schedule: respondent's age, the nature, length, and treatment of illnesses from January 1, 1975 to the time of the interview, and length of residence at the current address. The interviewer was instructed to speak with the respondent if possible, or to speak with the spouse if the respondent were not available. Three checks were conducted with respondents and seven with wives. Despite the fact that someone else was reporting for the respondent in most cases, there was exact duplication of 25 of the 30 items (83.3 percent) in the reliability check.

Logue's Study

This study was conducted in the spring of 1977, two years after Melick's investigation and five years post-disaster. The primary purpose of the study was to determine the long-term effects, both health and other, resulting from the disaster. The study was concerned with two time periods, the recovery period and the post-recovery period. The principal independent variable which differentiated "exposed" individuals from controls was the actual flooding of the respondent's homes (yes/no). However, the study was also designed to test the effects of other hypothesized independent variables such as stress due to the recovery period and major life events during the period 1972–1977.

Population and Sample

The population consisted of all females, 21 years of age or older, who lived in a portion of the Wyoming Valley, both in 1972 and 1977, as determined by appropriate city directories. The population, therefore, basically represented a post-disaster community which had elected to remain at the same location five years after the event. The specific communities selected for study included Kingston, Luzerne, Wilkes-Barre Township, Georgetown, Lee Park, Hanover

Township, and Newton. Much of the literature on the effects of Agnes in the Wyoming Valley has indicated that the city of Kingston experienced almost complete flooding. It was anticipated, therefore, that flood respondents would primarily be residents of this small city. The other communities were chosen since they were within a few miles of Kingston and they experienced little or no actual flooding. It was anticipated that most of the non-flood respondents would be residents of these areas.

This study was planned as an epidemiology study and large sample sizes were projected in order to allow greater flexibility in stratifying the data base. Therefore, only a lower bound was placed on the age requirement and no requirement was placed on social class. Females only were chosen for two reasons. First, only males were utilized in Melick's study, and Logue's study was initially planned to complement that study to some extent. Second, mental health status was viewed as an especially important health effect and females are at greater risk of mental disorders than males (Weissman and Klerman, 1977). In this respect, a disaster community represented by females defined a high risk group and this, we felt, provided Logue's study with greater power to detect mental health effects, if any in fact existed.

The sample for the Logue study was selected in the following way:

1. With the use of a street map of the Wyoming Valley, the names of all the streets for Kingston and the adjoining towns mentioned above were arranged in a notebook, one name to a page. The names and addresses for all families on each of these streets at the time of the flood were obtained from the *Greater Wilkes-Barre City Directory* (1972) and copied in the notebook. A street was skipped if it did not appear in the directory. Also, names and addresses for businesses or for families with a different legal address were deleted from this list.

2. Using a more recent edition of the *Greater Wilkes-Barre City Directory* (1976), the list was further modified to *include only those families who still lived at the same address since the flood*. This maneuver had the effect of limiting the study population to those families who had not moved after the flood.

3. A count was made of the number of families who remained in Kingston and the adjoining towns after the first two procedures were carried out. Approximately 3,500 families were counted for the city of Kingston and about the same number of families were counted for the adjoining towns from which the controls were to be chosen. The desired sample for this study was about 1,500 families or about 750 families from Kingston and about 750 families from the adjoining towns. A systematic random sample, using every fourth household on the list, was the procedure for obtaining the sample from both Kingston and the surrounding towns. However, if the family chosen, using the systematic procedure, did not happen to have an adult woman who was a member of the household both in 1972 and 1976, the family was simply skipped in the selection. The skipped family was still considered the "fourth" household and the procedure continued taking the next "fourth" household on the list.

4. The final count for the selected sample indicated 784 families from the city of Kingston (flood area) and 755 families from the adjoining towns (non-flood area) or a grand total of 1,539 families represented by adult women.

Overall, 407 women from the flooded city of Kingston (52 percent) and 155 women from the adjoining "non-flood" areas (21 percent) responded to the mail questionnaire utilized in the Logue study. However, a few respondents from either Kingston or the surrounding areas were reclassified based on their personal flood experience so that the study flood group consisted of 396 women who experienced flooding of their homes—392 residents of Kingston and four residents of the adjoining areas—and the non-flood group consisted of 166 women who did not experience flooding—15 Kingston residents and 151 residents of the adjoining areas.

A concern in Logue's study relates to potential bias because of the large number of non-respondents in the non-flood group (79 percent) and the flood group (48 percent). However, a number of analyses presented in the results section deal with internal comparisons of subgroups only in the flood group. Nonetheless, based on two analyses of respondents in the non-flood group, we determined that these individuals were a geographically representative sample of the target non-flood area.[1] We were able to contact almost all non-respondents in the flood group. Our impression based on this approach to follow-up was that many non-respondents in the flood group were elderly and reported that "health" was the reason they could not respond. Thus, overall health effects may have been underestimated in the final sample of flood respondents. Although we are only working with impressions, the overall effect of bias on flood/non-flood comparisons in Logue's study may well have been to minimize the actual effect of the flood on health.

Instrumentation

The study questionnaire was 30 pages in length and contained 105 questions including many multi-item questions dealing with such things as health, demography, personal and household characteristics, major life events, psychosocial assets, loss experiences following the 1972 flood, and other issues.

Prevalence of mental health symptoms in 1977 was primarily assessed with the following three self-rating scales: (1) Zung's 20-item Self-Rating Depression Scale (Zung, 1965a); (2) Langner's 22-item Screening Instrument (Langer, 1962); and (3) a modified version of the 90-item Self-Report Symptom Inventory (SCL-90), involving five subscales (Derogatis et al., 1973 and 1974; U.S. Department of Health, Education, and Welfare, 1976).

As implied, the Zung scale is a brief and reliable scale useful in measuring various symptoms of depression (Zung, 1965b, 1967). The Zung scale has been shown to correlate fairly strongly with the MMPI-D scale or depression scale (Zung, 1965a and 1967), thus supporting the content validity of the scale. Many of the items on the Zung scale correspond to commonly occuring symptoms of depression as viewed by experts in the field. Zung has also demonstrated that the scale is reliable based on different population studies (1965b, 1967).

It has been well documented in the literature that depression is much more common among women than men (Weissman and Klerman, 1977). Since the

Logue study applies only to female respondents, one might expect on a priori grounds to find depression as a frequent complaint among the study participants.

The Langner scale developed out of the Midtown Manhattan study (Srole et al., 1962) and is especially useful for assessing symtoms of the anxiety dimension.

We utilized the 54 items of the SCL-90 which constitute the first five factors of dimensions of that scale (U.S. Department of Health, Education, and Welfare, 1976): (1) Factor 1—Somatization (12 items); (2) Factor 2—Obsessive-Compulsive (10 items); (3) Factor 3—Interpersonal Sensitivity (9 items); (4) Factor 4—Depression (13 items); and (5) Factor 5—Anxiety (10 items). For each scale, a higher total score represented greater symptomatology along that dimension.

In addition, we developed a 50-item scale using various questions appearing on the U.S. Public Health Service Health Interview Survey (U.S. Department of Health, Education, and Welfare, 1975) in order to assess five-year incidence (1972–1977) of various health effects. The scale or checklist consisted of various conditions (e.g., cancer, accidents) as well as symptoms relating to the major body systems, especially the cardiovascular system, the digestive system, and the respiratory systems. The respondent was also asked to rate the perceived health status of herself and every member of her immediate family at the time of the survey. In addition to the dependent health variables just described, other "soft" indicators of health status corresponding to the time of the survey or the earlier recovery period were also utilized.

An issue which has not received adequate attention in the disaster literature is the concept that the family can be approached as a unit when conducting epidemiological studies (Miller, 1974; Fox, 1974). Hill and Hansen (1962) have contributed an entire chapter of a book on disasters to conceptual and methodological issues relating to families who are involved in disasters. Although Melick (1976) had defined her target population as working class, middle-age males, the questions asked of the study participants frequently dealt with the experience of the entire "family" in the long recovery period. In this paper, therefore, the family will be used as an epidemiological unit whenever possible.

Study Strategies

Five principal hypotheses will be considered in the next section dealing with study results. The hypotheses are illustrated in Figure 2, with accompanying Venn diagrams for Hypotheses 1–4. We have attempted to follow the advice of Susser (1973) on elaborating the association between an independent variable and a dependent variable by introducing other variables into the analyses. The first hypothesis deals exclusively with the effect of flooding on health and presents appropriate results from both Melick's study and Logue's study.

In Hypothesis 2, the association between flooding and health should be elaborated by introducing two additional variables into the analysis: stress due to major

Figure 2. Hierarchy of Elaboration with Respect to Association Among Important Study Variables

Hypothesis 1: the effect of flooding on health

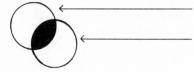

the dependent health variable, Y

the independent variable, X, stress due to the flood: flooding of dwelling unit

Hypothesis 2: the additive effect of flooding, perceived stress due to major life events, and present psychosocial assets on health

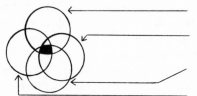

the dependent health variable, Y

the independent variable, X, flooding of dwelling unit

the 3rd variable, A, perceived stress due to major life events

the 4th variable, B, present psychosocial assets

Hypothesis 3: the effect of the recovery period on health

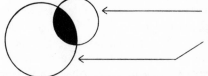

the dependent health variable, Y

the independent variable, X, stress due to the recovery period: various indices of loss for this period

Hypothesis 4: the additive effect of the recovery period, perceived stress due to major life events, and present psychosocial assets on health

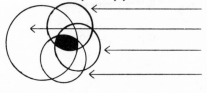

the dependent health variable, Y

the independent variable, X, the recovery period

the 3rd variable, A, perceived stress due to major life events

the 4th variable, B, present psychosocial assets

Hypothesis 5: the effects of many independent variables on health (multiple regression)

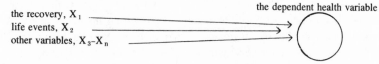

the dependent health variable

the recovery, X_1

life events, X_2

other variables, X_3-X_n

238

life events and present psychosocial assets. The test of the additive effect of these three variables on health corresponds to the second study hypothesis. Hypotheses 3 and 4 are identical to hypotheses 1 and 2 except that experiences in the recovery period serve as the independent variables rather than flooding. There is good reason to believe that the stress associated with losses in the recovery period is of much greater magnitude than that due only to the flooding experience (Erikson, 1976). We have indicated this assumption by using larger circles to represent loss in the recovery period. One of the best ways to elaborate the associations between many hypothetical independent variables and the dependent health variable is through the use of the multiple regression procedure. The fifth and last hypothesis relates to those results obtained using this approach.

RESULTS

Flood versus Non-flood Comparisons

Mental Health Status

Both Melick and Logue hypothesized that the mere flooding of one's dwelling unit would be a stressor of sufficient intensity as to have a long-term effect on mental health status. To test this theory, therefore, flood respondents were compared with non-flood respondents regarding total scores on the self-report mental health scales. The results of the analyses for both studies are displayed in Table 1. Although the flood respondents in Melick's study demonstrated more mental health symptoms than the non-flood respondents, the difference was not statistically significant. The flood respondents in Logue's study also demonstrated more mental health symptoms than the non-flood respondents for the five pertinent dimensions of mental health. Statistical trends ($p<.10$) were noted regarding total Langner (anxiety) and Factor 2 of the SCL-90 (obsessive-compulsive). Factor 2 of the SCL-90 appears to correspond to the state of "psychic numbing" described by Lifton and Olson (1976) in the studies of victims of the 1972 Buffalo Creek disaster. These authors noted that this condition is an important manifestation of the "disaster syndrome" described in the disaster literature.

The failure to find a stronger relationship between flood condition and mental/emotional status may, in part, be the result of the length of time which had elapsed since the disaster impact. On the other hand, our findings may be related more to our method of measurement than to the amount of mental or emotional distress experienced by the population at the time of measurement. Perry and Lindell (1978), based on their review of literature, observed that those researchers who have found a correlation between disaster and mental illness have tended to employ a psychodynamic perspective, being concerned with psychiatric diagnosis and relying on self-report and clinical interviews as measures of psychological consequences. Those studies which have not found a strong relationship tend to use a behavioral model of psychopathology and used rating scales, observers' reports or admission to psychiatric care. They note that these measures are sensitive to different aspects of human behavior and constitute different criteria for establishing the presence of the psychological consequences of disaster. Both of the present studies used such rating scales. The decision to use clinical interviews may have produced a stronger relationship between flooding and mental disorders.

In addition to the assessment of psychological status through the use of rating scales, in the Logue study, the respondent rated her own health and the health of every member of her immediate family at the time of the survey, using a six-point scale ranging from 1 (excellent) to 6 (very poor). Statistically significant flood versus non-flood differences were noted based on a statistical procedure identical to that described in Table 1.[2] The analysis pertaining to the respondent revealed "weighted" adjusted means of 2.81 and 2.63 (F = 3.77, d.f. 1,418, p = .05) for the flood and the non-flood groups respectively.[3] Similarly, the analysis pertaining to the immediate family revealed weighted adjusted means of

Table 1. Mental Health Symptoms

				Means (Total Score)*				
Study	Time Frame	Mental Health Dimension	Scale	Flood Group (n=)	Non-flood Group (n=)	Statistic	d.f.	Probability (2-tailed)
Melick	1975, 3 years post-disaster	Anxiety	Gurin Scale	72.2 (43)	71.0 (48)	t = 0.73	89	.46
Logue	1977, 5 years post-disaster	Anxiety	Langner Scale	3.93 (312)	3.28 (125)	F = 3.41	1,426	.07
		Depression	Zung Scale	37.0 (282)	35.4 (118)	F = 2.39	1,389	.12
		Somatization	Factor 1 of SCL-90	20.2 (286)	19.8 (118)	F = 0.77	1,393	.38
		Obsessive-Compulsive	Factor 2 of SCL-90	17.7 (286)	16.3 (118)	F = 3.01	1,393	.08
		Interpersonal Sensitivity	Factor 3 of SCL-90	14.6 (295)	14.1 (121)	F = 1.12	1,405	.29
		Depression	Factor 4 of SCL-90	23.7 (285)	22.4 (118)	F = 1.94	1,392	.16
		Anxiety	Factor 5 of SCL-90	16.6 (286)	16.1 (118)	F = 1.24	1,393	.27

*Adjusted means resulting from a 3-way analysis of covariance procedure: (1) 3 main effects—flooding of dwelling unit (Yes/No), age (< 60 vs. ≥ 60), Religion (Catholic vs. other); (2) 3 covariates—education, income, dependence on family or origin at time of flood (1972)

2.73 and 2.48 (F = 6.55, d.f. 1,420, p = .01) for the flood and the non-flood groups, respectively. Although the difference between means in both cases was not that striking, the flood group experienced significantly lower health ratings. The respondents were also asked to record the overall (perceived) effect of the flood on health over the five years up to the time of the survey. Based on a four-point scale from 1 (not at all) to 4 (very much), the flood group indicated a significantly greater association between the flood and ill health (mean score 2.18) than the non-flood group (mean score 1.28).

Approaching the perceptions of health in a slightly different way, Melick asked respondents about the number and duration of illnesses experienced by the male respondents before and after the flood. She then asked them to compare their present health status with one year ago, and finally, respondents were asked what influence, if any, they thought the flood had had on their general health.

Focusing on the self-perception of health, it was interesting to note that flood group respondents were more likely than non-flood respondents to state that their present health status was poorer than a year ago ($x^3 = 8.10$, 2 df, p<.02). In addition, flood group respondents more frequently cited specific effects that the flood had had on their health ($x^2 = 18.09$, 3 df, p<.001), while non-flood respondents overwhelmingly (94 percent) stated that the flood had no influence on their general health. The specific influences on health cited by flood group respondents included: fatigue or loss of pep (14 percent), anxiety or tension (16.3 percent), and causation of a specific disease condition (11.6 percent).

Specific Physical Symptoms

A 50-item symptom checklist, developed from the Health Interview Survey conducted by the National Center for Health Statistics (U.S. Department of Health, Education, and Welfare, 1975), was also utilized in Logue's study to assess five-year incidence of selected key symptoms (1972–1977) relating to the cardiovascular, digestive, and respiratory systems in addition to other major systems (neurological, genito-urinary, etc.) The incidence of some key conditions such as cancer and serious injuries/accidents was also assessed through the checklist. In addition to analyzing each of the 50 conditions, analyses were also performed regarding the occurrence of any of the 50 conditions, plus the occurrence of any of those conditions pertaining to the three major systems mentioned above. The respondent was instructed on the questionnaire to indicate the occurrence of any of the 50 conditions for both herself or members of her immediate family during the five-year period following the 1972 Agnes flood. This gave us the opportunity to assess incidence rates for the respondent, her husband (if applicable), and the entire family.

With respect to the respondent, statistically significant (p≤.05) flood versus non-flood differences were noted regarding severe headaches, bladder trouble, and the occurrence of at least one condition. A significant difference was noted in the incidence of hypertension for the husbands of the respondents. Finally, with respect to the entire family, a number of significant differences were noted: gastritis, frequent constipation, severe headaches, bladder trouble, disease of the bone or cartillage, conditions pertaining to the cardiovascular and digestive systems, and the occurrence of at least one condition. In each of these cases, the flood group experienced greater incidence rates than the non-flood group.

The finding of a significantly greater incidence rate of hypertension for husbands in the flood group is noteworthy. Hypertension has been linked to stressful life conditions by numerous investigators (Harburg et al., 1973; Henry and Cassel, 1969; James and Kleinbaum, 1976; Susser and Watson, 1971) and the descriptive epidemiology of hypertension suggests that white males are at much greater risk of the disease than white females. The conditions noted for the respondent and the entire family are, to a large extent, psychosomatic in nature. As noted earlier in this paper, the Agnes flood was one of the worst natural disasters experienced in this country and previous psychiatric assessments of disaster victims, at least in the early recovery period, have shown that the victims will frequently manifest such conditions. Although based on retrospective information, the significant differences noted in this study suggest that psychosomatic conditions may not be as short-lived as some have believed in the past, but may endure well beyond the projected recovery period.

Joint Effect of Flooding, Perceived Stress Associated with Major Life Events, and Psychosocial Assets

As illustrated in our earlier stress-disease model, mediating factors such as life events and other social stressors can exacerbate the stress resulting from some given stressor such as a natural disaster. Supportive factors such as social support systems which may be encompassed in the more general category of psychosocial assets, on the other hand, can lessen the overall effect. The work which has been done in the town of Rosetto, Pennsylvania (Bruhn *et al.*, 1966, 1968), demonstrates the stress buffering effect of strong social ties and social support. Nuckolls et al. (1972) investigated the joint effect of life events and social support systems with regard to final pregnancy outcome, and demonstrated that this approach proved more informative than one which is based on only one independent factor.

Although there is controversy concerning how to measure the stress resulting from major life events (Dohrenwend and Dohrenwend, 1974), Logue quantified stress for life events occurring between the 1972 flood and the 1977 survey by obtaining a "perceived" stress score self-reported for a select group of major life events. Melick relied primarily on the SRE which views the amount of life change, rather than the desirability of change or individual perception of stressfulness, as being a measure of stress experienced. A number of researchers have recommended a further refinement of the methods used to measure life events by concentrating on personal perception of life change rather than on life change itself. (Theorell et al., 1975; Goldberg and Comstock, 1976).

Item 97 of the Logue questionnaire consisted of 22 major life events, plus an open-ended question regarding some other major events not found on the checklist (Appendix 1). The item dealt specifically with life events occurring since the 1972 flood. The respondent was directed to check which of the listed life events may have happened to her and her immediate family, to fill in the date (month and year) of the event, and to note how stressful she perceived the event to be based on a six-point scale of 1 (not too stressful) to 6 (extremely stressful). Most of the items included in the set of major life events applicable to this study were extracted from a set of 32 crisis items utilized in a recent Australian study (Bazeley and Viney, 1976) of women experiencing various crisis situations and coping with these crises. These items were judged to be applicable to the Logue study since they were intended for use by women respondents only. The set of 22 questions covered many different areas important in a woman's life including marriage, children, work, and financial difficulties, to name a few.

An *average* perceived stress score was calculated for each respondent based on all the stress scores corresponding to the reported life events. If no stress ratings were marked by the respondent, the average stress score was simply marked "0." Based on an initial display of the stress scores, an average score of 0, 1, 2, or 3 was reclassified as a "1" (low stress) while a score of 4, 5, or 6 was reclassified as a "2" (high stress). It is worth noting that the average perceived stress score for the flood group was 3.78, while that for the non-flood group was 3.03. The difference between the two means is statistically significant ($p \leqslant .05$). Hence, the flood group demonstrated significantly more perceived stress than the non-flood group for those life events experienced between 1972 and 1977.

Melick's analysis of the stress experience of flood and non-flood respondents showed that during Period I (pre-flood), the two groups experienced approximately the same amount of life change. During Period II, extending from immediately post impact to January, 1975, the flood respondents reported significantly greater life change ($t = 3.32$, 82.03 df, $p = .001$). Although the life change unit (LCU) score for the flood respondents remained higher than that of the non-flood respondents during Period III, January to June, 1975, the difference between groups was not significant.

Ever since Durkheim's (1951) classic work on suicide (written in 1897) showing that suicide was not randomly distributed in the population, researchers have been interested in determining the relationships between psychosocial assets (such as social support and social position) and other behavioral variables, including illness (Levi, 1971; Andrews et al., 1978). Recently, the stress buffering role of social support has been highlighted by Dean and Lin (1978) who believe that increased awareness of the stress buffering functions of social support has important implications for primary prevention of illness, and by Rabkin and Struening (1976) who view individual characteristics, social supports, and social position as being mediating and potentially stress buffering factors in the stress equation (see Figure 1, Individual, Social and Economic Resources, Sections D, E, and F).

Both the Melick and Logue studies, particularly the latter, were interested in investigating the stress buffering role of psychosocial assets in a post-disaster population. In order to investigate this relationship, ten psychosocial items were selected from a larger group of such items (Logue, 1978, pp. 67–68). The items chosen were unique in that they pertained to the actual time of the survey (1977) and no mention of the 1972 flood was made in the wording of the items (to avoid a potential confounding effect with flooding of housing unit and perceived psychosocial assets at the time of the survey). (See Appendix 2 for a complete description). Intercorrelations among the ten psychosocial items were examined and the items were factor-analyzed, using a principal components analysis with varimax rotation. Four factors were identified. Only those variables which had loadings of .50 or greater were selected to represent a given factor. The factor loadings pertaining to each of the four factors obtained from the varimax rotation are displayed in Table 2. Those variables with loadings greater than or equal to .50 are identified by being *underlined* in the table. Items 85, 86, and 87 constitute Factor 1, the respondent's perception of self. Items 74 and 78 make up Factor 2, religious feelings. Items 94 and 96 constitute Factor 3, financial situation. Items 54, 79 and 86 constitute Factor 4, perceived satisfaction with life in general. Item 55 was not selected for any factor, so it was decided to consider this item as an independent variable presented here.

Psychosocial variables pertaining to marriage and children were not considered in the analyses since about 75 percent of both study groups were married and an even smaller percentage of respondents would find the questions on children applicable. It was felt that the ten variables chosen would apply to the largest possible group of respondents. This would assure that adequate sample sizes would be available to each of the eight subgroups to be examined in this section.

A total score for a factor was calculated by summing the actual values of the items constituting that factor. Thus, for Factor 1, a respondent's score on items 85, 86, and 87 was summed to obtain the total Factor 1 score.[4]

Table 2.   Factor Loadings for Psychosocial Items Based on Varimax Rotation

Items	Factor 1	Factor 2	Factor 3	Factor 4
54 Satisfaction with home life	.15	.11	.30	−.63
55 Friends	.47	.38	.28	.45
74 Perceived feelings about religion	.06	.87	−.01	−.11
78 Importance of religion	−.02	.89	−.02	−.11
79 Satisfaction with use of time	.25	.20	.18	−.72
85 Grade compared to others	.81	−.05	.11	−.00
86 Satisfaction with self	.71	.08	.09	−.51
87 Satisfaction with body	.71	.07	.12	−.30
94 Satisfaction with yearly income	.15	−.01	.87	−.15
96 Financial problems	.11	−.02	.87	−.19

The dependent variables chosen were the total Zung score, the total Langner score, and the respondent's rating of her own health and the "average" health rating for her immediate family. These variables were picked with the idea of being "representative" of both the physical health and the mental health questions. Obviously, the large number of health variables necessitated the selection of just a few health variables which would be used as the dependent variables in this section. The Zung and Langner scales appeared as adequate representative measurements of mental health, while the respondent's health rating was judged to be a representative measurement of either the respondent's physical health or the physical health of the immediate family in general.

To test the additive effects of the flood and other significant factors, a three-way analysis of covariance procedure assuming a fixed model was employed. The main effects were flooding of housing unit (yes/no), *average* perceived stress associated with life events which occurred since the 1972 flood (high/low), and perceived psychosocial assets at the time of the 1977 survey (high/low). Thus the design corresponded to a 2X2X2 factorial. Age, education, and income were used as covariates in the three-way analyses. Based on the three-way analyses reported earlier for the same dependent variables considered here, education and income both demonstrated significant regression slopes when used as covariates.[5] In addition, age was still judged an important variable to include in the model, but, rather than employ this variable as a main effect, the variable was used as a covariate. Since there was a priori interest in the results of the multiple comparisons among the eight resultant adjusted means using the three-way model, these comparisons were also performed despite the results of the F test corresponding to the three-way interaction term (Winer, 1971, p. 384). The complete results of the three-way analyses of covariance pertaining to this section are presented elsewhere (Logue, 1978; pp. 243–249). The Newman-Keuls method for multiple comparisons, using the harmonic mean of the eight subgroups, was the basis of testing the differences between all possible pairs of means (Winer, 1971, p. 216). The estimate of the variance used in the Newman-Keuls procedure corresponded to the mean square error term reported in the appropriate Analysis of Covariance table.

Displays of the adjusted means resulting from the three-way covariance procedure for all four dependent health variables are provided for review in Table 3. Tests of the three double interaction terms and the single triple interaction term revealed no statistically significant ($p < .05$) findings with regard to all of the analyses pertaining to Total Langner and Total Zung. (In the interest of conserving space, the complete analysis is not presented here. For additional information, see Logue, 1978, pp. 243–249). This failure to find significant interaction terms demonstrates that the model corresponded to a linear additive model and a review of Table 3 will demonstrate that the joint effect of the main factors yielded results in the expected direction.

The first column of the table represents the subgroup at "highest risk" of

Table 3.   Display of Means* For The 2 × 2 × 2 or Three-way Model Testing the Joint Effect of Flooding (Yes/No), Psychosocial Assets (Low/High), and Perceived Stress Associated with Major Life Events (High/Low)

D E P E N D E N T / V A R I A B L E	Psychosocial Variable	Flooding of Housing Unit							
		Yes				No			
		Psychosocial Assets							
		Low		High		Low		High	
		Perceived Stress for Major Life Events							
		High (n=)	Low (n=)	High (n=)	Low (n=)	High (n=)	Low (n=)	High (n=)	Low (n=)
T O T A L L A N G N E R	Factor 1— Perception of Self	5.92 (97)	3.53 (58)	3.66 (97)	2.23 (82)	5.67 (28)	4.28 (26)	2.73 (38)	1.78 (49)
	Factor 2— Religious Feelings	5.19 (101)	2.65 (74)	4.29 (99)	2.94 (69)	4.32 (29)	3.64 (30)	3.62 (38)	2.03 (48)
	Factor 3— Financial Situation	5.35 (96)	3.21 (37)	4.23 (102)	2.56 (104)	4.84 (37)	3.57 (28)	3.04 (29)	2.24 (49)
	Factor 4— Satisfaction With Life	6.14 (82)	4.42 (42)	3.65 (106)	2.00 (96)	6.92 (21)	4.99 (17)	2.60 (44)	1.95 (56)
	Item 55— Good Friends	4.98 (118)	3.12 (80)	4.47 (83)	2.39 (64)	4.55 (42)	3.31 (45)	2.90 (25)	1.83 (32)
T O T A L Z U N G	Factor 1— Perception of Self	40.40 (91)	37.15 (51)	36.09 (89)	33.41 (74)	40.88 (27)	38.55 (25)	33.91 (37)	33.33 (44)
	Factor 2— Religious Feelings	38.88 (96)	34.90 (67)	37.77 (88)	34.94 (61)	38.75 (27)	37.31 (27)	35.42 (38)	33.60 (43)
	Factor 3— Financial Situation	40.51 (90)	35.19 (35)	36.12 (93)	34.58 (91)	37.52 (36)	37.60 (23)	36.19 (28)	34.22 (45)
	Factor 4— Satisfaction With Life	41.78 (77)	40.37 (37)	35.13 (98)	32.38 (86)	42.19 (21)	40.70 (16)	34.23 (42)	33.39 (51)
	Item 55— Good Friends	38.99 (108)	36.04 (71)	37.21 (76)	33.27 (57)	36.96 (41)	36.59 (42)	36.69 (24)	32.79 (28)

Table 3—Continued

DEPENDENT VARIABLE

HEALTH OF RESPONDENT / AVERAGE HEALTH OF FAMILY

Psychosocial Variable	Flooding of Housing Unit							
	Yes				No			
	Psychosocial Assets							
	Low		High		Low		High	
	Perceived Stress For Major Life Events							
	High (n=)	Low (n=)	High (n=)	Low (n=)	High (n=)	Low (n=)	High (n=)	Low (n=)
Factor 1—Perception of Self	3.12 (95)	2.83 (57)	2.68 (96)	2.37 (80)	3.04 (27)	3.05 (26)	2.33 (36)	2.45 (48)
Factor 2—Religious Feelings	3.00 (101)	2.50 (73)	2.83 (96)	2.66 (68)	2.65 (28)	2.84 (30)	2.64 (36)	2.54 (46)
Factor 3—Financial Situation	2.95 (93)	2.49 (35)	2.89 (101)	2.62 (103)	2.87 (36)	2.98 (28)	2.37 (28)	2.49 (47)
Factor 4—Satisfaction With Life	3.05 (81)	2.96 (41)	2.82 (103)	2.43 (94)	2.93 (20)	3.40 (17)	2.52 (42)	2.44 (55)
Item 55—Good Friends	2.88 (116)	2.67 (78)	2.98 (81)	2.47 (63)	2.71 (41)	2.65 (44)	2.51 (23)	2.65 (31)
Factor 1—Perception of Self	2.98 (96)	2.72 (57)	2.63 (96)	2.38 (81)	2.70 (27)	2.76 (26)	2.31 (36)	2.38 (48)
Factor 2—Religious Feelings	2.86 (101)	2.51 (73)	2.79 (97)	2.55 (69)	2.53 (28)	2.65 (30)	2.47 (36)	2.42 (46)
Factor 3—Financial Situation	2.91 (93)	2.40 (36)	2.76 (102)	2.58 (103)	2.63 (36)	2.84 (28)	2.33 (28)	2.33 (47)
Factor 4—Satisfaction With Life	3.02 (81)	2.70 (41)	2.67 (104)	2.45 (95)	2.58 (20)	2.93 (17)	2.44 (42)	2.39 (55)
Item 55—Good Friends	2.80 (116)	2.58 (79)	2.86 (82)	2.47 (63)	2.45 (41)	2.54 (44)	2.56 (23)	2.45 (31)

*Adjusted means resulting from a 3-way analysis of covariance procedure: (1) 3 main effects—flooding of dwelling unit (Yes/No), *Average* perceived stress due to major life events (High/Low), perceived psychosocial assets (High/Low) at time of survey. (2) 3 covariates—age, education, income.

impairment based on the stress-disease model since this group experienced flooding, low psychosocial assets, and high perceived stress for major life events. It is noteworthy that, in most cases (exceptions: satisfaction with life for Total Langner and Total Zung and perception of self for Total Zung), respondents in this group demonstrated the most mental health symptoms. The last column represents the subgroup at "lowest risk," and in all but one of the cases (satisfaction with life for Total Zung) this group demonstrated the least mental health symptoms. The pair-wise comparisons of the groups in the first and last columns of Table 3 for the mental health dependent variables consistently showed statistically significant (p≤.05) group differences with only one exception (religious feelings for Total Zung).

It is noteworthy that the tests of the three main effects demonstrated that flooding was the least important main effect in the model, and in no case was the test of this main effect significant (p≤.05). Stress due to the flooding of one's home, therefore, was less responsible for mental health symptoms than stress due to life events or low psychosocial assets. However, the joint "stress" effect of these three factors generally revealed the lowest and highest risk subgroups for mental health symptoms which, in most cases, differed at what was noted to be a statistically significant level (p≤.05).

The linear additive model was, in general, not supported for the physical health dependent variables. Specifically, the test of the interaction between flooding and the stress of major life events proved to be either significant or approaching the significant level (p≤.10) in all 10 analyses. A review of Table 3 will, to some extent, help to explain the situation. The effects of stressful life events are of no significance for respondents not experiencing flooding (columns 5-8), but these effects do appear important for the flood victims (columns 1-4). The additive model appears to hold up for the analyses of flood respondents with respect to the following psychosocial variables: perception of self, satisfaction with life, and good friends. The effects of psychosocial assets, however, appears of little consequence with respect to religious feelings and financial situation. Findings from these analyses suggest, therefore, that other life stressors may affect the health status of disaster victims in different ways than they affect non-disaster individuals. General support for the linear additive model for the flood respondents in this study indicates that flood respondents who experience: (1) high stress regarding perception of life events; and (2) low psychosocial assets are at particular risk for physical health symptoms.

Having completed the comparison of flood and non-flood groups on mental and physical health, the flood group was examined in greater detail. The sections which follow further analyze the stress experience for those respondents who experienced flooding of their dwelling unit.

Internal Flood Group Comparisons

Flood respondents from the city of Kingston (N = 392) were further studied by dividing the group into various stress subgroups and conducting a series of internal contrasts. Stress was related to loss phenomena and various adjustments during the recovery period and was measured retrospectively at the time of the survey.[6] Fourteen key variables pertaining to the recovery period were factor analyzed after the matrix of intercorrelations was constructed and inspected (see Table 4). Two hundred and ninety-six respondents provided sufficient information for the factor analysis of these 14 variables. Complete details on these variables are provided in Appendix 3.

The primary factor emerging from the factor analysis subsumed seven of the variables and was regarded as a "subjective" factor measuring general distress. We refer to this factor as Factor 1. A second factor, Factor 2, was also identified. This factor consisted of two variables which both assessed the lack of medical care as perceived by the respondent for the recovery period. The five remaining variables were as follows: (1) damage to home and possessions; (2) use of alcoholic beverages; (3) monetary loss; (4) perceived stress associated with unemployment; and (5) stress associated with temporary living quarters. We viewed the two variables measuring damage to home and monetary loss as "objective" measures of loss in the recovery period. This distinction between subjective and objective was made because, referring to the stress-disease model, it is obvious that individuals are at different levels of sensitivity at the time they become victims of a natural disaster such as the 1972 Agnes flood. This is related to such considerations as levels of social support, internal threshold levels, the experience of major life events, etc. For this reason, a large group of victims, all experiencing the same degree of property damage or the same level of financial loss, will "react" to or perceive these "objective" types of losses in different ways. To illustrate the stressful nature of the recovery period, we will first review

Table 4. Factor Loadings for 14 Items Relating to the Recovery Based on Varimax Rotation

Item	Factor 1	Factor 2
8c Damage to home and possessions	.36	−.01
10 Use of tranquilizers/other Rx	−.54	.24
11 Use of alcoholic beverages	.07	−.06
15 State of mind	.76	.02
16 Estimate of monetary loss	−.09	.09
17 Perceived financial problems	.62	−.12
20 People "cheating" respondent	.63	−.10
21 Perception of physical work (strain)	.69	−.06
27 Stress due to unemployment	−.35	.04
36 Perception of distress, in general	−.72	.19
50 Stress associated with relocation	−.19	.11
70 Regular medical checkups hindered	−.20	.92
71 Required medical attention hindered	−.15	.93
100 Perceived length of recovery period	−.62	.18

some of the initial, univariate results in Logue's study pertaining to many of the experiences in this time period.

Results Relating to the Recovery Period

Most respondents in the flood group indicated that "everything was totally destroyed" or that they experienced "extremely severe damage" when they were asked about the amount of damage to home and possessions which was incurred by the flood. Concerning the "state of mind" of respondents in the flood group after the disaster struck, most women answered that they were "very discouraged" (44 percent). The average perceived property loss for the flood group was in the $10,000–$20,000 range. (The median value was $18,000 in Melick's study.) Most flood group respondents indicated that they experienced "moderate" financial problems as a result of the flood. It is noteworthy that 71 (19 percent) of the flood respondents felt that the work in the recovery period was so hard that someone in the immediate family became sick as a result. Although both the flood group and the non-flood group experienced similar rates of unemployment during the recovery period (about 20 percent for husbands and about 30 percent for respondents), the flood group demonstrated significantly longer rates of unemployment than the non-flood group (nine months versus six months for husbands on the average, and seven months versus four months for respondents on the average.) The average flood respondent indicated that the duration of emotional distress was two years and the duration of physical distress was two and one-half years for the particular family member mentioned as having suffered the most distress. For married respondents, it is interesting to note that, in both the Melick and Logue studies, husbands were most often mentioned as the family member who suffered the most emotional and physical distress. While husbands also demonstrated a longer duration of emotional distress than wives (not statistically significant), wives demonstrated a significantly longer duration (about three years on average) of physical distress than husband (about two and one-half years on average). Most respondents in the flood group indicated that they experienced "moderate" distress with respect to the overall rating of perceived distress in the recovery period. Many respondents in the flood group believed that the flood hindered them from obtaining regular medical check-ups (44 percent) and attention for specific medical problems (35 percent). It is noteworthy that both the mean and median perceived duration of the recovery period for the flood group was calculated to be *18 months*. Most flood respondents indicated that they were housed in one or two temporary living quarters before returning to their own homes and that these temporary living conditions were perceived as "somewhat" stressful.

Both the federal government and the American Red Cross were singled out as rendering the most aid to flood victims during the recovery period, other than the immediate family. Neighbors were identified as rendering the least help. Respondents were questioned about whether various types of social contacts were disrupted by the flood, and comparisons of the flood group and the non-flood group revealed that those in the flood group experienced significantly more disruption with respect to close friends, neighbors, and "the gang."

Two-Way Covariance Analyses

A two-way analysis of covariance procedure was utilized to test the effect of stress in the recovery period upon the longer term physical/mental health symptoms reported by the respondent at the time of the 1977 survey. In the model, age (<55, 55-64, ≥65) and stress (low, medium, or high for Factors 1 and 2; low or high for other variables) associated with the flood experience were the main effects and income and education served as covariates.[7] Total Langner and Total Zung were again selected as representative measures of mental health, while health of respondent and health of immediate family were selected as representative measures of physical health. The results of the analyses of covariance are presented elsewhere (Logue, 1978, pp. 250-255), but the adjusted means corresponding to the stress main effect are presented in Table 5, as well as the statistics pertaining to the tests of that main effect. Clearly, the overall distress factor was consistently related at a statistically significant level to stress in the recovery period. Factor 2, relating to the availability of medical care, demonstrated consistent results for the test of the stress main effect in all cases, with the exception of health of the immediate family. Other significant results were also noted, as can be seen by a review of Table 5. It is interesting, however, that the results for damage to the respondent's home and possessions and monetary loss were not significant for any of the four dependent health variables (a statistical trend was, however, noted regarding monetary loss for Total Langner). These items were viewed as the most "objective" loss variables, but appeared to be the least "sensitive" with respect to distinguishing long term high and low risk subgroups.

Joint Effect of Perceived Stress Associated with the Recovery, Perceived Stress Associated with Major Life Events, and Psychosocial Assets

To test the joint effect of: (1) experiences associated with the recovery period (1972-1974); (2) the presence of stressful life events over the past five years (1972-1977); and (3) the presence or absence of psychosocial assets at the time of the interview (1977), we used an approach somewhat similar to that described earlier in this paper. To simplify the analyses, only the general distress factor (Factor 1) described in Appendix 3 was chosen to represent loss in the recovery period. We adopted a three-way covariance model with loss in the recovery period, perceived stress associated with major life events, and psychosocial assets serving as main effects, and age, education, and income serving as covariates.[8] For the ten psychosocial variables, a factor analytic procedure was performed with respect to disaster victims only and the first three factors identified earlier in Table 2 were again detected. However, Factor 4, corresponding

Table 5.   The Relationship Between Stress Associated With the Recovery Period and Long-Term Mental/Physical Health Symptoms

Dependent Variable	Recovery Period Characteristic	Means (Total Score)*			Statistic	d.f.	Probability (2-tailed)
			Stress				
		Low (n=)	Medium (n=)	High (n=)			
Langner	Factor 1—Overall distress	2.55 (75)	3.70 (119)	6.42 (70)	F = 29.04	2,253	<.01
	Factor 2—Lack of medical care	2.98 (140)	4.96 (76)	5.95 (48)	F = 19.24	2,253	<.01
	Item 8c—Damage to home and possessions	3.78 (119)		4.34 (145)	F = 1.44	1,256	.23
	Item 11—Use of alcholic beverages	3.66 (193)		5.26 (71)	F = 10.45	1,256	<.01
	Item 16—Monetary loss	3.50 (100)		4.45 (164)	F = 3.64	1,256	<.06
	Item 27—Stress associated with unemployment	3.72 (201)		5.27 (63)	F = 7.73	1,256	<.01
	Item 50—Stress associated with temporary living quarters	3.55 (160)		4.92 (104)	F = 7.24	1,256	<.01
Zung	Factor 1—Overall distress	34.5 (75)	35.3 (119)	42.4 (70)	F = 17.17	2,253	<.01
	Factor 2—Lack of medical care	34.9 (140)	38.6 (76)	40.3 (48)	F = 10.29	2,253	<.01
	Item 8c—Damage to home and possessions	36.6 (119)		37.2 (145)	F = .32	1,256	.57
	Item 11—Use of alcoholic beverages	36.1 (193)		39.2 (71)	F = 8.08	1,256	<.01
	Item 16—Monetary loss	36.3 (100)		37.3 (164)	F = 1.48	1,256	.23
	Item 27—Stress associated with unemployment	36.5 (201)		38.4 (63)	F = 3.09	1,256	.08
	Item 50—Stress associated with temporary living quarters	36.6 (160)		37.5 (104)	F = 1.31	1,256	.25

to satisfaction with life, was not detected here. This factor included items 54 and 79. Therefore, psychosocial variables considered in this section correspond to Factors 1–3 and Items 54, 55, and 79.[9] Finally, the dependent health variables were represented by Total Langner and Total Zung (mental health) and by health of respondent and health of immediate family (physical health).

Displays of the adjusted means resulting from the three-way covariance proce-

Table 5—Continued

Dependent Variable	Recovery Period Characteristic	Means (Total Score)*			Statistic	d.f.	Probability (2-tailed)
		Stress					
		Low (n=)	Medium (n=)	High (n=)			
Health of Respondent	Factor 1—Overall distress	2.32 (76)	2.61 (120)	3.20 (71)	F = 16.56	2,256	<.01
	Factor 2—Lack of medical care	2.52 (140)	2.74 (77)	3.08 (50)	F = 7.10	2,256	<.01
	Item 8c—Damage to home and possessions	2.67 (120)		2.70 (147)	F = .05	1,259	.82
	Item 11—Use of alcoholic beverages	2.73 (195)		2.58 (71)	F = 1.44	1,259	.23
	Item 16—Monetary loss	2.63 (102)		2.72 (165)	F = .50	1,259	.48
	Item 27—Stress associated with unemployment	2.66 (204)		2.76 (63)	F = .27	1,259	.61
	Item 50—Stress associated with temporary living quarters	2.58 (162)		2.84 (105)	F = 4.19	1,259	.04
Health of Immediate Family	Factor 1—Overall distress	2.33 (76)	2.61 (120)	3.04 (71)	F = 12.41	2,256	<.01
	Factor 2—Lack of medical care	2.55 (140)	2.70 (77)	2.84 (50)	F = 2.50	2,256	.08
	Item 8c—Damage to home and possessions	2.63 (120)		2.66 (147)	F = .05	1,259	.83
	Item 11—Use of alcoholic beverages	2.69 (196)		2.54 (71)	F = 1.64	1,259	.20
	Item 16—Monetary loss	2.56 (102)		2.70 (165)	F = 1.80	1,259	.18
	Item 27—Stress associated with unemployment	2.61 (204)		2.75 (63)	F = 1.01	1,259	.31
	Item 50—Stress associated with temporary living quarters	2.60 (162)		2.72 (105)	F = 1.05	1,259	.31

*Adjusted means resulting from a 2-way analysis of covariance procedure: (1) 2 main effects—age (<55, 55-64, ≥65), stress associated with recovery period (LOW, MEDIUM, or HIGH for factors 1 & 2; LOW/HIGH for other items) (2) 2 covariates—education, income

dure (Logue, 1978, pp. 258-265) for all four dependent health variables are provided for review in Table 6.

The linear additive model was, in general, supported for the mental health dependent variables (exceptions were religious feelings or Factor 2 for both dependent variables with a significant (p≤.05) triple interaction term and good friends or Item 55 for Total Zung with a significant (p≤.05) triple interaction

Table 6.　　Display of Means* for The 2 × 2 × 2 or Three-way Model Testing the Joint Effect of Perceived Stress for the Recovery (High/Low), Psychosocial Assets (Low/High), and Perceived Stress Associated with Major Life Events (High/Low)

DEPENDENT VARIABLE

		Perception of Stress During the Recovery							
		High				Low			
		Psychosocial Assets							
		Low		High		Low		High	
		Perceived Stress for Major Life Events							
	Psychosocial Variable	High (n=)	Low (n=)	High (n=)	Low (n=)	High (n=)	Low (n=)	High (n=)	Low (n=)
TOTAL LANGNER	Factor 1—Perception of Self	6.67 (55)	5.09 (9)	4.55 (46)	3.78 (15)	4.39 (24)	3.11 (36)	2.00 (30)	1.76 (47)
	Factor 2—Religious Feelings	6.59 (51)	3.19 (19)	4.86 (50)	5.44 (11)	3.11 (33)	2.25 (45)	3.15 (21)	2.45 (38)
	Factor 3—Financial Situation	5.92 (58)	5.80 (10)	5.56 (43)	3.17 (14)	3.63 (18)	2.58 (22)	2.82 (36)	2.23 (61)
	Item 54—Satisfaction with Home Life	6.53 (36)	5.22 (12)	5.33 (65)	3.23 (12)	3.75 (12)	3.87 (12)	2.92 (42)	2.07 (71)
	Item 55—Good Friends	5.73 (61)	4.00 (15)	5.75 (40)	4.60 (9)	3.23 (31)	2.84 (42)	2.98 (23)	1.83 (41)
	Item 79—Satisfaction with the Way Time is Spent	7.34 (37)	5.28 (6)	4.82 (64)	3.86 (18)	4.22 (11)	3.75 (19)	2.82 (43)	1.93 (64)
TOTAL ZUNG	Factor 1—Perception of Self	40.78 (54)	42.07 (8)	37.63 (46)	37.00 (15)	37.14 (24)	36.63 (33)	33.41 (30)	32.01 (46)
	Factor 2—Religious Feelings	41.50 (51)	35.75 (12)	36.95 (49)	42.02 (11)	34.20 (33)	34.83 (43)	36.67 (21)	32.98 (36)
	Factor 3—Financial Situation	41.35 (58)	41.08 (10)	36.78 (42)	37.12 (13)	37.18 (18)	33.98 (21)	33.94 (36)	33.81 (58)
	Item 54—Satisfaction with Home Life	43.08 (36)	42.09 (11)	37.33 (64)	35.63 (12)	40.02 (12)	41.99 (11)	33.71 (42)	32.55 (68)
	Item 55—Good Friends	39.75 (60)	35.87 (14)	38.59 (40)	43.09 (9)	35.44 (31)	36.98 (41)	34.92 (23)	30.67 (38)
	Item 79—Satisfaction with the Way Time Is Spent	42.54 (37)	44.80 (5)	37.39 (63)	36.98 (18)	38.78 (11)	39.08 (19)	34.22 (43)	32.36 (60)

term). In all cases, a significant ($p \leqslant .05$) main effect was observed with respect to the factor of distress during the recovery period. Significant ($p \leqslant .05$) main effects for psychosocial assets and life events were also observed in many cases.

Although the high and low risk subgroups did not always correspond to columns 1 and 8 in Table 6, it is noteworthy that the subgroups appearing in

Table 6—Continued

DEPENDENT VARIABLE

Psychosocial Variable	Perception of Stress During the Recovery							
	High				Low			
	Psychosocial Assets							
	Low		High		Low		High	
	Perceived Stress for Major Life Events							
	High (n=)	Low (n=)	High (n=)	Low (n=)	High (n=)	Low (n=)	High (n=)	Low (n=)
HEALTH OF WOMAN								
Factor 1—Perception of Self	3.19 (54)	3.18 (9)	2.77 (46)	2.93 (15)	2.87 (23)	2.58 (36)	2.37 (30)	2.17 (45)
Factor 2—Religious Feelings	3.07 (51)	3.00 (13)	2.92 (49)	3.04 (11)	2.55 (33)	2.23 (44)	2.67 (20)	2.50 (37)
Factor 3—Financial Situation	3.05 (58)	2.95 (10)	2.90 (42)	3.06 (14)	2.52 (17)	2.17 (20)	2.64 (36)	2.42 (61)
Item 54—Satisfaction with Home Life	3.07 (36)	2.95 (12)	2.95 (64)	3.08 (12)	2.66 (11)	2.54 (12)	2.58 (42)	2.32 (69)
Item 55—Good Friends	2.89 (61)	2.93 (15)	3.15 (39)	3.15 (9)	2.52 (30)	2.43 (41)	2.71 (23)	2.28 (40)
Item 79—Satisfaction with the Way Time Is Spent	3.11 (37)	3.25 (6)	2.93 (63)	2.94 (18)	2.92 (11)	2.34 (19)	2.51 (42)	2.36 (62)
HEALTH OF FAMILY								
Factor 1—Perception of Self	3.06 (55)	2.97 (9)	2.69 (46)	2.99 (15)	2.69 (23)	2.45 (36)	2.30 (30)	2.16 (46)
Factor 2—Religious Feelings	2.84 (51)	2.88 (13)	2.94 (50)	3.08 (11)	2.53 (33)	2.28 (44)	2.39 (20)	2.29 (38)
Factor 3—Financial Situation	2.98 (58)	2.82 (10)	2.76 (43)	3.07 (14)	2.41 (17)	2.13 (21)	2.52 (36)	2.34 (61)
Item 54—Satisfaction with Home Life	2.92 (36)	2.73 (12)	2.87 (65)	3.21 (12)	2.51 (11)	2.19 (12)	2.47 (42)	2.31 (70)
Item 55—Good Friends	2.80 (61)	2.87 (15)	3.01 (40)	3.13 (9)	2.43 (30)	2.32 (42)	2.55 (23)	2.25 (40)
Item 79—Satisfaction with the Way Time Is Spent	3.13 (37)	2.93 (6)	2.75 (64)	2.99 (18)	2.77 (11)	2.29 (19)	2.40 (42)	2.29 (63)

*Adjusted means resulting from a 3-way analysis of covariance procedure: (1) 3 main effects—Factor 1 or general distress in recovery period (High/Low), *Average* perceived stress due to major life events (High/Low), perceived psychosocial assets (High/Low) at time of survey. (2) 3 covariates—age, education, income.

columns 1 and 8 demonstrated significant ($p \leq .05$) pairwise differences in the expected direction in all cases for Total Zung and in three out of six cases for Total Langner—perception of self, satisfaction with home life, and satisfaction with the way time is spent. The findings discussed here, therefore, tend to support an additive effect of three separate factors on the mental health dependent variables—stress associated with the recovery period, stressful life events, and psychosocial assets.

The tests of the interaction terms revealed no statistically significant ($p \le .05$) findings with regard to those analyses pertaining to health of the respondent and health of immediate family (physical health). This would tend to support the linear additive model. However, in most cases, a significant ($p \le .05$) main effect was only observed with respect to the factor of general distress in the recovery period. In other words, the effects due to stressful life events and psychosocial assets on the dependent physical health variables were minimal. These results do not agree with those obtained earlier (see Table 3) using the identical three way covariance model, but substituting, in this case, stress associated with the recovery period for flooding of the dwelling unit as one of the main effects. The results suggest that the most powerful predictor of current physical health status is stress experienced during the recovery period followed by the presence of stressful major life events over the past five years and by the lack of psychosocial assets at present. Flooding of one's dwelling unit appeared the least important predictor.

An inspection of columns 1 and 8 will verify that the high and low risk subgroups with respect to physical health symptoms were in most cases not found in these columns. Furthermore, only three significant ($p \le .05$) pairwise comparisons were noted for the subgroups appearing in columns 1 and 8—perception of self (Factor 2) for both dependent health variables and satisfaction with the way time is spent (Item 79) for health of immediate family. While many interpretations can be proposed to explain the results described in Table 6, the one which we would like to suggest is that the stress associated with the recovery period demonstrated a more consistent and important effect with respect to physical health symptoms than the stress associated with major life events or low psychosocial assets.

Delineating High Risk Groups

In view of the scarce mental health resources, treatment facilities and personnel which may be available in a post-disaster community, it seems prudent to identify groups at greater risk of developing mental health problems. Resources can then be directed toward prevention, particularly primary prevention, of health problems in this group.

To test the hypothesis that "high risk" groups could be identified based on high levels of mental/physical health problems and pre-survey characteristics such as demographic variables or other pertinent variables, multiple regression analyses (both backward and stepwise) were performed using the four dependent health variables also used in previous analyses: Total Langner and Total Zung (mental health); respondent's health and health of immediate family (physical health). Four categories of independent variables pertaining to 30 items on the questionnaire were identified as having a potentially important effect on the dependent health variables:[10]

(1) *social resources* (see Appendix 4—items 28, 29, 37, 39, 19, 46, 40, 41, 42, 31, 45 and 49)
(2) *loss and adjustment experiences* (see Appendix 3—Factor 1 (items 10, 15, 17, 20, 21, 36, 100), Factor 2 (items 70 and 71), and items 8c, 11, 16, 27 and 50)
(3) *stressful life events* (item 97)
(4) *demographic items*—items 91 (age), 80 (education), and 95 (income).

The independent variables which were chosen for the multiple regression procedures appeared to precede the dependent variables in time so that any significant relationship which would appear between a specific independent variable and dependent variable would suggest a possible cause and effect relationship.

A summary of the important results for the multiple regression analyses with respect to the four dependent health variables is provided in Table 7.[11] Both the backward and stepwise techniques produced identical results for all the dependent variables except health of the immediate family. In that case, the techniques gave identical results except for the backward technique which also identified items 29 (religious feelings) and 39 as being significantly (p≤.10) associated with the dependent variable.

A review of Table 7 will reveal that Factor 1 (general distress during the recovery period) was significantly associated with all four dependent health variables.

Factor 2 (medical attention hindered during recovery period), item 46 (financial problems before the flood), item 39 (how well the respondent and her family adjusted to changes resulting from the flood), and item 11 (how helpful alcoholic beverages were in the recovery period) were all significantly associated with three of the four dependent variables.

Item 45 (social contacts disrupted because of the flood) was shown to be significantly associated with the two physical health variables. Finally, item 8c (perceived damage to home and possessions from the flood) was significantly associated with the two mental health measures.

In summary, based on the multiple regression analyses discussed in this section, there is strong evidence to support the hypothesis that "high risk" groups can be identified. High levels of stress associated with Factor 1 (general distress during the recovery period) consistently characterized the "high risk" groups as measured by the four dependent health variables—Total Langner and Total Zung (mental health) and perceived health of the respondent and her immediate family (physical health).

Each of the four dependent health variables appeared to be significantly associated with a number of other independent items not common to both measures of mental health or physical health. A review of Table 7 will help to identify other high risk groups.

Table 7. Results of Stepwise Multiple Regression Analyses*

Dependent Variable	Association**	Variables included in the model***	Probability associated with inclusion in model	Cumulative R^2
Total Langner	−	Factor 1—Overall distress in recovery period†	.0001	.295
	+	Factor 2—Lack of medical care in recovery period	.0010	.328
	−	Item 11—Use of alcoholic beverages in recovery period	.0039	.354
	+	Item 80—Respondent's educational level	.0003	.383
	+	Item 39—Perceived adjustment to changes right after the flood	.0028	.403
	−	Item 46—Perception of financial problems before flood	.0391	.414
	+	Item 29—Perceived feelings about religion after flood	.0449	.425
	+	Item 27—Perceived stress due to unemployment after flood	.0364	.432
	+	Item 97—Perceived stress due to major life events since flood	.0714	.440
	+	Item 95—Annual family income (1976)	.0809	.446
	+	Item 8c—Perceived damage to home and possessions from flood†	.0893	.453
Total Zung	+	Item 39—Perceived adjustment to changes after the flood	.0001	.170
	−	Factor 1—Overall distress in recovery period†	.0002	.234
	+	Item 91—Respondent's age	.0002	.270
	+	Item 8c—Perceived damage to home and possessions from flood†	.0136	.294
	+	Item 11—Use of alcoholic beverages in recovery period	.0142	.312
	+	Factor 2—Lack of medical care in recovery period	.0113	.329
	+	Item 46—Perception of financial problems before flood	.0517	.339

258

Respondent's Health	−	Factor 1—Overall distress in recovery period†	.0001	.177
	+	Item 45—Disruption of social contacts in recovery period†	.0051	.237
	−	Item 29—Perceived feelings about religion after flood	.0092	.252
	−	Item 11—Use of alcoholic beverages in recovery period	.0220	.267
	+	Item 39—Perceived adjustment to changes after the flood	.0209	.279
	+	Factor 2—Lack of medical care in recovery period	.0264	.292
	−	Item 16—Estimate of monetary loss regarding property damage	.0307	.302
	−	Item 80—Respondent's educational level	.0357	.306
Health of Immediate Family	−	Item 95—Annual family income (1976)	.0001	.178
	−	Factor 1—Overall distress in recovery period†	.0001	.259
	−	Item 46—Perception of financial problems before flood	.0287	.274
	+	Item 45—Disruption of social contacts in recovery period†	.0394	.286

*Based on 23 variables (Factor 1 is a 7-item variable; Factor 2 is a 2-item variable) corresponding to social resources, the flood experience, major life events, and demographic items.

**Direction of correlation of the variable with the dependent health variable.

***Only those variables which were significant at the p ≤ .10 level were included in the model.

†Low score signifies greater distress.

Items in italics indicate results which show a trend in the direction opposite of "logical" expectation.

259

DISCUSSION

The research reported here and the previous research reviewed indicate that long-term health effects may be associated with disaster. These changes in physical and mental health may persist for several years following the initial impact of the disaster. Despite the frequency with which disasters occur and despite their potential for affecting life and health, critical research strategies useful for disaster preparedness and prevention of long-term consequences have not been implemented to any great extent. These strategies would include systematic assessment of long-term physical and mental health sequelae associated with the recovery and post-recovery periods and the identification of high risk groups.

In the past decade, the expression "disaster epidemiology" has appeared in numerous medical journals. However, the principal epidemiological concern has been with the effects of natural disasters in developing countries. Mortality has usually served as the primary criterion variable. An opportunity now exists to apply disaster epidemiology to disasters in the United States. Disasters occurring here may be the result of the forces of nature, but increasingly may also be the result of technological failures or the result of the interaction of technology and the forces of nature. Natural and man-made disasters have not been comparable in the past, preventing the prediction of long-term physical and mental health effects of natural disasters from the results obtained through follow-up investigations of victims of war-related disasters. Recent emphasis on man-made disasters due to technological failures, however, has demonstrated that in many cases the same type of "disaster community" can be identified as in natural disaster situations. Thus, people living in the vicinity of Three Mile Island were subjected to the same type of community stress as those who experienced the Agnes flood: people were evacuated, unemployment increased, people had to decide if moving back would be a prudent decision, and ultimately, some people had to decide to leave the area. There was in the Three Mile Island nuclear disaster, of course, the additional physical stress of low-level ionizing radiation which affected those living in the immediate area. Because of the similarities between natural and technological disasters, the disaster community may be approached as a common system in future disaster research. In other words, the disaster community may serve as an ideal epidemiological laboratory for study just as the general community has already served as such a laboratory in previous investigations (Kessler and Levin, 1970).

On a less macroanalytical level, the studies presented in this chapter provide considerable evidence to support the conclusion that the kind and quality of response by individuals experiencing the disruption of a major disaster are strongly associated with subsequent health and mental health status. While there is also evidence to support the long-term effects of a disaster, such as that of the Agnes flood, it appears that the person's appraisal or evaluation of the resulting disruption in normal living and, in particular, the person's method of coping with this crisis are salient factors in the future health and mental health of the individual. Measures of reaction to highly stressful conditions are, in effect, the results of a real life test of the person's ability to cope and have potentially strong implications for the future health and mental health status of individuals. Future research should regard the recovery period (that is, the period beginning with the impact of the disaster and continuing for approximately two years) as a crucial period in the individual's reaction to disaster and should attempt to comprehensively measure salient dimensions of appraisal and coping behavior as important predictors of subsequent health and mental health. In an epidemiological framework, those people who cope poorly with the conditions resulting from a major disaster may be at high risk of experiencing mental and physical disorders in later years. A yield of retrospective studies, such as those described in this chapter, help to identify high risk populations and important constructs to be considered in the planning of prospective studies designed to more fully understand the causal priorities of physical and mental disorders. Of course, the retrospective reports noted here may be distorted by subsequent events; thus, prospective studies would be valuable to verify our conclusions.

The studies presented also implicate other characteristics of individuals and their socioeconomic context as potential predictors of health and mental health status following the experience of a major disaster. The person's age, socioeconomic status, changes in religious beliefs, and the nature of support systems are examples of the variety of characteristics associated with health and mental health status. Although not presented here, the entire data base was stratified into two levels of age, income and education. Review of the outcome of statistical analyses showed that women with lower educational levels and incomes are high risk candidates, regardless of age, concerning their long-term health status. The group at highest risk, however, are women under 65 years with lower levels of education and income.

To identify the many factors which affect health status, and to establish the relative importance of their causal impact in a temporal sequence, would appear to be an important challenge to researchers. Retrospective studies, guided by a comprehensive but well defined theory of social stress, and complemented by empirical methods of high quality, can contribute much to our understanding of the impact of major disasters. In addition, such studies play a salient role in the identification of high risk populations for further study and of those constructs with potential for predicting subsequent health and mental health status. The ultimate outcome of such knowledge, hopefully, would be the planning and implementation of programs designed to prevent large scale physical and mental morbidity in post-disaster populations.

ACKNOWLEDGMENTS

This research was supported in part by a Special Nurse Fellowship, U.S. Public Health Service, Department of Health, Education and Welfare. We gratefully acknowledge the secretarial assistance of Gail Bullis and Leslie Long in the preparation of the manuscript.

NOTES

1. Responders and nonresponders for the control area were compared with respect to the four towns which constituted the control area. Response rates from each of these four towns were statistically similar (p<.50). In addition, the original sample of 755 households was divided into 19 consecutive blocks of households each containing 40 households. The results indicated that the response rates across 19 blocks were statistically similar (p<.25).

2. All analyses were performed using the "SAS 72" statistical package (Service, 1972) with the following procedures: (1) "REGR" procedure—analysis of variance and multiple covariance analysis; (2) "STEPWISE" and "BACKWARD" procedure—multiple regression; (3) "FACTOR" procedure—factor analysis.

3. We assigned the following scores or "weights" to the variable corresponding to perceived health status: 1 = excellent; 2 = better than most; 3 = average; 4 = below average; 5 = poor. "Weighted" means were thereby calculated corresponding to the appropriate assignment of weights. In essence, the variable was considered as a continuous rather than a discrete variable since we employed an ordered six-point scale, thus assuming a continuous underlying distribution. This approach allows the researcher to utilize the more powerful methods of analysis applicable to continuous variables and has been described by Snedecor and Cochran (1967, pp. 243–246) under a section on "ordered classification." The weighted means were also adjusted since the three-way analysis of covariance procedure described in Table 1 (three main effects: flooding of dwelling unit, age, and religion; three covariates: education, income, and dependence on family of origin at time of flood) was employed producing means for the "flood" main effect which were adjusted due to the inclusion of covariates in the model.

4. As with the average perceived stress scores, a display of the total scores for Factors 1–4 in addition to item 55 suggested suitable "cut-points" to dichotomize the scores for both groups. Briefly, scores equal to or greater than 8 for Factor 1, 4 for Factor 2, 6 for Factor 3, 7 for Factor 4, and 3 for item 55 were reclassified as "1" (low psychosocial assets) while scores less than the "cut-points" just mentioned were reclassified as "2" (high psychosocial assets).

5. Dependence on family of origin was not used as a covariate in the present three-way analyses since it failed to show a significant regression slope in the previous three-way analyses. Religion, which was used in the earlier analyses as a main effect, was not included in the present model since the earlier analyses showed no significant effect of this variable on the dependent variables.

6. Recovery period was defined as the time interval extending from impact to approximately two years post-impact.

7. Total scores for Factor 1 (items 10, 36, and 100 were inverted) and Factor 2 were calculated and trichotomized and the scores of the remaining five independent items were dichotomized as described in Appendix 3.

8. For the general distress factor, scores less than 21 were classified "high" stress while scores equal to or greater than 21 were classified "low" stress.

9. The same rules used earlier in this paper to define high and low stress for psychosocial assets and major life events were used again in this section (Items 54 and 79 were classified in the same manner as Item 55).

10. In conducting the analyses, the actual weighted scores obtained for a particular item were, in general, utilized. The total score obtained by summing items 10, 15, 17, 20, 21, 36 and 100 (converted into a five-point scale as described in Appendix 3) corresponded to Factor 1 and the sum of items 70 and 71 corresponded to Factor 2. Items 10, 36 and 100 demonstrated negative loadings in the factor analysis and were inverted before the total score for Factor 1 was obtained. It should be noted that items 45 and 49 were actually "multiple" items on the questionnaire and, in performing the multiple regression analyses, the average score obtained for item 45 and item 49 only was used. The average "stress" score associated with life events was used to represent item 97 while the average "stress" score associated with temporary housing during the recovery period was used to

represent item 50. Finally, with respect to item 11, a score of 5 (I don't drink) was classified 1 (not at all helpful) to simplify the analyses.

11. Results in a direction opposite to what would be "logically" expected are italicized.

REFERENCES

Abrahams, M. J., J. Price, F. A. Whitback, and G. Williams (1976), "The Brisbane floods, January 1974: Their impact on health," *The Medical Journal of Australia* 2:936–939.

Andrews, G., C. Tennant, D. Hewson, and M. Schonell (1978), "The relation of social factors to physical and psychiatric illness," *American Journal of Epidemiology* 108:27–35.

Barton, Allen H. (1970), *Communities in Disaster*. New York: Anchor Books.

Bates, F. L., C. W. Fogelman, V. J. Parenton, R. H. Pittman, and G. S. Tracy (1963), "The social and psychological consequences of a natural disaster: a longitudinal study of Hurricane Audrey," unpublished manuscript, Disaster Research Group, National Academy of Sciences - National Research Council, Disaster Study Number 18, Publication 108.

Bazley, P., and L. L. Viney (1974), "Women coping with crisis: a preliminary community study," *Journal of Community Psychology* 2:321–329.

Bennett, G. (1970), "Bristol floods 1968: Controlled survey of effects on health of local community disaster," *British Medical Journal* 3:454–458.

Bolin, Robert, and Patricia Trainer (1978), "Modes of family recovery following disaster: A cross-national study," pp. 233–247 in E. L. Quarantelli (Ed.), *Disasters: Theory and Research*. Beverly Hills: Sage.

Bruhn, J. et al. (1966), "Social aspects of coronary heart disease in two adjacent, ethnically different communities," *American Journal of Public Health* 56:1493–1506.

Bruhn, John G. et al. (1968), "Social aspects of coronary heart disease in a Pennsylvania German community," *Social Science and Medicine* 2:201–212.

Chapman, Dwight W. (1962), "A brief introduction to contemporary disaster research," pp. 3–22 in George W. Baker and Dwight W. Chapman (Eds.), *Man and Society in Disaster*. New York: Basic Books.

Chodoff, Paul (1970), "Psychological response to concentration camp survival," in Harry S. Abram (Ed.), *Psychological Aspects of Stress*. Springfield, Illinois: Charles C. Thomas.

Cohen, Bernard M., and Maurice Z. Cooper (1954), "A follow-up study of World War II P.O.W.s," Doc. #VA 1.2 (19743). Washington, D.C.: U.S. Government Printing Office, Medical Monograph.

Cohen, Elie A. (1953), *Human Behavior in the Concentration Camp* (translated by M. H. Braaksma). New York: Grosset and Dunlop.

Dansbury, C. W. (1973), "Map of flooded area, Wilkes-Barre and Kingston, Pennsylvania," in David Krantz, *Trouble with Agnes*, Wilkes-Barre, Pa.: D.L.K. Associates.

Dean, Alfred, and Nan Lin (1977), "The stress-buffering role of social support," *Journal of Nervous and Mental Disease* 165:403–417.

Derogatis, L. R., R. S. Lipman, and L. Covi (1973) "SCL-90: an outpatient psychiatric rating scale—preliminary report," *Psychopharmacology Bulletin* 9:13–28.

Derogatis, L. R., R. S. Lipman, K. Rickels, E. H. Uhlenhuth, and L. Covi (1974) "The Hopkins Symptom Checklist (HSCL): a self-report symptom inventory," *Behavioral Science* 19:1–15.

Dohrenwend, Barbara Snell, and Bruce P. Dohrenwend (Eds.), (1974), *Stressful Life Events: Their Nature and Effects*. New York: Wiley.

Durkheim, Emile (1951), *Suicide*. New York: Free Press.

Eitinger, Leo (1971), "Organic and psychosomatic aftereffects of concentration camp imprisonment," *International Psychiatry Clinics* 8:205–215.

Elson, K. A. et al. (1960), "Periodic health examination: nature and distribution of newly diagnosed diseases in executives," *Journal of the American Medical Association*, 172:55–60.

Erikson, Kai T. (1976), *Everything in Its Path: Destruction of Community in the Buffalo Creek Flood*. New York: Simon and Schuster.

Erikson, Kai T. (1976), "Loss of communality at Buffalo Creek," *American Journal of Psychiatry* 133:302–305.

Farberow, Norman L., and Calvin J. Frederick (1978), "Human problems in disasters: pamphlet for government emergency disaster services personnel," Washington, D.C.: DHEW Publication No. (ADM) 78–539, Government Printing Office.

Fox, J. P. (1974), "Family-based epidemiological studies," *American Journal of Epidemiology* 99:165–179.

Franke, David (1974), *America's Fifty Safest Cities*. New Rochelle, New York: Arlington House Publishers.

Friedsam, H. J. (1962), "Older persons in disaster," pp. 151–182 in George W. Baker and Dwight W. Chapman (Eds.), *Man and Society in Disaster*. New York: Basic Books.

Goldberg, E. L., and G. W. Comstock (1976), "Life events and subsequent illness," *American Journal of Epidemiology* 104:146–158.

Greater Wilkes-Barre City Directory (1972), Boston: R. L. Polk.

Greater Wilkes-Barre City Directory (1974), Boston: R. L. Polk.

Greenson, Ralph R., and Thomas Mintz (1972), "California earthquake 1971: some psychoanalytic observations," *International Journal of Psychoanalytic Psychotherapy* 1:7–23.

Gurin, Gerald, Joseph Veroff, and Sheila Feld (1960), *Americans View Their Mental Health*. New York: Basic Books.

Harburg, E., J. C. Erfurt, L. S. Hauenstein, W. J. Schull, and M. A. Schork (1973), "Socioecological stressor areas and black-white blood pressure: Detroit," *Journal of Chronic Diseases* 26:595–611.

Henry, J. P., and J. C. Cassel (1969), "Psychosocial factors in essential hypertension," *American Journal of Epidemiology* 90:171–200.

Hocking, F. (1970), "Extreme environmental stress and its significance for psychopathology," *American Journal of Psychopathology* 24:4–26.

Hocking, Frederick (1970), "Psychiatric aspects of extreme environmental stress," *Diseases of the Nervous System* 31:542–545.

Hocking, F. H. (1971), "Stress and psychiatry," *Medical Journal of Australia* 2:837–840.

Hollingshead, August B. (1957), "Two factor index of social position," Mimeograph, Department of Sociology, Yale University, New Haven, Connecticut.

Holmes, Thomas H., and Richard H. Rahe (1967), "Schedule of Recent Experience," Seattle: University of Washington, School of Medicine, Department of Psychiatry.

Hill, R., and D. A. Hansen (1962), "Families in disaster," pp. 185–221 in G. W. Baker and D. W. Chapman (Eds.), *Man and Society in Disaster,* New York: Basic Books.

James, S. A., and D. G. Kleinbaum (1976), "Socioecologic stress and hypertension-related mortality rates in North Carolina," *American Journal of Public Health* 66:354–358.

Janis, Irving L. (1971), *Stress and Frustration*. New York: Harcourt, Brace, Jovanovich.

Janney, James G., Minoru Masuda, and Thomas H. Holmes (1977), "Impact of a natural catastrophe on life events," *Journal of Human Stress* 3:22–34.

Kafrissen, Steven R., Edward F. Heffron, and Jack Zusman (1975), "Mental health problems in environmental disasters," pp. 157–170 in H. L. P. Resnick and Harvey L. Ruben (Eds.), *Emergency Psychiatric Care: The Management of Mental Health Crisis*. Bowie, Maryland: Charles Press Publishers.

Kessler, Irving I., and Morton L. Levin (1970), "The community as an epidemiologic laboratory," pp. 1–22, in I. I. Kessler and M. L. Levin (Eds.), *The Community as an Epidemiologic Laboratory: A Caseload of Community Studies*. Baltimore: Johns Hopkins Press.

Kinston, Warren, and Rachel Rosser (1974), "Disaster: effects on mental and physical state," *Journal of Psychosomatic Research* 18:437–456.

Klein, Hilel (1971), "Families of holocaust survivors in the kibbutz: psychological studies," *International Psychiatry Clinics,* 8:67–92.

Knaus, R. L. (1975), "Crisis intervention in a disaster area: the Pennsylvania flood in Wilkes-Barre," *Journal of the American Osteopathic Association* 75:297–301.

Krantz, David (1973), *Trouble with Agnes.* Wilkes-Barre, Pa.: D. L. K. Associates.

Krystal, Henry (1971), "Trauma: considerations of its intensity and chronicity," *International Psychiatry Clinics* 8:11–28.

Langner, Thomas S. (1962), "A 22 item screening score of psychiatric symptoms indicating impairment," *Journal of Health and Human Behavior* 3:269–276.

Lazarus, Richard H. (1966), *Psychological Stress and the Coping Process.* New York: McGraw-Hill.

Lazarus, Richard S. (1978), "A strategy for research on psychological and social factors in hypertension," *Journal of Human Stress* 4:35–40.

Lazerwitz, Bernard (1968), "Sampling theory and procedures," pp. 278–328 in Hubert M. Blalock and Ann B. Blalock (Eds), *Methodology in Social Research.* New York: McGraw-Hill.

Levi, Lennart (ed.) (1971), *Psychosocial Environment and Psychosomatic Diseases,* Vol. I. Oxford: Oxford University Press.

Lifton, Robert Jay (1967), *Death in Life.* New York: Random House.

Lifton, Robert Jay, and Eric Olson (1976), "The human meaning of total disaster: the Buffalo Creek experience," *Psychiatry* 39:1–18.

Logue, James Nicholas (1978), "Long-term effects of a major natural disaster: the hurricane Agnes flood in the Wyoming Valley of Pennsylvania, June, 1972. Ph.D. dissertation submitted to School of Public Health, Columbia University.

Lorraine, N. S. R. (1954), In *Medical Officer* 91:59.

MacMillan, Allister M. (1957), "The health opinion survey: technique for estimating prevalance of psychoneurotic and related types of disorder in communities," *Psychological Reports,* 3:325–339.

Melick, Mary Evans (1976), "Social, psychological and medical aspects of stress-related illness in the recovery period of a natural disaster." Ph.D. dissertation submitted to State University of New York at Albany.

Metropolitan Life Insurance Company (March 1977), "Catastrophic accidents—a 35 year review," *Statistical Bulletin* 58:2–4.

Miller, F. J. W. (1974), "The epidemiology approach to the family as a unit in health statistics and the measurement of community health," *Social Science and Medicine* 8:479–482.

Moore, Harry Estill, and H. J. Friedsam (1959), "Reported emotional stress following a disaster," *Social Forces* 38:135–139.

Mussari, Anthony J. (1974), *Appointment with Disaster: The Swelling of the Flood.* Wilkes-Barre, Pa.: Northeast Publishers.

Newland, C. A., W. E. Waters, A. P. Standford, and B. G. Batchelor (1977), "A study of mail survey method," *International Journal of Epidemiology* 6:65–67.

Newman, C. Janet (1976), "Children of disaster: clinical observations at Buffalo Creek," *American Journal of Psychiatry* 133:306–312.

Nuckolls, C., J. Cassel, and B. Kaplan (1972), "Psycho-social assets, life crises and the prognosis of pregnancy," *American Journal of Epidemiology* 95:431–441.

Okura, K. P. (1975), "Mobilizing in response to a major disaster," *Community Mental Health Journal* 11:136–144.

Parker, Gordon (1977), "Cyclone Tracy and Darwin evacuees: on the restoration of the species," *British Journal of Psychiatry* 130:548–555.

Penick, Elizabeth C., Barbara J. Powell, and William A. Sieck (1976), "Mental health problems and natural disaster: tornado victims," *Journal of Community Psychology* 4:64–67.

Perry, Ronald W., and Michael K. Lindell (1978), "The psychological consequences of natural disaster: a review of research on American communities," *Mass Emergencies* 3:105-115.

Poulshouch, S. Walter, and Elias S. Cohen (1975), "The elderly in the aftermath of a disaster," *The Gerontologist* 15:357-361.

Powell, J. W., and Jeanette Rayner (1952), *Progress Notes: Disaster Investigation July 1, 1951-June 30, 1952*. Edgewood, Maryland: Army Chemical Center, Chemical Corps Medical Laboratories.

Price, John (1978), "Some age-related effects of the 1974 Brisbane floods," *Australian and New Zealand Journal of Psychiatry* 12:55-58.

Rabkin, Judith Godwin, and Elmer L. Struening (1976), "Social change, stress, and illness: a selective literature review," *Psychoanalysis and Contemporary Science* 5:573-624.

Rangell, Leo (1976), "Discussions of the Buffalo Creek disaster: the course of psychic trauma," *American Journal of Psychiatry* 133:313-316.

Rennie, Thomas A. C. (1953), "The Yorkville community mental health research study," in Millbank Conference, *Interrelations between the Social Environment and Psychiatric Disorders*. New York: Millbank Memorial Fund.

Richardson, Arthur H., and Howard E. Freeman (1972), "Evaluation of medical care utilization by interview surveys," *Medical Care* 10:357-362.

Romanelli, Carl J., and William M. Griffith (1972), *The Wrath of Agnes*. Wilkes-Barre, Pa.: Media Affiliates.

Schor, S. T. et al. (1964), "An evaluation of periodic health examinations: the findings of 350 examinees who died," *Annals of Internal Medicine*, 61:999-1005.

Service, J. A. (1972), *User's Guide to the Statistical Analysis System*. Raleigh: North Carolina State University Student Supply Stores.

Sigal, John J. (1971), "Second generation effects of massive psychic trauma," *International Psychiatry Clinics* 8:55-65.

Silverman, C. (1968), *The Epidemiology of Depression*. Baltimore: The Johns Hopkins Press.

Snedecor, G. W., and Cochran, W. G. (1967), *Statistical Methods*, 6th ed. Iowa: The Iowa State University Press.

Spiegal, John P. (1957), "The English flood of 1953," *Human Organization* 16:3-5.

Srole, Leo, T. S. Langner, S. T. Michael, M. K. Opler, and T. A. C. Rennie (1962), *Mental Health in the Metropolis: The Midtown Manhattan Study*. New York: McGraw Hill.

Susser, Mervyn (1973), *Causal Thinking in the Health Sciences: Concepts and Strategies of Epidemiology*. New York: Oxford University Press.

Susser, M. W., and W. Watson (1971), *Sociology in Medicine*. New York: Oxford University Press.

Takuma, Taketoshi (1978), "Human behavior in the event of earthquakes," pp. 159-172 in E. L. Quarantelli (Ed.), *Disasters: Theory and Research*. Beverly Hills, California: Sage.

Theorell, T., E. Lind, and B. Flodreus (1975), "The relationship of disturbing life-changes and emotions to the early development of myocardial infarctions and other serious illnesses," *International Journal of Epidemiology* 4:281-293.

Titchener, James L., and Frederick T. Kapp (1976), "Family and character change at Buffalo Creek," *American Journal of Psychiatry* 133:295-299.

U.S. Department of the Army, Corps of Engineers (Baltimore District), (1972), *Wyoming Valley Flood Control, Susquehanna River, Pennsylvania*. Baltimore, Maryland.

U.S. Department of the Army, Corps of Engineers (Undated), *Tropical Storm Agnes*. Washington, D.C.

U.S. Department of Commerce, National Oceanic and Atmospheric Administration (1972), *Final Report of the Disaster Research Team on the Events of Agnes*. Washington, D.C.

U.S. Department of Commerce, Bureau of the Census (1972), *1970 Census of Population and Housing: Census Tracts. Wilkes-Barre and Hazelton, Pennsylvania*, Washington, D.C.

U.S. Department of Health, Education and Welfare, Public Health Service, National Center for

Health Statistics, Publication in Vital and Health Statistics Series (1975), *Health Interview Survey Procedure 1957–1974,* Washington, D.C.: U.S. Government Printing Office.

U.S. Department of Health, Education and Welfare, Public Health Service, National Institute of Mental Health, Psychopharmacology Research Branch (1976), *ECDEU Assessment Manual for Psychopharmacology.* W. Guy (Ed.), Rockville, Maryland: DHEW Publication Number (ADM) 76-338.

Wallace, A. F. C. (1956), "Tornado in Worcester: An explanatory study of individual and community behavior in an extreme situation." Committee on Disaster Studies. National Academy of Science-National Research Council Publication 392, Washington, D.C.

Weissman, Myrna M., and Gerald L. Klerman (1977), "Sex differences and the epidemiology of depression," *Archives of General Psychiatry* 34:98–111.

Wilson, Robert N. (1962), "Disaster and mental health," pp. 124–150, in George W. Baker and Dwight W. Chapman (Eds.), *Man and Society in Disaster.* New York: Basic Books.

Winer, B. J. (1971), *Statistical Principles in Experimental Design.* 2nd ed., New York: McGraw-Hill.

Zung, W. W. K. (1965a), "A self-rating depression scale," *Archives of General Psychiatry* 12:63–70.

———— (1965b), "Self-rating depression scale in an outpatient clinic," *Archives of General Psychiatry* 13:508–515.

————(1967), "Factors influencing the self-rating depression scale," *Archives of General Psychiatry* 16:543–547.

APPENDIX 1

Presence or Absence of Stressful Life Events Over the Last Five Years

Y E S	N O	EVENT	Date the Event Happened?	
			MONTH	YEAR
		Retirement		
		Lengthy separation from loved ones		
		Falling out with your family of upbringing for any reason		
		A death in your family or among your close relatives (WHO)		
		The flood of 1972		
		Serious personal illness or injury (WHO)		
		Severe job dissatisfaction		
		Severe financial problems		
		A broken engagement or romance		
		A broken marriage		
		A miscarriage		
		Loss of job		
		A major disappointment or conflict with any member of your family		
		Serious marital conflicts		
		Heavy drinking by someone in your family		
		Heavy gambling by someone in your family		
		A nervous disorder in a member of the family		
		Severe upsets with children or close relatives		
		Legal problems		
		Birth of a child		
		Family member leaving home		
		Close friends or relatives leaving the area		
		Something else you can think of (WHAT)		

Respondents were given the following directions on the questionnaire for item 97:

"Over the *last 5 years,* which of the following life events have your and your immediate family experienced? (*Check YES or NO* for each event.) If *YES,* provide the *additional* information which is requested in the *spaces provided* to the immediate *right* of the event."

Respondents were further directed to rate the stressfulness of each event using the six-point scale 1=not too stressfull, 2=just a bit, 3=somewhat, 4=quite a bit, 5=very stressful, 6=extremely stressful:

"How 'stressful' for your and/or your immediate family would you say this particular event was?"

APPENDIX 2

Select Psychosocial Questions (Items) Pertaining to the Time of the Survey in 1977 and not Associated with the Flood Experience

Item 54 How satisfied are you with your home life at present?
(Scale) 1=Very satisfied, 2=Moderately satisfied, 3=Somewhat satisfied, 4=Not sure but probably satisfied, 5=Not sure but proba-

bly dissatisfied, 6=Somewhat dissatisfied, 7=Moderately dissatisfied, 8=Very dissatisfied.

Item 55 How many good, close personal friends would you say you have?
(Scale) 1=Large number, 2=Good number, 3=Some, 4=Just a few, 5=No close friends.

Item 74 Would you describe yourself as:
(Scale) 1=Very religious, 2=Moderately religious, 3=Somewhat religious, 4=Not at all religious.

Item 78 Aside from going to church, how important would you say religion is to you in your own life?
(Scale) 1=Very important, 2=Moderately important, 3=Somewhat, 4=Not at all.

Item 79 Would you say that you are satisfied with the way you spend most of your time right now? In other words, if you are working for a living, how satisfied are you with the job? If you are a housewife, are you satisfied with doing this? If you are unemployed, retired, disabled, etc., how satisfied are you with the way most of your time is spent?
(Scale) 1=Very satisfied, 2=Moderately satisfied, 3=Somewhat satisfied, 4=Not sure but probably satisfied, 5=Not sure but probably dissatisfied, 6=Somewhat dissatisfied, 7=Moderately dissatisfied, 8=Very dissatisfied.

Item 85 In general, if you had to compare yourself with the average woman your age, what grade would you give yourself, would you say:
(Scale) 1=Excellent, 2=Very good, 3=Good, 4=Average, 5=Below average, 6=A lot below average.

Item 86 In general, how satisfied are you with yourself? Would you say:
(Scale) 1=Very satisfied, 2=Somewhat satisfied, 3=Not sure but probably satisfied, 4=Not sure but probably dissatisfied, 5=Somewhat dissatisfied, 6=Very dissatisfied.

Item 87 In general, how satisfied are you with your body? Would you say:
(Scale) 1=Very satisfied, 2=Somewhat satisfied, 3=Not sure but probably satisfied, 4=Not sure but probably dissatisfied, 5=Somewhat dissatisfied, 6=Very dissatisfied.

Item 94 How satisfied are you with your immediate family's present total yearly income? Would you say:
(Scale) 1=Very satisfied, 2=Somewhat satisfied, 3=Not sure but probably satisfied, 4=Not sure but probably dissatisfied, 5=Somewhat dissatisfied, 6=Very dissatisfied.

Item 96   Lately how easy or difficult has it been for you (or your spouse) to pay for the expenses that come up from month to month?

(Scale) 1=Very easy, 2=Somewhat easy, 3=Not too easy, 4= Somewhat difficult, 5=Very difficult.

APPENDIX 3

Questions (Items) Specifically Relating to Loss and Adjustment Experiences

Factor 1 - General Distress During Recovery Period

Item 10*   Did you find that you were using tranquilizers or other medications to help you calm down after the 1972 flood?

(Scale) 1=Not at all, 2=Some of the time, 3=Quite a bit of the time, 4=Most of the time.

Item 15   Which of the following statements best describes your state of mind after the flood occurred?

(Scale) 1=So discouraged felt like giving up completely, 2=Very discouraged, 3=Moderately discouraged, 4=Somewhat discouraged, 5=Not at all discouraged.

Item 17   Which one of the following statements best describes how much of a financial problem you and your immediate family experienced because of the flood?

(Scale) 1=Severe financial problems, 2=Moderate problems, 3= Some problems, 4=No financial problems.

Item 20   How many times in the recovery period after the flood did you feel that people were trying to cheat you?

(Scale) 1=All of the time, 2=Practically all of the time, 3=Very often, 4=Fairly often, 5=Sometimes, 6=Just a few times, 7=Not at all.

Item 21   If your home was flooded, how do you feel about the physical work you and your immediate family had to do after the flood to get your home back in shape?

(Scale) 1=Work was so hard someone in family became sick, 2-Very hard work (really wore us out), 3=Hard work (proceeded without many problems), 4=Worked consistently (very few problems), 5=Worked at own pace (things went along smoothly), 6=Did not work that hard, 7=Someone else did most of the work.

Item 36*   Which of the following best describes the amount of distress you and your immediate family experienced, in general, in the long recovery period after the flood?

(Scale) 1=None, 2=Slight, 3=Moderate, 4=Severe, 5=Very severe.

Item 100* It took some families a long time to get things "back to normal" after the 1972 flood occurred while other families may have recovered in a short period of time. The time period which is necessary to restore things back to normal is defined as the "recovery period". In terms of your own personal experiences, which of the following best describes how long the "recovery period" lasted for you and your own immediate family?
(Scale) 1=1 to 6 months, 2=7 to 12 months, 3=13 to 17 months, 4=19 to 24 months, 5=more than 24 months.

Factor 2 - Lack of Medical Care During Recovery:

Item 70 How much did the flood hinder you and your immediate family from getting regular medical check-ups?
(Scale) 1=Not at all, 2=Somewhat, 3=Moderately, 4=Very much.

Item 71 How much did the flood hinder you and your immediate family from seeing a medical doctor for a specific problem or problems which required medical attention?
(Scale) 1=Not at all, 2=Somewhat, 3=Moderately, 4=Very much.

Other Items:

Item 8c Which of the following best describes the damage which was done to your home and possessions as a result of the flood?
(Scale) 1=Everything totally destroyed, 2=Extremely severe damage, 3=Very severe damage, 4=Severe damage, 5=Moderate damage, 6=Some damage.

Item 11 How helpful would you say that drinking wine, beer, or liquor was to you after the flood to help you relax and forget your problems?
(Scale) 1=I don't drink or Not at all helpful, 2=Somewhat helpful, 3=Moderately helpful, 4=Very helpful.

Item 16 Try to estimate the total amount of property damage you experienced as a result of the flood in terms of money lost.
(Scale) 1=None, 2=Under $10,000, 3=$10,000 to $20,000, 4=$20,000 to $30,000, 5=$30,000 to $40,000, 6=$40,000 to $50,000, 7=Over $50,000.

Item 27 If either you or your husband (if you were married at the time of the

*These items were inverted before summing to calculate Factor 1

flood) or both of you were unemployed due to the flood, how ''stress-ful'' was the situation for you and your family?
(Scale) 1=Not at all stressful, 2=Somewhat, 3=Moderately, 4= Very stressful.

Item 50   How ''stressful'' for you and your family would you say it was living at this location (each temporary living quarters after the flood)?
(Scale) 1=Not too stressful, 2=Somewhat, 3=Moderately, 4= Very, 5=Extremely stressful.

Stress

For factor 1, scores less than 18 corresponded to ''high'' stress, scores between 18 and 24 corresponded to ''medium'' stress, and scores greater than 24 corresponded to ''low'' stress.

For Factor 2, scores less than 3 corresponded to ''low'' stress, scores of either 3 or 4 corresponded to ''medium'' stress, and scores greater than 4 corresponded to ''high'' stress.

For variables 8c, 11, 16, 27 and 50, low and high stress groups were defined using the following rules: for variable 8c, scores less than 3 corresponded to high stress while scores equal to or greater than 3 corresponded to low stress; for variable 11, scores equal to 1 corresponded to low stress while scores of 2, 3, or 4 corresponded to high stress; for variable 16, scores equal to or less than 3 corresponded to low stress while scores greater than 3 corresponded to high stress; for variable 27, scores of 1 or 0 (if not applicable) corresponded to low stress while scores greater than 1 corresponded to high stress; for variable 50, an average stress score less than or equal to 2 corresponded to low stress while an average score greater than 2 corresponded to high stress.

APPENDIX 4

Select Pre-Survey (1972–1977) Social Resources Questions (Items)
Associated with the Flood Experience

Item 19 Are you still in debt because of the flood?
(Scale) 1=Yes, deeply in debt, 2=Yes, moderately in debt, 3=Yes, somewhat in debt, 4=Yes, but the debt is small, 5=No, we paid off the debt, 6=No, we never had a debt because of the flood.

Item 28 In general, how religious were you just before the Agnes flood? Would you say:
(Scale) 1=Very religious, 2=Religious, 3=Somewhat religious, 4=Not religious.

Item 29 Which of the following best describes what effect the Agnes flood had on your feelings about religion?
(Scale) 1=Became much more religious, 2=Became somewhat more religious, 3=Stayed about as religious as before the flood, 4=Became somewhat less religious, 5=Became much less religious.

Item 31 In terms of your own family experiences, do you think your community has improved or deteriorated since the flood of 1972?
(Scale) 1=Very much improved, 2=Moderately improved, 3=Somewhat improved, 4=No noticeable change, 5=Somewhat worse, 6=Moderately worse, 7=Very much worse.

Item 37 Do you think that, because of the flood, your family grew closer together or became farther apart?
(Scale) 1=Grew much closer, 2=Grew somewhat closer, 3=Grew just a little closer, 4=No noticeable change, 5=Grew a little farther apart, 6=Grew somewhat farther apart, 7=Grew much farther apart.

Item 39 In general, how well do you think you and your family have adjusted to the changes in your community and in your own lives resulting from the 1972 flood?
(Scale) 1=Very well, 2=Fairly well, 3=Not too well but not too poorly either, 4=Somewhat poorly, 5=Very poorly.

Item 40 Would you say you had a good relationship with your family of origin (your mother, father, and any sisters or brothers you may have had) before the 1972 flood?
(Scale) 1=Very good, 2=Good, 3=Not good but not poor either, 4=Poor, 5=Very poor.

Item 41 How much did you depend on your family of origin for such things as love, companionship, and help in general when the flood occurred in 1972?
(Scale) 1=Very much, 2=Moderate amount, 3=Somewhat, 4=Just a little, 5=Not at all.

Item 42 What effect, if any, did the flood have on your relationship with your family of origin?
(Scale) 1=We grew much closer, 2=We grew somewhat closer, 3=We grew just a little closer, 4=No noticeable change, 5=We grew a little farther apart, 6=We grew somewhat further apart, 7=We grew much farther apart.

Item 45 After the flood, did you find that your social contacts were disrupted regarding the following groups (relatives who lived close when the flood happened, other relatives, close friends, neighbors, the "gang", friendly acquaintances)?

(Scale) 1=Very much, 2=Quite a bit, 3=Somewhat, 4=Just a little, 5=Not much at all, 6=Not at all.

Item 46 Were you and your immediate family having financial problems just before the flood of 1972?

(Scale) 1=Not at all, 2=Just a little, 3=Some problems, 4=Moderate problems, 5=Very many problems, 6=Severe problems.

Item 49 How much did the following people or groups help you and your family out in terms of getting you "back on your feet" after the flood occurred? (Eleven groups were specifically rated: (1) the respondent and her immediate family, (2) other relatives, (3) close friends, (4) neighbors, (5) American Red Cross, (6) Salvation Army, (7) the Church, (8) strangers, (9) the federal government, (10) state government, (11) local government. Two additional spaces were also available for "write in" groups who offered help.)

(Scale) 1=Helped very much, 2=Moderately, 3=Somewhat, 4=Just a little, 5=Not help at all.

FAMILIES OF HYPERACTIVES

Lily Hechtman

INTRODUCTION

In recent years, there have been several studies that have addressed themselves to the problem of psychiatric illness in families of hyperactive children. Morrison and Stewart (1971) interviewed parents of 59 hyperactives and 41 control children and showed a high prevalence of alcoholism, sociopathy, and hysteria in fathers and mothers of hyperactive children. They also found that significantly more parents of hyperactive than control children had probably been hyperactive as children themselves. This suggested associations of adult and childhood psychiatric disorders and they questioned whether childhood hyperactivity might be related to alcoholism, hysteria, and sociopathy and whether the hyperactive child syndrome was transmitted genetically or socially from parent to child.

Cantwell's (1972) findings were similar. He gave a systematic psychiatric examination to parents of 50 hyperactive children and 50 matched controls. Increased prevalence rates for alcoholism, sociopathy, and hysteria, but not affective disorders, were found in parents of hyperactive children. Ten percent of the parents of hyperactive children were thought to be hyperactive as children

Research in Community and Mental Health, Volume 2, pages 275–292
Copyright © 1981 by JAI Press, Inc.
All rights of reproduction in any form reserved.
ISBN: 0-89232-152-0

themselves; and of this 10 percent, all were psychiatrically ill with alcoholism, sociopathy or hysteria. Cantwell felt that the hyperactive child syndrome is passed from generation to generation and may be a precursor for certain adult psychiatric illness. Whether this transmission was environmental or genetic remained unclear.

In a later study, Cantwell (1975) discusses the evidence of a genetic component in the hyperactive child syndrome and concludes that further family studies, including twins and adoptees, are needed. One such study, involving a comparison of adoptive and biological parents of hyperactive children was carried out by Morrison and Stewart (1973a). They interviewed the legal parents of 35 adopted hyperactive children. These children had almost no contact with their biological parents, having been cared for by hospital nurseries, adoption agencies, or foster homes prior to placement at an average age of 15.7 weeks. The high prevalence of hysteria, sociopathy, and alcoholism found in biological parents of hyperactive children was not found in adopting parents. Also, adopting parents were not as likely to have been hyperactive themselves.

Morrison concluded that this supported a genetic transmission. In two subsequent papers (Morrison and Stewart, 1973b, 1974), the authors tried to make a case for a polygenic mode of inheritance.

In another study involving adoptees, Goodwin et al. (1975) connect alcoholism with the hyperactive child syndrome by showing that alcoholics as children were more often hyperactive, truant, antisocial, shy, aggressive, disobedient, and friendless. The authors acknowledged the limitation of the retrospective approach to the problem, but cited literature suggesting the relationship between the hyperactive child syndrome and subsequent alcoholism, as well as a possible relationship between these disorders and antisocial behavior.

Thus, although several studies (Morrison, 1971; Cantwell, 1972) have linked the hyperactive child syndrome with the prevalence of alcoholism, sociopathy, and hysteria in biological parents, the association with affective disorders is less pronounced. Stewart and Morrison (1973) determined the incidence of bipolar and unipolar[1] affective disorder among natural relatives of 59 hyperactive children, legal relatives of 35 adopted hyperactive children, and relatives of 41 control children. There were no significant differences in the incidence of the two conditions between the groups of relatives, except for a greater incidence of unipolar affective disorder in the combined second degree blood relatives of hyperactive children compared to relatives of controls. Moreover, the incidence of bipolar affective disorder in natural parents of hyperactive children was much lower than figures reported for parents of patients with this type of affective disorder. Therefore, the data did not support a connection between hyperactivity in childhood and adult manic depressive affective disorder.

In a recent paper, Stewart (1979) has pointed out that earlier family studies (Morrison and Stewart, 1971; Cantwell, 1972) have suffered from three limitations. Firstly, investigators used normal children as controls rather than children attending a psychiatric clinic for reasons other than hyperactivity. Thus, the increased psychopathology seen in relatives of hyperactive children may be seen in all families who bring their children to child psychiatric clinics for emotional problems and may not be particularly related to hyperactivity. Secondly, hyperactivity is generally very broadly defined. Other behaviors—for example, resistance to discipline, aggression, and specific antisocial behaviors—have been included in the criteria for diagnosing this syndrome. The adult disorders found associated with hyperactivity in children may actually be related to some other dimension of the children's behavior—for example, aggressiveness or antisocial behavior.

Finally, many of the studies were not done "blind." Interviewers were aware that the parents were relatives of a hyperactive or a control child and this may have affected their ratings.

Stewart and his group have sought to show that when the above limitations are corrected, different results are obtained regarding psychiatric illness in parents of hyperactive children.

The group has focused on the "unsocialized aggressive" boy, and has found (Stewart, 1978a) that relatives of these boys (for example, fathers, uncles, siblings) had a higher incidence of antisocial personality disorders than a matched control group of boys coming for psychiatric help for other problems.

Unfortunately, 14 of 17 boys in the "unsocialized aggressive" group were also diagnosed as being hyperkinetic. It is thus unclear if the results reflect a connection with unsocialized aggression of the boys or a combination of hyperactivity *and* unsocialized aggression.

Stewart (1978b) distinguished between the two groups in the following way:

> To qualify as hyperactive, a boy had to be described as being unusually active, energetic, and having difficulties concentrating or finishing tasks, both to a marked degree and persisting over at least the past year. To qualify as unsocialized aggressive, a boy had to have the following items: aggressiveness (shown by fighting, extreme competitiveness, attacks on adults or verbally abusing adults), resistance to discipline (not following directions, impossible to control, out late at night, or doing the opposite of what parents want), and either destructiveness (fire setting, destroying private property or destroying public property), or meanness (frequent quarrels, taking revenge or bullying). Again, these symptoms had to have been present to a marked degree for longer than a year.

Stewart (1978b) re-examined the prevalence of alcoholism and antisocial disorders in parents of hyperactive and unsocialized aggressive boys. His finding that antisocial personality and alcoholism occurs more frequently in the fathers of unsocialized aggressive boys, is not surprising. However, 27 of the 38 subjects classified as unsocialized aggressive were *also* hyperactive—so again, it may well be this combination which is significant.

We thus see that earlier studies (Cantwell, 1972; Morrison et al., 1971, 1973) have suggested a strong relationship between childhood hyperactivity and parental problems with alcoholism, antisocial disorders, and hysteria. More recent work (Stewart et al., 1978a, 1978b, 1979) which is somewhat better controlled, has questioned the relative significance of hyperactivity in children versus unsocialized aggression in connection with this adult psychopathology. However, the very significant overlap, with many children showing both these symptoms, leaves the issues unclear. Obviously, larger, more distinct samples with less overlap need to be studied to clarify these issues.

Preliminary findings of our ten-year prospective follow-up study of hyperactives as young adults (Hechtman, Weiss, Finkelstein et al., 1976) indicated that although these subjects continued to have problems in a number of areas (e.g., restlessness, cognitive style, social skills, and emotional well being) they do not load the psychiatric or antisocial population as reported by others (Menkes, Rowe, and Menkes, 1967). It thus became important to assess if the families of our group of hyperactive subjects were also functioning differently (better) than has generally been reported by Cantwell (1972) and others (Morrison et al., 1971).

The first part of our study, therefore, consisted of a comparison of 65 families of hyperactive young adult subjects and 43 families of control subjects matched for socioeconomic class. In addition to the socioeconomic factors, areas such as child rearing practices, physical and mental health of family members, and family relationships were assessed. The families of our hyperactive subjects had had similar assessments initially and at five-year follow-up in the areas outlined above. We thus had an opportunity to evaluate if and how families had changed in these areas with time, and whether these changes had any relationship to the hyperactives' functioning. This sequential evaluation of families of hyperactives constituted a second part of our study.

The preliminary report on hyperactives as young adults (Hechtman et al., 1976) indicated that their functioning had improved when compared to the five-year follow-up study during adolescence. We were also surprised to see many of the subjects still living at home in spite of previous marked conflicts with families. It thus became important to assess the families' view of the subjects' current functioning. Did the families also perceive their children's improvement? Had past conflicts between the hyperactives and families subsided, or have the past negative experiences and expectations of the families made it difficult for improvements to register with them? Thus, the families' view of the subjects' current functioning constitutes the third part of the study.

Finally, we compared the parents' view of their children's functioning at different ages in their development. What improvements or difficulties did they perceive at these various stages? This was the fourth and final part of the study.

METHOD

Subjects

Sixty-five families of hyperactives being assessed in a ten-year follow-up study (Hechtman et al., 1976) were compared with 43 families of normal control subjects matched with the hyperactives for age (range 17 to 24 years), sex, I.Q. (all above 85), and socioeconomic class (each group having equal representation from each class.

Subjects in the hyperactive group had been referred to the Montreal Children's Hospital Department of Psychiatry 10 to 13 years ago with a major problem of sustained chronic hyperactivity, both at school and at home. They were then six to 12 years of age, all of normal intelligence, free of epilepsy, cerebral palsy and psychosis, and living at home with at least one parent. Shortly after their initial evaluation, the group (numbering 104) took part in a short-term drug study to determine the effect of chlorpromazine and dextroamphetamine on behavior and learning (Werry et al., 1966; Weiss et al., 1968). Ninety one of the 104 children were re-evaluated in a series of follow-up studies during their adolescence five to six years after initial assessment (Weiss et al., 1971; Minde et al., 1971, 1972).

In the present study, 76 of these 91 subjects agreed to participate once more while nine subjects refused. The most common reason for refusal given over the telephone was that they were "doing well" and did not wish to be reminded of their problems. All nine who refused to come for follow-up stated that they were living at home and were working or going to school. Six subjects could not be traced.

Twenty-eight subjects who were seen initially but not evaluated at ten-year follow-up (either because they could not be traced or because they refused evaluation) were compared to the 76 hyperactive subjects who were evaluated with respect to initial I.Q., socioeconomic class, sex, and initial measurements of hyperactivity. Findings showed that there was no difference between the two groups.

In general, the hyperactive subjects represent a relatively untreated group, with few receiving adequate counselling or drug therapy. Therefore, the group provides good baseline data for comparison with data from groups who have received prolonged specific treatment.

Sixty-five of the 76 families of hyperactives participated in the family evaluations. The 11 missing families were not included either because the families had moved out of town or refused to participate.

The control group consisted of 44 subjects. Thirty-five of these were selected in 1968 at the time of the five-year follow-up study of hyperactive children. At that time, notices were posted in three high schools asking for volunteers to participate in some studies on adolescents in which they would be required to talk with a psychiatrist and do some pencil and paper tasks. Payment was offered for volunteers who were selected. The three high schools were selected to represent a range of economic classes. Many students volunteered and we included those who met the following criteria: (1) they matched individually with a hyperactive subject on age, I.Q. (Wechsler Intelligence Scale for Children), socioeconomic class, and sex; (2) they had never failed a grade; (3) neither teachers nor parents complained that they were or had been a behavior problem.

At the beginning of the ten-year follow-up study, we decided to enlarge the control group from 35 to 45. The additional subjects included were generally referred to us by another control subject as being someone they knew at work or at school. The same inclusion criteria already described were used to select amongst these additional volunteers. Forty-three families of control subjects agreed to participate in the family interviews. Unfortunately, control families were not interviewed at five-year follow-up, so only the current assessments are available for these families.

Family Interview

One of the parents, usually the mother (but occasionally the father or both parents), was interviewed in a well-outlined though open-ended interview by a psychologist or social worker. During the early part of the training of a new interviewer, two interviewers saw a family together, with one doing the interview and the other sitting in. The roles of the two interviewers were reversed for the next family. After the interview was completed, each interviewer independently scored all relevant variables in the family interview. The training process ended when the agreement on scores was high, and the interviewing style was similar. At the beginning of the interview, examiners were "blind" as to whether this was the family of a hyperactive or control subject. Families were thus assessed on socio-cultural factors, child rearing practices, physical and mental health of family members, and family relationships (Table 1). The same questionnaire was used to assess families of hyperactives initially, at five-year follow-up and at ten-year follow-up. Scores on various items were compared at each of these three stages (Table 3).

Following the interview, families were asked to complete a number of forms which dealt with their view of their children's functioning, past and present. These forms included:

Family's Current Assessment of Young Adult's Functioning
   1. Katz family rating of subject's psychopathology (Hogarty and Katz, 1971). This scale measured the family's impressions of its child on various psychopathological parameters, on a four-point scale (Table 4).
   2. Form outlining the family's current view of the child's functioning vis-a-vis plans, work, school, friends, money, drugs, etc. Possible areas of conflict were also noted (Table 5).

Family's View of Child's Functioning at Various Stages of Development
   Three questionnaires—one for the preschool, one for the elementary school, and one for the high school period—were designed to tap social, academic, and hyperkinetic parameters. Parents were asked to complete these questionnaires. Most items required that they score them on a five-point scale (1, Hardly ever; 2, Sometimes; 3, Usually; 4, Nearly always; 5, Always).
   Data which included the assessment of families of hyperactive and control subjects and their responses on the various questionnaires outlined above, was analysed via chi squares or analysis of variance, whichever was most appropriate.

RESULTS

Current Assessment of Families of Hyperactive and Control Subjects at 10 Year Follow-Up (Table 1)

1. *Socio-Cultural Factors.* In view of the fact that both groups were matched for socioeconomic class (each group having an equal representation from each class), most of the sociocultural factors reflecting socioeconomic class were, as expected, not significantly different for the families of hyperactives and

Table 1. Current Evaluation of Families of Controls versus Hyperactives
Ten-year Follow-up

	Mean (HA) (N = 61-65)	Mean (Control) (N = 41-43)		
o Cultural Parameters				
vel of Education				
(Mother)	10.32	10.88		
(Father)	10.6	12.2		
	Chi²	*Df*	*Significance*	*Direction*
ther's Working Status (Hollingshead)	4.8	6	—	—
other's Working Status (Hollinghsead)	5.82	6	—	—
other Working	.21	1	—	—
ysical Qualities of Home	6.12	4	—	—
mily Size	4.2	5	—	—
hild Offspring of Previous Marriage	.57	1	—	—
hild Adopted	2.6	1	—	—
bling Order	12.19	4	p = .01	More HA's Eldest
d Rearing Practices				
ontinued Presence of Mother or Stable Substitute	3.36	4	—	—
consistent	6.7	4	—	—
ck Control	2.4	4	—	—
nitive-Authoritative	8.4	4	p = .07	Controls Better
ver-Protective	2.9	4	—	—
lth of Family Members				
ysical Illness in Family	.09	1	—	—
eath in Family	.06	1	—	—
ental Health of Family Members	8.9	4	p = .06	Controls Better
tionships				
arital Relationship	9.2	5	p = .09	Controls Better
motional Climate of Home	3.4	4	p = .009	Controls Better
of Scores of Family Scale:	34.4 (Mean HA)	37.8 (Mean Control)	p = .004	Controls Better

controls. No significant differences were seen also in other social factors such as family size, whether the subject was adopted or an offspring of a previous marriage. With respect to sibling order, hyperactives were significantly more frequently the eldest (p = .01).

2. *Child Rearing Practices.* Of the child rearing parameters assessed which included inconsistency, lack of controls, punitive-authoritative, and over-protective styles, only the punitive-authoritative parameter tended to be more marked in families of hyperactive subjects (p = .07).

3. *Health of Family Members (Tables 1 and 2).* There was no difference in the prevalence of physical illness or deaths in the two groups of families, but parents of hyperactives tended to have more mental health problems (p = .06). Unfortunately, the types of mental health problems which prevailed were not specifically categorized. However, the severity was categorized on a five-point scale. "Severe" referred to any condition which required psychiatric hospitalization, psychotic conditions, character disorders with multiple offences, or drug addiction including alcoholism. "Mild" referred to any neurotic condition.

We see (Table 2) that seven of 41, or 17 percent, of families of controls had psychiatric treatment compared to 18 of 65, or 28 percent, of families of hyperactives. However, when one examines a history of psychiatric symptoms in family

Table 2. Mental Health of Family Members
Ten-year Follow-up

	Hyperactives (N = 65)		Controls (N = 41)	
Item	Number	Grouped Percent	Number	Grouped Percent
Psychiatric treatment for severe mental disorder of both parents	1		0	
Psychiatric treatment for severe mental disorder of one parent or milder disorder of both parents	8	28%	3	17%
Psychiatric treatment for mild disorder of one parent	9		4	
No treatment but symptoms present on and off in one or both parents	27	41%	10	24%
Good dynamic integration of both parents	20 / 65	31% / 100%	24 / 41	59% / 100%

(a) Significance of Table: Chi^2 = 7.99; 2df; p < .05

members with no treatment having been received, we see that 10 of 41, or 24 percent, of control families had such symptoms compared to 27 of 65, or 41 percent, of hyperactive families. We thus see that the striking difference in the mental health of family members in the two groups lies not in severe psychiatric pathology which requires treatment, but in milder symptoms which usually go untreated. Finally, a significantly higher proportion of parents of controls versus hyperactives showed good dynamic integration (Table 2: p = .05).

4. *Relationship.* Marital relationship also tended to be worse in families of hyperactives (p = .09). However, the two most significant findings indicated that the emotional climate of the home (p = .009) and the overall family score (p = .004) were considerably worse in families of hyperactives when compared to those of controls. Emotional climate of the home referred to the degree of positive versus negative interactions amongst family members; e.g., arguments, quiet talks, etc., giving rise to a general level of tension or tranquility.

Sequential Evaluation of Families of Hyperactive Subjects (Table 3)

1. *Socio-Cultural Parameters.* There appears to be little change in factors which reflect socioeconomic class during the three assessment periods. Parents' education and work status appears to have changed little although, as one would expect, more mothers are working at the ten-year follow-up period.

2. *Child Rearing Practices.* Child rearing practices remained the same in the three time periods except for a less punitive-authoritative approach at the ten-year follow-up.

3. *Health of Family Members.* Families had experienced more medical illnesses and deaths at ten-year follow-up than at initial or five-year follow-up. However, the mental health of family members was better at ten-year follow-up than initially. This trend was seen at five-year, but was not as yet significant at that time.

4. *Relationship.* Emotional climate of the home, marital relationship, and total family score were not significantly different during the three assessments. However, when one analyzed those families where the hyperactive subjects were no longer at home, we see that at five-year follow-up, the emotional climate at home was considerably worse than initially or at ten-year follow-up, even though the marital relationship remained unchanged. It would thus seem that the emotional climate of the home improved when the adolescent left.

Families' Current Assessment of Young Adults' Functioning—Katz Scale of Psychopathology (Table 4)
Only two of the 18 parameters tapped by this scale were scored significantly differently by the families of hyperactives versus control subjects. These two

Table 3.   Sequential Evaluation of Families of Hyperactive Subjects

Scored Means
(N = 35)*

	Initial	Five-year Follow-up	Ten-year Follow-up	f	Direction
Socio Cultural Parameters					
Level of Education of Mother	9.25	10.50	9.25	—	—
Level of Education of Father	10.25	9.00	10.50	—	—
Father's Working Status	3.68	3.44	3.28	—	—
Mother's Working Status	3.00	3.00	3.00	—	—
Mother Working	1.77	1.80	1.40	p = .001	Ten-year More than Initial and Five-Year
Physical Qualities of Home	4.09	4.33	4.29	—	—
Family Size	5.03	5.06	5.12	—	—
Child Adopted	1.89	1.89	1.91	—	—
Sibling Order	2.45	2.64	2.58	—	—
Child Rearing Practices					
Continued Presence of Mother or Stable Substitute	4.52	4.68	4.68	—	—
Inconsistent	1.14	1.21	1.21	—	—
Lack Controls	3.94	3.96	3.86	—	—
Punitive-Authoritative	3.43	3.50	4.07	p = .003	Ten-year Better than Initial or Five-year
Over-Protective	3.83	9.09	3.88	—	—
Health of Family Members					
Physical Illness in Family	1.68	1.80	1.40	p = .001	Ten-year More than Initial or Five-year
Death in Family	1.93	1.89	1.42	p = .001	Ten-year More than Initial or Five-year
Mental Health of Family Members	3.25	3.52	3.89	p = .003	Ten-year Better Than Initial but Same as Five-year
Relationships					
Marital Relationship	3.42	3.30	3.36	—	—
Emotional Climate of Home	3.01	3.15	3.07	—	—
TOTAL Family Score	32.65	33.78	34.45	—	—
Subject No Longer at Home					
Marital Relationship	3.16	2.50	3.00	—	—
Emotional Climate of Home	3.33	2.00	3.16	p = .007	Five-year Worse Than Initial and Ten-year

*N represents the number of subjects on whom all measures were obtained at all three time periods.

Table 4. Current View of Young Adult by His Family
Katz Scale of Psychopathology

Item	Families of Hyperactives N = 63 Mean	Families of Controls N = 43 Mean	Significance
Belligerence	6.0	6.3	—
Verbal expansiveness	8.0	7.3	—
Negativism	16.1	13.9	$p = .05$
Helplessness	6.3	6.3	—
Suspiciousness	5.2	5.6	—
Anxiety	6.6	7.4	—
Withdrawal	9.2	10.4	—
Nervousness	8.1	7.7	—
Confusion	3.2	4.4	—
Bizarreness	5.8	6.4	—
Hyperactivity	6.0	5.1	—
Stability	32.1	32.2	—
General psychopathology	36.1	34.4	—
Performed household chores	33.2	33.8	—
Expected to perform household chores	35.3	35.5	—
Discrepancy between performance and expectation	10.4	9.6	—
Leisure activities	47.4	46.1	—
Satisfaction	32.1	27.6	$p = .001$ (Controls better)

items were negativism ($p = .05$) and ability to derive satisfaction ($p = .0001$). In both instances, families of hyperactives scored their offspring as doing worse on these parameters than families of control subjects.

Other measures, such as belligerence, verbal expansion, nervousness, suspicion, confusion, hyperactivity, stability, bizarreness, and compulsion with household chores, were not scored differently by the two groups.

Questionnaire: Current Functioning and Conflicts (Table 5)

There seemed to be no differences in the families' views about their children's futures; i.e. their optimism about offspring's future, whether he was making plans for the future, or if these plans were realistic. There were also no differences with regard to whether they thought the child used money wisely. Families of hyperactive subjects perceived that their child worked for his money more than did families of control subjects ($p = .02$).

Main areas of conflict which distinguished the two groups included conflicts

Table 5. Current View of Young Adult by His Family—Questionnaire
(Hyperactives: N = 62–64; Controls: N = 41–42)

Item	Chi²	Df	Significance	Direction
Parent optimistic about child's future	5.1	4	—	—
Child making plans for future	2.9	4	—	—
Are plans realistic?	4.8	4	—	—
Does he use money wisely?	7.5	4	—	—
Works for money	11.6	4	p = .02	HA's more
Parents and offspring agree re:				
money	6.9	4	—	—
school or work	13.0	4	p = .01	Controls more
drug use	5.5	4	—	—
keeping rules	7.4	4	—	—
friends	8.9	4	p = .06	Controls more
friends of opposite sex	3.6	4	—	—
tidiness	10.8	4	p = .02	Controls
noise levels	2.9	4	—	—

Item	Mean (HA)	Mean (Control)	Significance	Direction
Sum of Scores on General Questionnaire	43.78	49.45	p = .015	Controls more

around school or work (p = .01), tidiness (p = .02), and friends (generally) (p = .06). In each case, families of hyperactive subjects reported more conflicts than those of controls. However, the two groups did not differ with respect to conflicts around drug abuse, keeping rules, friends of the opposite sex, and noise level.

The sum of the scores on the questionnaire was worse for families of hyperactives than control subjects (p = .015).

Families' Retrospective View of Their Children at Different Developmental Stages (Table 6)

Comparison of retrospective family ratings of hyperactives versus controls on all parameters (similar to Table 6) at all three time periods—i.e., preschool, elementary, and high school—indicated that families of hyperactives viewed their children as functioning significantly worse on almost all parameters. This was less marked in the preschool period than in the elementary and high school periods.

1. Parental Concern. We see that the main areas of parental concern shift from medical problems and activity level per se in the preschool period, to predominantly social concerns in the elementary and high school period. There was no difference in concern with regard to emotional, intellectual, or school difficulties during the three periods. Parents tended to seek more help during the elementary school period than during preschool or high school.

2. *Restlessness.* Most parents of hyperactives see their children as being less restless as they get older, with the high school period being scored better than preschool or elementary school.

3. *Relationship.* Parents of hyperactives perceive their children's relationship with peers and adults to be similar in the elementary and high school period with the exception of teachers. Parents feel they related to teachers better in elementary school than in high school.

4. *Socially Positive Behavior.* Again, no difference was rated by parents of hyperactives in parameters such as stealing or lying, between the elementary and high school period.

5. *Schooling.* No clear-cut picture emerges as to whether the family perceived their hyperactive child as functioning better in the elementary or high school period. Some factors were scored better in elementary school (e.g., Did he like school?), while others scored better in the high school period (e.g., school behavior and independent homework).

DISCUSSION

Assessment of Families

Generally, our findings suggest that even though families of hyperactives and control subjects were matched for socioeconomic class, the families of hyperactives tended to have more difficulties. These difficulties were mainly in the areas of mental health of family members, marital relationship and, most particularly, the emotional climate of the home.

Our findings support those of Cantwell (1972), who found increased incidence of psychiatric difficulties in families of hyperactives. However, the severity of these problems, particularly with regard to mental health of family members, appears much milder. It has also been shown that having a disabled child causes a great deal of stress for families (Kelman, 1964). Thus, whether the hyperactive child's difficulties were accentuated because of family problems, or whether the family's stress was amplified by his disabilities, is difficult to evaluate. It is likely that they eventually worked synergistically in causing the situation to deteriorate. It points out the importance of focusing on both the child's and family's problems in the comprehensive treatment of the condition and thus preventing this negative synergism.

Families of hyperactives tended to use more punitive authoritative approaches in child rearing than families of control subjects. It is unclear as to what is the origin or effect of this approach. It is hoped that current research in various behavioral strategies with these children will provide useful guidelines to parents as to which approach is more beneficial with their child.

Table 6. Families' Retrospective View of Their Hyperactive Children at Different Developmental Stages
(N = 51)

	Preschool	Elementary school	High school	f	Direction
Parental Concern					
Sought professional help	1.78	1.04	1.54	p = .001	More in elementary than preschool or high school
Areas of concern:					
emotional	1.83	1.63	1.70	—	—
social	1.79	1.58	1.54	.001	High school and elementary more than preschool
intellectual	1.95	1.97	1.97	—	—
medical	1.89	2.00	2.00	.002	Preschool more than elementary or high school
activity level	1.50	1.66	1.91	.001	Preschool more than elementary, elementary more than high school
				t-test	
school	—	1.70	1.74	—	—

				t-test	
Restlessness					
Sits through meal	2.72	2.90	3.64	p = .001	High school better than preschool or elementary
Sleeps well	3.42	3.52	3.84	.026	High school better than preschool or elementary
Occupies spare time	—	3.24	3.64	.006	High school better
Relationships					
Peers—generally	—	3.28	3.50	—	—
Teachers	—	3.82	3.56	.06	Elementary better
Close continuous friendships with peers	—	3.14	3.26	—	—
Considerate of others	—	2.80	3.04	—	—
Socially positive behaviour					
Considerate of others' property	—	3.10	3.26	—	—
Trusted not to steal	—	4.32	4.40	—	—
Truthful	—	3.82	3.80	—	—
Schooling					
Did subject like school?	—	3.11	2.84	p = .09	Elementary better
Academic performance	—	2.60	2.50	—	—
Grades failed	—	1.26	1.28	—	—
School behavior	—	2.83	3.35	.01	High school better
Expelled	—	2.78	2.46	.01	Elementary better
Does homework independently	—	2.34	3.00	.001	High school better

It should be pointed out that even though the questionnaires were similar at initial, five-year and ten-year assessments, the interviewers differed. However, all the interviewers were trained on interview style and scoring methods with another interviewer who had made assessments five years earlier. It is unfortunate that we lack these sequential measures for families of control subjects. We can, therefore, only discuss changes with time in families of hyperactives and not whether these changes differ from families of control subjects.

In the sequential view of how families of hyperactives function, it is of importance to point out that the punitive child rearing approach decreases at the ten-year follow-up and the mental health of the family members improves. However, the emotional climate of the home improves only when the hyperactive has left home.

Other findings which differ at ten-year follow-up, such as more mothers working, more physical illness and death in the family, can be explained by the aging of parents and children.

Factors pertaining to socioeconomic class—e.g., fathers' and mothers' education and physical quality of the home—have remained stable throughout,

We thus see that though families of hyperactives do not function as well as families of control subjects at ten-year follow-up, they seem to show some improvement when compared to initial and five-year follow-up measures. This may be due to the decreasing demands of their hyperactive child as he matures and improves or leaves home.

Families' Current Assessment of Young Adults' Functioning

Generally, families of hyperactive and control subjects did not score their offspring differently on the Katz Scale of Psychopathology. This is supported by our own assessment of the subjects which indicated that although they still had problems, they did not load the psychiatric or antisocial population (Hechtman et al., 1976). Parents of hyperactives did see problems—e.g., in increased negativism and decreased ability to derive satisfaction—but generally they were not significantly more concerned about their future than parents of control subjects. We thus see that positive changes in the hyperactives' functioning did register with the families, too. Nonetheless, some conflicts between the hyperactive and his family remain, namely, in the area of school or work, friends and tidiness, but these tend to be managed fairly well by both the hyperactive and his family, enabling many hyperactives to remain in fairly close contact with their families.

Families' View of their Children at Different Developmental Stages

These findings (reported by parents at ten-year follow-up) are subject to all the limitations of retrospective parental reports, and therefore need to be evaluated in that light (Langhorne, Loney, Paternite, and Bechtolt, 1976).

At each stage of development, families of hyperactives viewed their children more negatively than did families of controls on social, academic, and hyperkinetic parameters. These differences are particularly pronounced during the elementary and high school period and somewhat less so in the preschool period.

This finding is expected in light of the difficulties these families experienced with their hyperactive children at all developmental stages. However, this does not necessarily represent a general negative halo effect by parents of hyperactive subjects with regard to their children.

We see that not only do these areas of concern change (e.g., medical and activity level in the preschool period to social concerns in the elementary and high school period), but that parents can see improvements in various areas of functioning at various developmental stages; for example, improvement of restlessness with age.

It is interesting that despite considerable antisocial behavior in hyperactive subjects during adolescence, their parents do not score them differently on this type of behavior in elementary or high school. It may be that some of the antisocial behavior (e.g., lying, stealing) had begun at home during the elementary school period and only become a problem in the community during adolescence and the parents did not distinguish between the two. An alternative explanation may lie in the fact that adolescents are more skilled in keeping such misdeeds from their parents.

It is important to note that families do not view their hyperactive offspring in a static, globally negative light, but perceive changes, positive and negative, on various parameters with time.

SUMMARY

In summary, families of hyperactive children have more difficulties than those of normal controls. These difficulties were mainly in the areas of mental health of family members, marital relationships, and, most particularly, emotional climate of the home. They also tended to use a more punitive-authoritative child rearing approach to their children.

However, in the sequential evaluation of families, we see that this punitive child rearing tendency decreases at ten-year follow-up. Mental health of family members also improves at ten-year follow-up as does the emotional climate in the home, the latter only if the hyperactive has moved out.

Generally, families of hyperactive subjects tend to improve in their function with time, even though they do not equal the functioning of families of matched controls.

Even though families of hyperactives see their offspring as having more difficulties currently than controls, they are on the whole not more pessimistic about their current or future functioning. Conflicts that remain appear tolerable to both the families and the hyperactive young adult.

Finally, families of hyperactive subjects can, despite many problems with their children, still appreciate shifts in both their achievements and difficulties at each developmental stage.

In view of the above findings, more concentrated work with the families of hyperactives as part of the comprehensive treatment of this condition seems highly indicated.

ACKNOWLEDGMENTS

The study reported in this chapter was supported by a grant from the National Institute of Mental Health (U.S.A.) and a National Health Grant (Department of Health and Welfare, Canada) to Dr. Gabrielle Weiss.

These findings were presented at the Annual Meeting of the Canadian Psychiatric Association, September 27-30, 1977, Saskatoon, Saskatchewan.

NOTE

1. Bipolar and unipolar affective disorder refers to a psychiatric condition characterized by recurrent cyclical periods of both marked depression and mania (bipolar), or recurrence of only one of these states, usually depression (unipolar).

REFERENCES

Cantwell, D. P. (1972), "Psychiatric illness in the families of hyperactive children," *Archives of General Psychiatry* 27:414.

——— (1975), "Genetics of hyperactivity," *Journal of Child Psychology and Psychiatry* 16(3):261.

Goodwin, D. W., F. Schulsinger, L. Hermansen, S. Guze and G. Winokur (1975), "Alcoholism and the hyperactive child syndrome," *Journal of Nervous and Mental Disease* 160(5):349.

Hechtman, L., G. Weiss, J. Finkelstein, A. Wener and R. Benn (1976), "Hyperactives as young adults: Preliminary report," *Canadian Medical Association Journal* 115:625.

Hogarty, G. E. and M. M. Katz (1971), "Norms of adjustment and social behaviour," *Archives of General Psychiatry* 25:470.

Kelman, H. R. (1964), "The effect of the brain-damaged child on the family," in H. C. Birch (Ed.), *Brain Damage in Children: The Biological and Social Aspects.* New York: William and Wilkins.

Langhorne, J. E., S. Loney, C. F. Paternite and H. P. Bechtolt (1976), "Childhood hyperkinesis: A return to source," *Journal of Abnormal Psychology* 85(2):201.

Menkes, M. M., J. Rowe and J. Menkes (1967), "A twenty-five year follow-up study on the hyperactive child with minimal brain dysfunction," *Pediatrics* 29:393.

Morrison, J. R. and M. A. Stewart (1971), "A family study of the hyperactive child syndrome," *Biological Psychiatry* 3:189.

——— (1973a), "The psychiatric status of legal families of adopted hyperactives," *Archives of General Psychiatry,* 28(6):888.

——— (1973b), "Evidence for polygentic inheritance in the hyperactive child syndrome," *American Journal of Psychiatry* 130(7):791.

——— (1974), "Bilateral inheritance as evidence for polygeneticity in the hyperactive child syndrome," *Journal of Nervous and Mental Disease* 158(3):226-228.

Stewart, M. A. and J. R. Morrison (1973), "Affective disorder among the relatives of hyperactive children," *Journal of Child Psychology and Psychiatry* 14:209.

Stewart, M. A. and L. Leone (1978a), "A family study of unsocialized aggressive boys," *Biological Psychiatry* 13(1):107-117.

Stewart, M. A., C. S. de Blois and C. C. Adams (1979), "Psychiatric disorder in parents of hyperactive boys and those with conduct disorder," Submitted to Archives of General Psychiatry.

Stewart, M. A., C. S. de Blois and S. Singer (1978b), "Alcoholism and hyperactivity revisited: A preliminary report," *Currents in alcoholism* Vol. 5:349-57.

Part III

ISSUES OF MEASUREMENT

TOWARD THE DEVELOPMENT OF A TWO-STAGE PROCEDURE FOR CASE IDENTIFICATION AND CLASSIFICATION IN PSYCHIATRIC EPIDEMIOLOGY

Bruce P. Dohrenwend and Patrick E. Shrout

INTRODUCTION

Most morbidity data on psychiatric disorders are based on records of patients admitted to mental hospitals and other psychiatric facilities. It has long been known, however, that such data are biased by a host of selective factors that determine who among those suffering from a particular disorder actually receive treatment (Dohrenwend and Dohrenwend, 1969: 3–7). The consequences, as Kramer (1976) has strongly described them, are that:

> . . . systematic morbidity statistics on the incidence and prevalence of the mental disorders as a group, or of individual disorders within the group, do not exist for the U.S. or any other

Research in Community and Mental Health, Volume 2, pages 295–323
Copyright © 1981 by JAI Press, Inc.
All rights of reproduction in any form reserved.
ISBN: 0-89232-152-0

country. Major impediments to their development continue to be the absence of standard case finding technique that can be used in a uniform and consistent fashion in population surveys to detect persons with mental disorders, and reliable differential diagnostic techniques for assigning each case to a specific diagnostic category with a high degree of reliability (p. 188).

The General Argument for a Two-Stage Procedure for Case Identification and Classification

Against this background, it is interesting and instructive to review the general procedure recommended by the first and only textbook in this field:

> Few surveys have been based on personal examination of all members of a population, or even of a random sample by psychiatrists. Occasionally, in small rural communities it has been possible to adopt this approach, but in the conditions of modern urban society it is hardly feasible. In consequence, a two-stage process of case-identification becomes essential for large-scale field surveys (Cooper and Morgan, 1973: 40).

The first stage is the screening stage and it is related to the second stage as follows:

> Psychiatric screening is the presumptive identification of previously unrecognized or unreported psychiatric disorder by the application of tests, examinations or other appropriate procedures to defined population samples. Psychiatric screening procedures differentiate between those members of the population who probably have a clinically significant mental or emotional disturbance and those who do not. Such screening tests are not intended to be diagnostic. Persons with positive or suspicious findings will require more intensive examination for definite identification and diagnosis (Cooper and Morgan, 1973: 41).

Sensible as this recommendation sounds, there have been only a handful of systematic attempts to use a multi-stage procedure for case identification and classification in psychiatric epidemiology. Notable among them is the approach of Rutter and his colleagues in their research on children (e.g., Rutter, Tizard, and Whitmore, 1970). Goldberg (1972) and Eastwood (1975) have developed and used two-stage approaches for studying psychiatric disturbances in patients of general practitioners. More recently, Duncan-Jones and Henderson (1978) have used Goldberg's General Health Questionnaire (GH) (1973) together with Wing, Cooper, and Sartorius' (1974) Present State Examination (PSE) in a two-stage procedure for studying psychiatric disorders in a general population.

Duncan-Jones and Henderson (1978) speculate that use of two-stage procedures is so rare because of fear of loss of respondents between the first screening stage and the follow-up diagnostic stage. They themselves found, however, that with careful planning, they were able to conduct interviews with 91 percent of the respondents designated for follow-up on the basis of initial screening.

Despite the rarity of sophisticated two-stage approaches to case identification and classification in psychiatric epidemiology since Cooper and Morgan published their recommendation five years ago, there have been a number of new developments in the field, plus new understandings of some of the older developments that should make it possible to design and implement rigorous tests of the two-stage approach. For example, several older instruments that were developed and used for research with psychiatric patients (and sometimes medical patients as well) over the past 10 or 15 years, have begun to be used with samples from the general population. These instruments are of two general types. First, there are instruments of the self-report variety such as the Johns Hopkins Symptom Check List which, in its most developed form, is called the SCL-90 (Derogatis, 1977). A variation of this has been used with a general population sample in Chicago (Ilfeld, 1978). Second, there are instruments with scores based on rating scales utilizing clinical judgments by the interviewer rather than the subject's self-reports; two examples of these are Wing, Cooper, and Sartorius' (1974) Present State Examination (PSE) and Spitzer, Endicott, Fleiss, and Cohen's (1970) Psychiatric Status Schedule (PSS). Wing, Mann, Leff, and Nixon (1978), as well as Brown, Harris, and Copeland (1977), have used the PSE with general population samples, and our own group has tested the PSS on such a sample (Dohrenwend, Yager, Egri, and Mendelsohn, 1978). Moreover, new interview instruments of these two types have been developed and used with general population samples. One of them is the Psychiatric Epidemiology Research Interview (PERI) that we constructed largely out of structured questions with fixed alternative response formats like most self-report instruments (Dohrenwend, Shrout, Egri, and Mendelsohn, in press). Another, the Schedule for Affective Disorders and Schizophrenia (SADS) was constructed by Endicott and Spitzer (1978) and has much in common with their earlier PSS and with the PSE. A brief version of SADS called SADS-L has been used with a sample from the general population (Weissman, Myers, and Harding, 1978).

Possible First Stage Screening Instruments and Second Stage Diagnostic Instruments.

Whether the first-stage instrument should be a clinical rating scale or a self-report measure is a matter of controversy. The argument for the rating scale approach which relies on clinical judgment to score such interviews as the PSE and SADS has been stated by Wing, Mann, Leff, and Nixon (1978) as follows:

> The clinical diagnostic examination is conducted in order to discover whether specific symptoms (the definitions of which are carried in the examiner's memory) are present, and an affirmative answer to a question about, for example, depressed mood, will be discounted if the clinician does not regard the evidence as sufficient. The questionnaire approach leaves interpretation of the questions to the subject and necessarily accepts the subject's positive answers as indicating the presence of "symptoms" (p. 204).

In contrast to Wing et al., proponents of what was called "the questionnaire approach" might argue, as does Derogatis (1977), that:

> The self report mode of psychological measurement contains much to recommend it. Particularly concerning psychopathology, self-report provides certain exclusive information that is

simply unavailable through other assessment channels. To begin with, self-report possesses the singular advantage of reflecting information from the "experiencing self"—the person directly experiencing the phenomena. No external observer can share this experience except through its public manifestations—the clinical observer is limited to reporting "apparent" versions of the patient's experience, based on his behavior and verbal report (p. 3).

In point of fact, we think that the two approaches may prove to be not as antagonistic as it would appear from the above descriptions if the approaches are developed within the framework of a two-stage screening and diagnostic sequence for case identification and classification in psychiatric epidemiology. Our understanding of these contrasting approaches and their strengths and weaknesses for research in psychiatric epidemiology is strongly conditioned by the research conducted at our Social Psychiatry Research Unit at Columbia University. Let us, therefore, fill in this background of our investigations of the different types of interview approach to date.

A comparison of self-report and rating scale approaches: The Structured Interview Schedule (SIS) and the Psychiatric Status Schedule (PSS). A basic assumption of our program of methodological research has been that the first step toward reliable and valid case identification and diagnosis is the collection of reliable and valid data on which they can be based. One way to throw light on how to secure such data is to test the reliability and validity of the main types of interview approaches that have been used in epidemiological studies. In previous research, we attempted to do just that; we tested two sharply contrasting interview approaches as illustrated by two sharply contrasting interview instruments.

The first of these interview instruments we have called the Structured Interview Schedule or SIS. The SIS relies for the most part on self-reports to closed questions with fixed alternative response categories (true-false; often-sometimes-never). It is based on the kind of interview approach used in the Midtown Study (Srole, Langner, Michael, Opler, and Rennie, 1962), the Stirling County Study (D. C. Leighton, Harding, Macklin, Macmillan, and A. H. Leighton, 1963) and in the earlier research of one author in Washington Heights (B. P. Dohrenwend and B. S. Dohrenwend, 1969). The general approach is strongly influenced by the work of the Research Branch of the U.S. Army in Selective Service screening during World War II, and the symptom questions in the SIS come for the most part from the Psychosomatic Scale developed by the Research Branch (Star, 1950) and from the MMPI (Dahlstrom and Welsh, 1960). Unlike these previous instruments, however, the SIS contained a large number of items on role functioning in the areas of work, marriage, parenting, and social relations which were developed from such sources as the nationwide survey by Gurin, Veroff, and Feld (1960) and surveys of specific communities by Bradburn and Caplowitz (1965).

The second instrument was the Psychiatric Status Schedule or PSS developed out of the rating scale tradition by investigators in the Biometrics Department of the New York State Psychiatric Institute (Spitzer, Endicott, Fleiss, and Cohen, 1970). The PSS is an attempt to standardize interviews of the kinds used for intake and diagnosis in clinical settings. It consists of fixed questions, many of them open-ended, together with suggested probes. The actual responses to these questions and probes, however, are not recorded. Rather, they form the basis for judgments by the interviewer as to whether each of the several hundred carefully described signs or symptoms is "true" or "false" of the subject. These clinical judgments then become the basic data resulting from the interview. We chose this instrument on the grounds that it is likely to have much in common with the less explicit and less reproducible types of clinical interviews used by a number of epidemiological investigators, especially those working in Europe and Asia rather than in North America (e.g., Bash, 1967; Hagnell, 1966; Lin, 1953). It is similar in type to the PSE and SADS which, as was mentioned above, have only recently been used with samples from the general population. Like these instruments, and in sharp contrast to instruments such as the SIS, the PSS requires considerable clinical experience and considerable training on the part of the interviewer in order for the clinical judgments to be made properly. Thus, the interviewer of choice with such instruments is an experienced psychiatrist or clinical psychologist.

The subjects used in our tests of the PSS and SIS were 528 adults between the ages of 21 and 64 in the Washington Heights section of New York City. These respondents consisted of 67 community leaders and a community sample of 257 adult heads of families (both men and women, married and single) drawn on a strict probability basis from the general population. The remaining subjects will be called the "patient sample"; they are 118 outpatients from various psychiatric clinics, 62 psychiatric inpatients, and 24 prisoners. The community sample and patient sample were drawn in roughly equal proportions from five ethnic groups: relatively advantaged white Protestants of European ancestry, Jews, and Irish; relatively disadvantaged blacks, and Puerto Ricans. Within each ethnic group in the community sample, an attempt was made to balance educational levels in order to unconfound class and ethnic status. The psychiatric patients were selected in such a way as to insure a diagnostically heterogeneous sample. A random half of the 528 subjects were used in the tests of the PSS; the other half in tests of the SIS. The interviewers with both the PSS and the SIS consisted of 15 psychiatrists, all but one of whom had completed residency training.

The results that most directly indicated the strengths and weaknesses of the two instruments were the estimates of the internal consistency reliability of the symptom scales. These scales were constructed by placing items a priori into non-overlapping and clinically meaningful groupings on the basis of a consensus of two our of three psychiatrists. The groupings bore such names as "anxiety," "suspiciousness," and "delusions and hallucinations." They represented what we hoped would be the yield of reliable and valid measures of a large number of important dimensions of psychopathology in the different sex, class, and ethnic groups from the general population. The yield of reliable and valid measures, however, proved small indeed. Moreover, there was sharp contrast in the strengths and weaknesses of the two interview instruments in this regard.

From the SIS (the self-report approach) it was possible to develop a high ratio of reliable symptom scales to symptom groups tested for both general population and patient samples; however, these scales lacked discriminant validity in both samples—that is, each scale tended to correlate as highly with every other as their reliabilities would permit. What these scales measured, we concluded, was one thing only—something that, we think, is best described by Jerome Frank's construct of "demoralization" (Frank, 1973). In Frank's formulation, "... a person becomes demoralized when he finds that he cannot meet the demands placed on him by the environment, and cannot extricate himself from his predicament" (1973: p. 316). In this view, demoralization may or may not accompany clinical psychiatric disorders (p. 315). More often, it is related to a large variety of other things, such as: situations of extreme environmental stress (p. 316); physical illnesses, especially those that are chronic (pp. 46-47); or "existential despair" (p. 317). Our findings are consistent with this formulation; demoralization, while interesting in its own right, is only weakly and often indirectly related to clinical psychiatric disorders (Dohrenwend, Oksenberg, Shrout, Dohrenwend, and Cook, in press).

From the PSS (the clinical rating scale approach), by contrast, we were able to develop from the large number of scales tested—and we tested scales developed by the Biometrics group as well as our own a priori symptom groups—only a few scales with satisfactory reliabilities in the general population. Moreover, unlike the SIS, the reliable PSS scales showed satisfactory discriminant validity. While the presence of discriminant validity was encouraging, the most striking result of the PSS analysis was the contrast between the PSS results for psychiatric patient and non-patient samples. Using the patient sample, we were able to replicate the finding of Spitzer and his colleagues (1970) that a large number of Biometrics PSS scales were internally consistent; using the general population sample, however, we found that most of those scales were not adequately reliable.

Note that, as formulated in terms of an intraclass correlation, internal consistency is a function of both the true score variance and the amount of error in the scores: $\rho = \sigma_T^2/(\sigma_T^2 + \sigma_E^2)$, where σ_T^2 is the true score variance and σ_E^2 is the error variance. When, as with symptoms of relatively severe psychopathology in the general population, the phenomenon being measured is rare, error is particularly likely to swamp the true score variance. Our analysis of interrater agreement on individual symptoms indicated that there was simply too much error in the clinical judgments and too little correlation among the items in most of the PSS scales for the reliabilities obtained with patients to hold up in the general population (Dohrenwend, Yager, Egri, and Mendelsohn 1978). As it stands, an instrument such as the PSS is likely to yield reliably measured dimensions of psychopathology only in symptomatic groups. If this is so, such an instrument can function adequately only as a second stage instrument for research with general populations. We will come back to this point a few pages further on with reference to our discussion of SADS and the PSE, instruments that are similar in important respects to the PSS.

The Psychiatric Epidemiology Research Interview (PERI).   Since our studies with the SIS and PSS, we have made major progress in developing an interview approach that, we think, will prove suitable for first-stage screening of virtually the full range and variety of functional psychiatric disorders. As noted earlier, it is called the Psychiatric Epidemiology Research Interview (PERI) and relies, for the most part, on closed questions with fixed alternative responses, as did the SIS. PERI was developed in an attempt to borrow the strengths but avoid the weaknesses of the SIS and the PSS. Thus, we aimed to develop a number of reliable scales which measured dimensions in addition to Frank's demoralization.

We tested these scales using a new sample of subjects, 200 male and female household heads from the general population of adults in New York City, who were given different parts of the interview at three points in time. This sample was constructed to contain substantial numbers of Blacks and Puerto Ricans, as well as non-Puerto Rican whites, and to contain representatives of three education levels—non-high school graduates, high school graduates, and college graduates—within each of these ethnic groups. Because the sample was constructed from a four-year-old enumeration of subjects, and because the interview completion rate was poor (50 percent), this sample cannot be considered a probability sample of New York adults, but it economically provided non-patient respondents from contrasting sex, ethnic, and education groups for the testing of our new PERI scales. Our results were encouraging; PERI provides not only extremely reliable measures of Demoralization, it also provides—as our prior SIS instrument did not—reliable measures of 17 other distinct dimensions of psychopathology, to be described briefly below. As can be seen in Table 1, these scales are reliable in the general population sample as a whole and in subsamples of both sexes, higher and lower social classes, blacks and Puerto Ricans, as well as members of more advantaged ethnic groups. While our data from PERI on psychiatric patients is still very limited, results from two patient samples provide some additional evidence on reliability and criterion validity that is encouraging.

A complete description of these scales has been presented elsewhere. (Dohrenwend, Shrout, Egri, and Mendelsohn, in press). In brief summary, PERI contains 25 symptom scales, eight of which, when combined, form a Demoralization Composite. These eight are Poor Self Esteem, Helplessness-Hopelessness, Sadness, Anxiety, Dread, Confused Thinking, Psychophysiological Symptoms, and Perceived Physical Health. While the eight scales include a total of 42 items, a subset of 27 of the items can provide a highly reliable (about .90 or close to it in all subgroups) brief measure of demoralization. The

BRUCE P. DOHRENWEND and PATRICK E. SHROUT

Table 1.   Internal Consistencies of 25 PERI Scales

	Number of Items	Total Sample	Sex		Ethnic Group			Years of Education		
			M	F	Black	Puerto Rican	Other	≤12	12–15	≥16
1) Dread	4	74	63	75	*39*	80	80	76	76	56
2) Anxiety	10	82	75	83	77	85	73	84	82	72
3) Sadness	4	72	61	73	77	68	68	68	76	71
4) Helplessness-Hopelessness	4	72	51	76	*49*	67	80	65	74	83
5) Psychophysiological Symptoms	6	59	70	53	*37*	63	56	62	52	55
6) Perceived Physical Health	2	59	57	61	52	54	62	61	58	54
7) Poor Self Esteem	8*	68	70	67	*49*	80	60	68	68	74
8) Somatic Problems (likely to be related to physical illness)	10	72	73	73	70	79	53	73	76	*45*
9) Confused Thinking	4	74	79	70	65	70	78	68	78	79
10) Guilt	4	73	76	61	66	65	79	71	68	86
11) Enervation	7	79	73	80	73	78	80	78	71	76
12) False Beliefs and Perceptions	9	75	73	79	58	78	70	64	86	76
13) Manic Characteristics	3**	64	60	66	*44*	70	61	63	61	69
14) Suicide: Ideation and Behavior	1***	n.a.								
15) Insomnia	3	80	83	80	74	75	86	73	82	92
16) Distrust	6	79	70	81	*43*	79	83	65	83	84
17) Perceived Hostility from Others	5	72	57	72	67	78	75	68	74	83
18) Rigidity	13	75	78	72	67	78	75	68	74	83
19) Passive Aggressive Behavior	3	65	63	66	66	65	64	62	63	78
20) Active Expression of Hostility	10	61	63	60	52	57	67	*48*	64	79
21) Antisocial History	8	64	66	62	61	55	70	*49*	59	79
22) Approval of Rulebreaking	20	87	91	87	79	92	87	86	82	90
23) Sex Problems	4****	71	84	67	67	74	70	73	67	75
24) Reasons for Drinking	6	70	65	74	64	72	75	65	75	64
25) Problems due to Drinking	5	80	82	79	84	*30*	87	80	57	93

Decimal points have been dropped for all internal consistency estimates. These numbers are known as alphas (Cronbach 1951); they indicate what proportion of the total variance is reliable. Thus, an alpha of .75 indicates that 75 percent of the variance is reliable, while 25 percent of the variance is random variation. Values of less than .50 are in italics.
*There were two additional items in the follow-up data set version;
**There were two additional items in the follow-up data set version;
***Not applicable—No internal consistency can be estimated from only one item;
****There are 4 items for males, 3 items for females.

other 17 scales consist of the following: False Beliefs and Perceptions, Manic Characteristics, Suicidal Ideation and Behavior, Guilt, Enervation, Insomnia, Perceived Hostility from Others, Rigidity, Passive Agressive Behavior, Active Expression of Hostility, Approval of Rule Breaking, Antisocial History, Reasons for Drinking, Problems Due to Drinking, Sex Problems, and Somatic Problems (likely to be related to physical illness). There are also items on frequency of drinking and of drug use.

In order to convey a feeling for PERI scales, Table 2 shows scale means for our sample, broken down by sex, education, and ethnicity. Because we did not have equal numbers of subjects in each of the cells of our three-way cross classified design, the means in Table 2 cannot be considered to be independent. In fact, the Puerto Rican sample is predominantly female, and thus the elevated Puerto Rican means and the elevated female means are often due to the same persons. While a statistically rigorous analysis of these data is available (Shrout and Dohrenwend, 1979), the detail of that analysis exceeds the scope of this chapter. Nevertheless, one can see from Table 2 that ethnic and sex differences are often apparent (the scores of Puerto Ricans tend to be most elevated on most scales and those of blacks least elevated; women are more elevated than men on most of these scales), but that education differences are less than one would expect. This latter result may be due to the fact that our sample consisted of a residentially stable group of respondents. Given that the PERI scales were each measured on a five point gradation (with the exception of Approval of Rule Breaking, which had six points), one can observe from Table 2 the relative frequency of the measured characteristics, Suicidal Ideation and Behavior being the most rare and Rigidity being the most common.

PERI also contains measures of role functioning (B. S. Dohrenwend, Cook, and B. P. Dohrenwend, in press) and an inventory of items to investigate recent experience with stressful life events (B. S. Dohrenwend, Krasnoff, Askenasy, 1978; B. P. Dohrenwend, 1977). The measures of role functioning include scales of Job Stability, Job Satisfaction, Job Performance, Housework, Marriage, Parenthood, and Single Heterosexual Relations. The inventory of stressful life events includes lists of 102 events, magnitude scores for each event, and probes to establish the time the event occurred, whether it was anticipated, and whether its occurrence was seen as within or outside the control of the subject.

Two sets of factors make PERI unique among instruments of its type that have been used in psychiatric epidemiology. The first is that all of its symptom and role measures have had to show not only content validity but high internal consistency reliability in samples of nonpatients as well as patients, and in contrasting sex, class, and ethnic groups within both types of samples. Second, PERI contains measures of far more dimensions of psychopathology than other measures of this type that have been used in epidemiological research.

As we mentioned, while the data on the validity of PERI are not as extensive as those available from the samples of patients studied with the PSS and SIS, what we do have is encouraging. For example, Tessler (1977) included five of the PERI symptom scales in a study of psychiatric inpatients at Northhampton State Hospital in Massachusetts. As Table 3 shows, these scales discriminate sharply between our community sample and Tessler's inpatients. Note the especially strong contrast on False Beliefs and Perceptions; it is just the difference one would expect if the scale were sensitive to delusions and hallucinations, given that the large majority of Tessler's patients had been diagnosed as psychotic.

Table 2. Means of PERI Symptom Scales Broken Down by Ethnicity, Education and Sex

| | Ethnic Breakdown | | | | | | | | |
| | Black | | | Puerto Rican | | | Other White | | |
Scale	$\bar{X}$	SD	N	$\bar{X}$	SD	N	$\bar{X}$	SD	N
1) False Beliefs and Perceptions	.10	.21	30	.26	.43	36	.10	.22	53
2) Manic Characteristics	.59	.66	49	1.14	.84	49	.95	.71	71
3) Suicide: Ideation and Behavior	.08	.33	62	.25	.76	52	.15	.48	84
4) Guilt	.53	.61	49	.75	.65	49	.88	.71	71
5) Enervation	.82	.68	61	1.37	.82	53	1.05	.71	82
6) Insomnia	.81	1.14	62	1.34	1.01	53	1.25	.99	85
7) Distrust	1.21	.87	29	1.44	.78	36	1.17	.80	53
8) Perception of Hostility	.56	.71	62	.74	.73	53	.56	.62	82
9) Rigidity	1.73	.65	48	1.93	.75	46	1.65	.64	68
10) Passive Aggressive Behavior	1.73	.98	61	1.51	.85	50	1.29	.74	82
11) Expression of Hostility	1.20	.54	62	1.23	.55	51	1.43	.56	84
12) Antisocial History	.21	.35	61	.23	.37	53	.21	.47	83
13) Attitude toward Rulebreaking	.81	.58	49	.54	.64	49	.87	.65	68
14) Sex Problems	.64	.66	59	.78	.86	52	.96	.72	76
15) Reasons for Drinking	.20	.45	58	.26	.50	50	.32	.53	81
16) Problems due to Drinking	.23	.68	29	.16	.30	35	.12	.44	53
17) Demoralization	.74	.47	49	1.22	.69	48	.90	.52	70
18) Somatic Problems	.50	.55	62	1.00	.81	53	.51	.47	85

| | Education Breakdown | | | | | | | | |
| | Less than 12 Years of Education | | | High School Graduate | | | College Graduate | | |
Scale	$\bar{X}$	SD	N	$\bar{X}$	SD	N	$\bar{X}$	SD	N
1) False Beliefs and Perceptions	.17	.30	48	.16	.33	42	.10	.26	29
2) Manic Characteristics	.82	.77	75	1.00	.76	57	.91	.74	34
3) Suicide: Ideation and Behavior	.14	.61	90	.14	.38	73	.23	.60	35
4) Guilt	.68	.67	75	.74	.66	60	.88	.72	34
5) Enervation	1.10	.82	88	1.04	.75	73	1.01	.60	35
6) Insomnia	1.17	1.06	92	1.15	1.11	73	1.02	.97	35
7) Distrust	1.32	.79	47	1.27	.89	42	1.16	.77	29
8) Perception of Hostility	.64	.72	89	.65	.72	73	.43	.45	35
9) Rigidity	1.87	.65	71	1.75	.65	59	1.49	.74	32

Table 2—Continued

| | Education Breakdown | | | | | | | | |
| Scale | Less than 12 Years of Education | | | High School Graduate | | | College Graduate | | |
	$\bar{X}$	SD	N	$\bar{X}$	SD	N	$\bar{X}$	SD	N
10) Passive Aggressive Behavior	1.67	.90	88	1.34	.86	72	1.31	.71	33
11) Expression of Hostility	1.27	.52	90	1.27	.56	72	1.45	.62	35
12) Antisocial History	.20	.31	91	.22	.41	71	.26	.61	35
13) Attitude toward Rulebreaking	.62	.63	73	.74	.53	60	1.04	.76	33
14) Sex Problems	.81	.80	83	.78	.70	69	.86	.76	35
15) Reasons for Drinking	.18	.42	84	.35	.60	71	.29	.45	34
16) Problems due to Drinking	.17	.53	46	.15	.37	42	.16	.56	29
17) Demoralization	1.02	.64	73	.94	.58	60	.80	.49	34
18) Somatic Problems	.77	.71	92	.55	.60	73	.47	.40	35

| | Sex Breakdown | | | | | |
| Scale | Males | | | Females | | |
	$\bar{X}$	SD	N	$\bar{X}$	SD	N
1) False Beliefs and Perceptions	.13	.20	41	.16	.34	78
2) Manic Characteristics	.88	.71	65	.92	.79	104
3) Suicide: Ideation and Behavior	.04	.20	74	.22	.65	124
4) Guilt	.68	.66	65	.78	.69	104
5) Enervation	.91	.64	73	1.16	.80	123
6) Insomnia	1.03	.94	75	1.20	1.13	125
7) Distrust	1.47	.86	41	1.15	.78	77
8) Perception of Hostility	.65	.68	73	.58	.68	124
9) Rigidity	1.75	.73	60	1.76	.66	102
10) Passive Aggressive Behavior	1.54	.86	70	1.46	.88	123
11) Expression of Hostility	1.26	.53	73	1.33	.58	124
12) Antisocial History	.33	.50	73	.15	.33	124
13) Attitude toward Rulebreaking	.80	.76	62	.72	.56	104
14) Sex Problems	.75	.86	69	.84	.68	118
15) Reasons for Drinking	.30	.50	72	.24	.50	117
16) Problems due to Drinking	.21	.55	40	.14	.43	77
17) Demoralization	.75	.47	64	1.07	.62	103
18) Somatic Problems	.54	.59	75	.69	.65	125

Table 3. Comparisons of Means from Massachusetts
Clinical Sample to New York Community Sample

	Massachusetts Clinical Sample		New York Community Sample	
	Mean	SD	Mean	SD
False Beliefs and Perceptions	1.42	1.05	0.15	0.30
Guilt	1.52	1.11	0.74	0.68
Components of Demoralization				
Sadness	2.47	0.96	1.33	0.94
Confused Thinking	2.07	1.22	1.04	0.84
Perceived Physical Health	1.54	1.26	1.09	0.90
Average	2.03	—	1.15	—

N's for New York Sample range from 168–110
N's for Massachusetts Clinical Sample is 147
All differences between samples are significantly different from zero, $p < .01$

In addition, Stokes (1976) used most of PERI in a study of samples of drug addicts in a treatment program conducted at Eagleville Hospital in Pennsylvania. Note in Table 4 that there is far less of a difference between the scores of the addict sample and our community sample on False Beliefs and Perceptions than there was between our sample and the inpatients in Table 3. The largest contrast in Table 4, as we would expect, is on the scale of Antisocial History. Note also the contrast on two other scales designed to measure antisocial tendencies and symptoms: Attitude toward Rulebreaking and Expression of Hostility.

PERI is not, however, designed to yield diagnoses. Rather, it is designed to screen probable cases and supply leads as to whether they are more likely to be of some diagnostic types than of others. The precise details of inclusion and exclusion criteria required for diagnoses of individuals within the screened groups according to current diagnostic criteria are beyond its scope. Table 5 shows how PERI scales are presumed to be related to likely diagnostic classifications according to either the third edition of the Diagnostic and Statistical Manual of the American Psychiatric Association (DSM-III) or International Classification of Diseases of the World Health Organization (ICD-9).

The Schedule for Affective Disorders and Schizophrenia (SADS) and the Present State Examination (PSE). As we also mentioned, considerable new work has been done—not by us, but by other research groups—with clinical interview and rating approaches similar in many respects to that represented by the PSS. Prominent examples of this work are the *Schedule for Affective Disorders* (SADS) and the *Present State Examination* (PSE). In the remainder of this chapter, we will focus on these two instruments, not only because they represent the best examples of the standardized clinical interview approach, but also be-

Table 4. Comparison of Means from New York
Community Sample and Eagleville Sample

	New York Sample		Eagleville Sample	
Scale	Mean	Standard Deviation	Mean	Standard Deviation
1. False Beliefs and Perceptions	0.148	0.302	0.323**	0.569
2. Manic	0.903	0.762	1.304**	0.728
3. Suicide: Ideation and Behavior	0.157	0.534	2.323**	3.654
4. Guilt	0.742	0.676	0.978*	1.114
5. Enervation	1.067	0.757	1.701**	0.866
6. Insomnia	1.138	1.062	1.364	0.888
7. Distrust	1.265	0.818	2.089**	0.804
8. Perception of Hostility	0.609	0.681	1.258**	0.773
9. Rigidity	1.753	0.683	2.224**	0.536
10. Passive Aggressive Behavior	1.487	0.868	2.039**	0.913
11. Expression of Hostility	1.274	0.528	1.666**	0.618
12. Antisocial History	0.218	0.411	1.770**	0.894
13. Attitude Toward Rulebreaking	0.752	0.640	1.639**	1.034
14. Sex Problems	0.809	0.754	0.979	1.021
15. Reasons for Drinking	0.228	0.428	0.598**	0.836
16. Problems due to Drinking	0.161	0.473	0.220	0.576
17. Demoralization	0.915	0.572	1.291**	0.593

N's for New York sample range from 168 to 110
N's for Eagleville sample range from 77 to 68
*Eagleville mean significantly larger than NY mean p < .05.
**Eagleville mean significantly larger than NY mean p < .01.

cause they are being used by more and more researchers and because they are likely to be influential in the development of new instruments in the years to come.[1]

The SADS has emerged from the Biometrics Department at the New York State Psychiatric Institute—the same group that constructed the PSS. This new instrument is explicitly linked to the work by Spitzer and his colleagues on DSM-III and their related Research Diagnostic Criteria (RDC) (Spitzer, Endicott, and Robbins, 1978). As Endicott and Spitzer (1978) point out:

> The SADS, SADS-L [a short version of SADS], and RDC are being used in a large number of studies to investigate a wide variety of research questions having to do with genetics, psychobiology, response to treatment, and clinical description of different mental disorders. . . . Investigators who are now using SADS and RDC know that they will be able to relate their findings to many of the diagnostic categories that are to be included in the third edition of the American Psychiatric Association's *Diagnostic and Statistical Manual* (DSM-III). DSM-III will contain operational criteria for all of its diagnostic categories, many of which will be virtually identical with or slight modifications of those contained in the RDC (p. 844).

Table 5. Hypotheses about How PERI Symptom and Role Scales are Related to DSM-III Diagnoses and to ICD-9 Diagnoses

Types to be differentiated	Relevant DSM-III categories	Relevant ICD-9 categories	Relevant PERI screening scales
Schizophrenia	Schizophrenic disorders (295.1, .2, .3, .5, .9) Paranoid disorders (297) Schizoaffective disorders (295.7) Schizophreniform disorder (295.4)	Schizophrenic psychoses (295) Paranoid states (297)	False Beliefs and Perceptions Manic (if above also) Perceived hostility Demoralization Role functioning
Affective	Major affective disorders (296.0–6) —psychotic level of severity	Affective psychoses (296)	Manic False Beliefs and Perceptions (if above also) Demoralization Enervation Insomnia Distrust Guilt Sex problems Suicide Problems with drinking Role functioning
Psychopathic or sociopathic or antisocial personality	Antisocial personality disorder (301.7) Disorders of impulse control not elsewhere classified (312.31–.35, .39)	Personality disorder with predominantly sociopathic or asocial manifestations (301.7) Disturbance of conduct not elsewhere classified (312)	Active expression of hostility Role functioning Antisocial history Approval of rule breaking

Category	DSM-III disorder (ICD-9 no.)	ICD-9 category	Symptoms
Alcoholism	Alcohol abuse (305.0)*	... syndrome (303)	Active expression of hostility Role functioning Antisocial history Approval of rule breaking Problems with drinking Reasons for drinking
Drug abuse	Drug abuse specified by type of drug—exclude tobacco (305.2–.7, .9)*	Drug dependence	Drug use index Role functioning
Neuroses	Episodic affective disorders (296.0–.6) —moderate, marked, or severe level of severity Chronic affective disorders (301.11–.13) Atypical affective disorders (296.70, .81, .82) Anxiety disorders (300.00–.02, .21–.23, .29, .30) Somatoform disorders (300.12–.15, .60)	Neurotic disorders (300) Psychophysiological malfunction arising from mental factors (306) Depressive disorder, not elsewhere classified (311)	Enervation Insomnia Active expression of hostility Role functioning Guilt Sex problems Suicide Problems with drinking Rigidity** Perceived physical health
Reaction to psychosocial stressor	Post-traumatic stress disorder (308.30, 309.81) Adjustment disorders (309.00, .24, .28, .30, .40, .83, .90)	Acute reaction to stress (308) Adjustment reaction (309)	Demoralization Role functioning

N.B. Numbers in parentheses are IC 9 classification numbers.

*DSM-III "Abuse" category includes criterion of "either psychological dependence or pathological pattern of use" but ICD 305 is "Nondependent abuse of drugs" involving "maladaptive use of a drug on which he is not dependent"

**Only for PSE Obsessional neurosis syndrome

The PSE developed by Wing and his colleagues is also a widely used instrument. In contrast to SADS, the PSE has a less wide coverage; it applies solely to functional psychoses and neuroses, and focuses on current disorder within the past four weeks rather than on current disorder within the past year or past disorder at any time. The authors claim, however, that like the SADS, the PSE has the advantage of providing "... a system of clinical classification based upon precisely specified rules and closely related to a diagnostic system in wide current use" (Wing, Cooper, and Sartorius, 1974: 134). In the case of the PSE, the diagnostic system is the psychiatric section of the ninth edition of the International Classification of Diseases (ICD-9) which is widely used outside of the United States. In fact, ICD-9 diagnoses can be made from the PSE protocol using a computer program called CATEGO (Wing, Cooper and Sartorius, 1974). What Endicott and Spitzer (1978) conclude of SADS and RDC at their present stage of development might well be said as well of the PSE:

> Within the next few years, evidence of the value of the SADS and RDC for different purposes will be available. To some extent, current users of these procedures are assuming that they are at least as valid as many of the previously developed assessment procedures and that they have the potential for having even greater usefulness.... (p. 844).

Recall, however, that both sets of instruments were developed on the basis of research with psychiatric patients. What of their potential for epidemiological investigations of general populations?

It has long been known that individual test items in the measurement of personality in general and psychopathology in particular are highly ambiguous in their implications (cf. Fiske, 1971: pp. 228–232; Nunnally, 1967). Summing conceptually related items to form scale scores is a straightforward and effective way of dealing with the limited scope and unreliability of single items. When this is done, moreover, there are mathematical procedures such as coefficient alpha (Cronbach, 1951) available for estimating the degree of internal consistency reliability achieved with such a scale. However, such approaches require that each item be asked independently of the responses to or scores of the preceding items.

The PSE and, to a lesser extent, SADS, rely on a series of "obligatory" questions that are followed up by sequences of other questions only if they are scored in a particular way. Wing et al. (1974) describe the "obligatory" questions this way:

> These must be asked if the interview is conducted at all. Thus subjects with no symptoms, who ask clarifying questions of their own and who answer clearly and decisively, can be screened very quickly indeed. Whenever there is any doubt, however, and certainly whenever a symptom needs clarification, the second kind of questions [i.e., the nonobligatory follow-ups designed to 'define the nature and extent of a symptom' and the examiner's own questions or probes] should be asked (p. 190).

Clearly, in this type of approach, reliance is being placed on the skilled clinical interviewer to deal with and to correct the errors that arise in the answers of subjects to individual questions.

Recall that we found that another rating scale instrument, the PSS, was far more adequate with psychiatric patients than with samples from the general population. On this basis, we do not think that skillful probes and expert judgments by clinical interviewers will adequately deal with the problem of measurement error in representative samples from the general population. We do think, on the other hand, that it is reasonable to hypothesize that SADS and PSE will perform adequately as second stage diagnostic instruments when focused on segments of the general population that have been screened to be highly symptomatic.

The authors of SADS and of the PSE, however, argue that these instruments will function adequately as both the initial screening and the final diagnostic stages in epidemiological research with the general population—in sum, that they can do the case identification and classification job in one stage (Wing, Mann, Leff, and Nixon, 1978; Spitzer, personal communication). While SADS and PSE purportedly can be used directly in community samples, both instruments have shorter measures associated with them which might be used in community samples for reasons of economy. Thus, Endicott and Spitzer (1978) suggest that SADS-L, an instrument focusing less on current disorder than on disorders over the lifetime, be used with populations containing large proportions of subjects who are unlikely to be current cases. For their part, Wing and his colleagues have developed an Index of Definition to classify general population subjects interviewed with the PSE into cases and noncases; only the former are then further categorized by CATEGO according to diagnostically meaningful syndromes (Wing, et al., 1978). The relatively brief SADS-L and the PSE's Index of Definition have been developed for practical reasons only; the authors of these instruments have not questioned the ability of either the SADS or PSE to provide adequate data for the division of general population samples into cases and noncases.

To date, the claims that SADS or SADS-L and the PSE can adequately perform both the screening and diagnostic functions in a one-stage interview with subjects from the general population have not been thoroughly investigated. The use of SADS-L in a recent study in New Haven (Weissman, Myers, and Harding, 1978) has proceeded without anything approaching a rigorous test of this claim. No evidence has been provided, for example, as to whether these instruments measure the same things in men and women, higher and lower social classes, advantaged and disadvantaged ethnic groups, and patient and nonpatient subjects. That such questions are pressing is underlined by some recent results reported by Wing et al. (1978) on differences between "cases" of depression in a sample from the general population and cases of depression in samples of psychiatric patients. Let us consider this study and its findings in some detail.

By contrast with the study done with SADS-L in New Haven (Weissman et al., 1978), the interviewers in this research by Wing and his colleagues were all trained psychiatrists (the New Haven study employed two interviewers, one of whom had a master's degree and one of whom had a bachelor's degree; both had had previous clinical experience). Their general population sample consisted of 123 women, ages 18–65, from a district of London, excluding immigrants and short-term residents. Of these, 22 were cases of "depressive disorders" on the basis of their identification as being above the threshold on the Index of Definition and their categorization as depressive disorders by CATEGO. However, when Wing and his colleagues examined the PSE scores in terms of widely used criteria for depressive disorders developed by Feighner, Robins, Guze, Woodruff, Winokur, and Munoz (1972), the results were as follows:

> One of the 22 "depressive disorders" in the general population series meets the standard, while 2 are probable. On the other hand, 16 of the 23 above threshold depressive disorders found in the in-patient series are definite and three are probable, while one patient with severe depressive retardation could not be rated on the subjective symptoms. Of the 14 above threshold depressive disorders in the out-patient series, 7 are definite, 5 are probable, and 2 show only 3 of the [Feighner] criteria (p. 213).

This is, of course, an extremely sharp contrast which would probably also hold if RDC criteria were applied, since the development of RDC has been strongly influenced by the work of Feighner et al. (1972). So far as the depressive disorders are concerned, the PSE and its Index of Definition and CATEGO system of case identification and classification are clearly not measuring the same thing in general population samples as they are in samples of psychiatric patients. Our hypothesis is that what the PSE was reliably measuring in the general population was demoralization, which can coincide with but is not the same thing as clinical depression. An important question is whether all the true cases of clinical depression were detected; if, due to a misunderstanding, a response bias or some other source of error, a depressed person was not picked up by the "obligatory" questions discussed earlier, that person might be missed. Until the reliability and validity of the PSE, as well as that of SADS and SADS-L, has been demonstrated in the general population, we feel that these instruments are adequate only for research with either psychiatric patients or with segments of the general population who have been previously screened to insure that the phenomena being measured by the PSE or SADS are not rare.

THE PROBLEM

In the abstract, the advantages of a first-stage screening test on the one hand and a second-stage diagnostic evaluation on the other for research in psychiatric epidemiology are clear and very similar to those described by Cooper and Morgan (1973). The screening measures should be economical and, accordingly, capable of being administered by nonclinicians without lengthy prior experience and training. By contrast, the second stage, diagnostic evaluation of a limited number of persons, should utilize the skills and abilities of highly trained clinicians.

These apparently clear considerations, however, have become blurred by the actual state of affairs in psychiatric epidemiology. The major problem is that there are unanswered questions about instruments that now exist and their relation to each other. For example, PERI was not developed with reference to either of the two major nomenclatures, DSM-III or ICD-9. Rather, its strengths are that it contains a large number of measures of important dimensions of psychopathology and role functioning and that these measures are reliable in contrasting sex, class, and ethnic groups in both nonpatient and patient samples. It is thus, potentially, a good candidate to be a first-stage screening instrument. Though we believe the measured dimensions are relevant to DSM-III, ICD-9 and the related RDC and CATEGO classifications (see Table 5), to date this belief has not been tested.

By contrast to PERI, both the PSE and SADS have been explicitly developed with reference to each of the two main diagnostic systems. Moreover, their authors believe that they can perform both the screening and diagnostic function in samples from the general population. Like the beliefs about PERI, however, these beliefs about SADS and PSE have not been adequately tested.

It would seem, then, that the time has come for a test of the ability of these various instruments to do the things claimed for them: To test whether PERI can screen demographically complex samples from the general population for different types of psychiatric disorder; and whether SADS, and the PSE can both screen and diagnose such disorders in such samples.

In the next section, we will outline a strategy for testing these instruments. This strategy involves a two-stage procedure for case identification and classification, plus an additional stage to evaluate the adequacy of the two-stage results. If SADS and PSE can be effectively used in a single stage to screen and diagnose disorders in samples from the general population, our strategy will document this ability as well. If, on the other hand, it is discovered that a one-stage procedure is deficient, our strategy should prove to be useful to researchers who wish to use a multistage approach for substantive research in psychiatric epidemiology in the future.

A STRATEGY FOR TESTING FIRST STAGE INSTRUMENTS IN A TWO-STAGE PROCEDURE FOR CASE IDENTIFICATION AND CLASSIFICATION.

The need for modification and calibration of PERI

Before PERI can be tested against PSE and SADS as a first stage instrument, some preliminary work is needed in order to make its time frame comparable to each of these instruments, and in order to calibrate it using known groups of psychiatric patients. Let us briefly discuss this necessary work before we go on to the strategy for actually testing PERI, SADS, and PSE.

The Problem of Time-sets.   In the research we have done so far with PERI, the time span referred to for most of the symptom items is the year prior to the interview. While this matches well with the half of SADS that focuses on current disorder during the preceding year, it is a poor match for both the second half of SADS that investigates past disorder, and SADS-L that is designed to investigate lifetime prevalence. It is also a poor match for the PSE which focuses on symptoms during the four weeks preceding the interview. Theoretically, the problem of one year versus four weeks is easy to solve, since most PERI questions begin with either "During the past_____ (time period) . . . "or "Since _____, . . . " When we use PERI to screen for SADS diagnosed current disorder, we can fill in a one-year temporal reference; by contrast, when we develop PERI to screen for PSE diagnosed current disorder, we can fill in a four-week temporal reference. However, we have tested the reliabilities of PERI scales only for the 12-month time reference. The shorter the interval, the more likely we are to tap state rather than trait; transient episode rather than chronic condition. It is possible that the reliabilities will be different and/or that scales will be related differently to each other depending on the temporal reference. In any case, the implications of the changes in temporal reference must be tested.

Calibration of PERI scales.   As we noted earlier, we were able to obtain valuable data on a sample of drug addicts in Pennsylvania and on a sample of inpatients at a psychiatric hospital in New Hampshire. These enabled us to compare PERI scale scores on, for example, Antisocial History obtained from our general population sample in New York with the scores on the same scale for the addicts and get an empirical example of what might reasonably be meant by a high score (see Tables 3 & 4). Unfortunately, however, these patient data are highly limited for our purposes. For example, all of the Massachusetts inpatients were white, and the researcher with whom we were collaborating was able to included only five of our 25 symptom scales. At the opposite extreme, almost all the addicts were black or Puerto Rican and young. These patient data are, therefore, too limited for the purposes of calibrating PERI scales.

Thus, new data are needed for the calibration of PERI scales. Ideally, those data would be from a sample of psychiatric patients from different sex, class, and ethnic groups and with DSM-III and ICD-9 equivalents to the diagnoses of schizophrenia, affective psychosis, neurosis, antisocial personality, and other personality disorders. Both timesets for PERI need calibration which could be accomplished during a single field operation with the assignment to one or the other form determined randomly.

Data from the patient samples can be used in two ways: (a) to provide assessment of PERI criterion validity; and (b) to provide a basis for estimation of discriminant functions for use in later classification of respondents. Means and standard deviations for each of the PERI scales can be calculated using each of the five patient samples described above, in order to establish values for the PERI scales which are considered extreme.

A multiple discriminant analysis can be performed on the community and patient samples in order to obtain a function of PERI scales which discriminates patients from nonpatients.[2] Using the estimated discriminant functions and the PERI scores from the patient and community samples, misclassification rates should be estimated via the jackknife-like techniques described in Lachenbruch (1975). These rates can be used as a rough indication of the adequacy of PERI as a screening instrument for psychiatric cases in general and they will also give some indication of how much diagnostic detail the screening instrument can provide. In the analysis of misclassifications from the discriminant function, special attention should be given to those members of the nonpatient community sample who were misclassified as patients. It is likely that some of these persons will actually be untreated cases. In a post-hoc clinical investigation of these subjects' responses to PERI, an attempt could be made to identify such untreated cases, and then to remove them from the nonpatient calibration group. A new discriminant function should then be estimated by using this purified sample. Through this analysis, efforts should be made not only to maximize the discriminant ability of PERI, but also to identify the smallest set of screening variables which provides the needed discrimination. When this work is completed, a rigorous test of PERI, PSE and SADS along the lines we will describe shortly will be possible.

A note on types of interviewers that can be used in a two-stage procedure for case identification and classification.

In a previous study, we found some tendency for respondents from the general population to report more symptoms to psychiatrists during PERI interviews than to regular interviewers employed by the New York Office of the National Opinion Research Center (see Riessman, 1977). The problem was not one of mastering the technical procedures of PERI which relies for the most part on closed questions with fixed alternative response categories that are pre-coded. Since the effect took place when the psychiatrists were not identified as physicians or "doctors," we infer that it was probably lack of comfort on the part of the lay interviewers in asking questions about psychopathology that somehow was communicated to respondents and inhibited their responses. If so, other health professionals should do as well as psychiatrists. For first-stage interviews, therefore, we recommend using health professionals at pre-doctoral levels of training and experience. These interviewers might typically be Masters-level psychologists, social workers or psychiatric nurses. We shall refer to these first-stage interviewers as "non-diagnosticians."

With regard to second-stage interviews, there is some controversy as to what level of training the interviewer should have. Wing and his colleagues developed the PSE mainly for use by psychiatrists and appear to be cautious about the circumstances in which it might be effectively used by others (Wing, Henderson, and Winckle, 1977). Endicott and Spitzer (1978) have a broader group of interviewers in mind as appropriate. Here is how they describe their position:

> The most suitable personnel for administering the SADS and the SADS-L, and for using RDC, are individuals with experience in interviewing and making judgments about manifest psychopathology. Although questions are provided to assist in collecting the information and all of the items are defined to assure uniform criteria for all raters, the types of judgments called for require more knowledge of psychiatric concepts than do many of the more commonly used rating scales. For this reason, raters should usually be limited to psychiatrists, clinical psychologists, or psychiatric social workers. If other research personnel are to be used much more training is generally necessary (Endicott and Spitzer, 1978: p. 838).

In the context of these opinions, it seems to us to make the most sense to have all second-stage interviews conducted by persons who have doctoral degrees in the fields of psychiatry, clinical psychology, and psychiatric social work. We will call these interviewers "diagnosticians."

Testing the Sensitivity and Specificity of PERI, SADS-L and PSE-ID

The major test of PERI, SADS-L and PSE-ID should be in terms of the sensitivity and specificity of those instruments as first-stage screening instruments for case identification and classification. To assess the adequacy of these instruments for identifying likely cases of different types of functional psychiatric disorders when they are administered by nondiagnosticians, they should be tested against second-stage diagnoses made on the basis of SADS and PSE interviews conducted by diagnosticians.

The Identification of True Positives and True Negatives. As Galen and Gambino (1975: p. 42) point out, it is rare in all of medicine to base a final decision on the result of a single test. Few would disagree with the desirability of multiple tests, perhaps especially in the field of mental health where there is so much controversy about individual procedures. Yet systematic multimethod determinations of what constitutes a case are extremely rare in psychiatric epidemiology. We would advocate and follow a multimethod strategy, developed within a two-stage approach, in order to maximize the likelihood that we ultimately identify cases as cases and non-cases as non-cases. In practice, where the results obtained by two contrasting interview methods such as PERI and PSE are found to converge, we would have added confidence in the validity of both. Where their results are seen to diverge, we would have questions to answer as to why this was the case and we would conduct additional follow-up interviews in the search for answers. The results of this process would provide us with our criterion for defining what we will call "true positives" and "true negatives." This general strategy is spelled out for two screening instruments and one diagnostic instrument in a flow chart in Figure I.

When one takes into account time frame, there are four first-stage instruments which are of interest to test: PERI with a four-week temporal reference; PERI with a one-year temporal reference; the PSE-ID; and SADS-L. The sample for this test should be a full probability sample consisting of subjects from a well specified population composed of persons from diverse social and cultural backgrounds to insure generality of the results. In order to test all four screening instruments, the subjects could be divided randomly among the four first-stage instruments, with four subsamples defined in terms of which first stage instrument is used. In addition, it would be a good idea to include a number of persons in the sample who have a history of severe psychotic disorder. These could be former patients or current outpatients who have been released into the community. Like the large sample, these would be distributed evenly among the four instruments, and interviewers would be initially blind to their origin. Figure 1 outlines the two-stage strategy for a single comparison between two screening tests. We have shown the comparison of PERI to SADS-L. The diagram which shows the comparison of PERI to PSE-ID would be identical, except PSE-ID would be substituted for SADS-L, PSE would be substituted for SADS, and the four-week version of PERI would be substituted for the year version of PERI. In either case, Figure 1 shows how subjects screened as positive on any one of the first stage instruments administered by non-diagnosticians would be followed up by either SADS or PSE conducted by diagnosticians.

Where the first and second stage results converge, we have defined the subject to be a "true positive." Where there is a discrepancy between the first-stage designation of a subject as positive and the second-stage diagnostic interview, we would not consider the matter decided on the basis of the second-stage result. Rather, other clinicians should review all the available evidence from both first- and second-stage interviews and conduct a third-stage follow-up interview to decide whether the subject is a true positive. We have had some experience with this type of follow-up and believe that it can be effective (Mendelsohn, Egri, and Dohrenwend, 1978). Note that the discrepancies themselves are of considerable interest, particularly with regard to the different information collected by the various screening instruments.

We have hypothesized on the basis of our analyses of existing data from epidemiological studies of true prevalence that, on the average, it is likely that the true prevalence rate of functional psychiatric disorders in the United States for a given period of a few months to a year is between about 16 percent and 25 percent (Dohrenwend, Dohrenwend, Gould, Link, Neugebauer, and Wunsch-Hitzig, 1980). The current prevalence for all functional disorders in the New Haven Study by Weissman et al. (1978) was close to 18 percent, based on SADS-L interviews and RDC diagnoses. Brown et al. (1977) have reported a

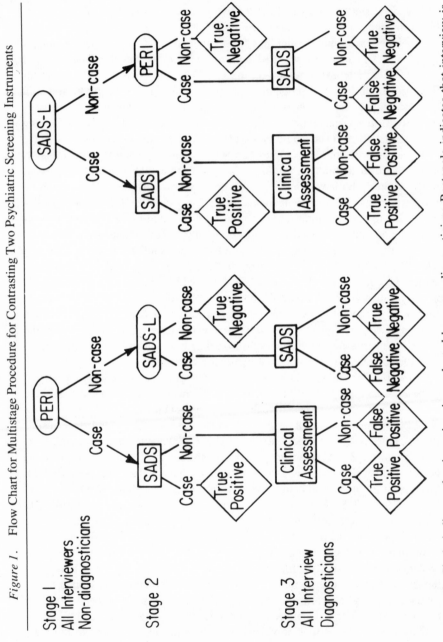

Figure 1. Flow Chart for Multistage Procedure for Contrasting Two Psychiatric Screening Instruments

Legend: Circle indicates that interview is conducted by a non-diagnostician. Rectangle indicates that interview is conducted by a diagnostician. Diamond marks decision relative to the first stage screening interview.

318

prevalence rate of 15 percent for a period of three months, based on PSE interviews with a sample of women from the general population of a section of London. If the true prevalence rate in the community being studied for all types of functional psychiatric disorders over the period of the study proved to be around 15 percent, the lowest of the figures mentioned above, one would expect a minimum of 50 true current cases if each sample contained, say, 350 subjects (above and beyond those patients added to the sample in this phase), although one should probably screen considerably more than this number for follow-up on the basis of PERI interviews to insure high sensitivity.

As is evident in Figure 1, our scheme also calls for a follow-up of subjects who are negative on the first stage, but with a somewhat different procedure than used for follow-ups of positives. Subjects who are negative on one screening test are followed up by a non-diagnostician using the competing screening instrument. Thus, our procedure clearly pits PERI against its competitors. Where PERI and its SADS-L or PSE-ID first-stage counterpart give the same results, we would define that subject to be a "true negative." the validity of this operational definition would be tested by noting whether any former patients are screened as negative by both instruments. Where the competing instruments do not agree, we would attempt to resolve the controversy by sending a diagnostician to do a second-stage interview with either SADS or the PSE in order to decide between true negative and false negative.

Let us summarize the design of the test of the first-stage instruments. For purposes of convenience, we will limit ourselves in this summary to two screening instruments, PERI and SADS-L, and one diagnostic instrument, SADS. The screening instruments would be applied to equivalent random samples and would be used to classify respondents as cases and noncases. For PERI, this classification would be based on the discriminant function developed in the prior calibration research. For SADS-L, classification would be based on published criteria (e.g., Spitzer, Endicott, and Robins, 1978). The second stage (and where necessary, the third stage) provides the criterion needed to assess the accuracy of the initial screening. As Figure 1 shows, respondents screened as cases would be interviewed by diagnosticians using SADS and would be reclassified as cases or noncases using formal diagnostic criteria (e.g., RDC). As a result of this second wave, persons screened as cases would be designated "true positives" or "false positives." Persons screened as noncases would be followed up by the alternative screening instrument (administered by a non-diagnostician); if these persons were again classified as noncases, they would be designated "true negatives." For those persons initially screened as noncases, but classified as cases by the follow-up test, a third interview would be ordered; this interview would be done by diagnosticians using the formal diagnostic criteria described above. Depending on the outcome of this third interview, these respondents will be designated either true negatives or false negatives. As a result of these designations, within each test, respondents could be classified into one of eight cells shown in Table 6.

Associated with each 2x2 table in Table 6 would be an odds ratio which reflects the association of the screening measure to the criterion. The formal comparison of PERI and the alternative measure can be done by statistically comparing the odds ratios corresponding to each measure to see if one measure has a significantly greater association with the criterion. This test could be done by applying the log-linear techniques described in Bishop, Fienberg, and Holland (1975).

Besides the formal test of PERI and the alternative measures, the strategy we have outlined would provide abundant qualitative data concerning the discrepancies between interview instruments. Thus, it might be possible to characterize the type of person who is a false positive; i.e., screened as a case, but subsequently classified as having no diagnosable disorder. Moreover, the design would also allow a comparison of the misclassifications made by one screening instrument, but not the other, since a portion of each sample would be administered two screening measures.

Further tests of the validity of the identifications or true positives and true negatives by means of follow-up measures over time. A major test of the validity of the assessments of true and false positives and negatives at any one point in time is their future course. It is devastating, for example, if those assessed as one diagnostic type at a particular time turn out to be another diagnostic type a year or two later. In studies of the sort we have outlined, therefore, it would be important to make provisions for follow-up study of the subjects in, say, about a year from the time of the baseline field work. On the basis of such a follow-up, it should be possible to identify the most valid of the procedures, summarized in Figure 1, for identifying and classifying cases. Since the samples shown in Figure 1 would have been rigorously drawn, this further test would make it possible to describe the nature and magnitude of problems of psychopathology in the community being studied with the most demonstrably valid measurement procedures yet devised for such a purpose.

Table 6. Classification of Screening Results

PERI

	Criterion Case	*Diagnosis Non-Case*
Case	True Positive	False Positive
Non-Case	False Negative	True Negative

SADS-L

	Criterion Case	*Diagnosis Non-Case*
Case	True Positive	False Positive
Non-Case	False Negative	True Negative

IN SUMMARY

The central unsolved problem in psychiatric epidemiology is how to measure psychiatric disorders independently of treatment status in general populations. We have argued that the next logical step toward this end is the development of two-stage procedures for case identification and classification. Our purpose in this paper has been to set forth a blueprint for how this might be done with leading instruments that have grown out of contrasting self-report and rating scale traditions in the assessment of psychopathology and the psychiatric disorders. Underlying our design for the development of this two-stage procedure is the belief that all instruments must be tested and validated before being applied to substantive research. We have proposed that in our present state of knowledge about the psychiatric disorders, a rigorous test of sensitivity and specificity requires the use of multiple methods (instruments) to ascertain the true psychiatric status of the respondents.

ACKNOWLEDGMENTS

Throughout this chapter results are reported of research conducted at the Social Psychiatry Research Unit at Columbia University. When we refer to "our" research, we mean the research of one or both of the authors in collaboration with our colleagues at the Research Unit: Barbara Snell Dohrenwend, Alexander Askenasy, Diana Cook, Gladys Egri, Frederick Mendelsohn, and Thomas Yager. Support for this work has come from Research Grant MH 10328 and Research Scientist Award K05 MH 14663, and from the Foundations' Fund for Research in Psychiatry. We would like to express our gratitude to Richard Tessler and to Janet Stokes who provided the data on patients that are reported in Table 1 and Table 2. We are also grateful to Barbara Dohrenwend and Barry Gurland for the classifications shown in Table 5.

NOTES

1. For example, at the time of the preparation of this chapter, the Center for Epidemiologic Studies of the National Institute of Mental Health is developing a new instrument called the Diagnostic Interview Schedule (DIS) based in part on SADS.

2. With one community sample and five patient samples, up to five functions might be needed for maximal discrimination, but it is our expectation that the first canonical vector will discriminate all patients from nonpatients.

REFERENCES

Bash, K. W. (1975), "Untersuchungen über die Epidemiologie neuropsychiatrischer Erkrankungen unter der Landbevoelkerung der Provinz Fars, Iran," *Aktuel. Fragen Psychiat. Neurol.* 5: 162.

Bishop, Y. M. M., S. E. Fienberg, and P. W. Holland (1975), *Discrete Multivariate Analysis: Theory and Practice*. Cambridge: M.I.T. Press.

Bradburn, N. M., and D. Caplowitz (1965), *Reports on Happiness*. Chicago: Aldine.

322   BRUCE P. DOHRENWEND and PATRICK E. SHROUT

Brown, G. W., T. Harris, and J. R. Copeland (1977), "Depression and Loss," *Brit. J. Psychiatry* 130:1.

Cooper, B., and H. G. Morgan (1973), *Epidemiological Psychiatry*. Springfield, IL: C.C. Thomas.

Cronbach, L. J. (1951), "Coefficient alpha and the internal structure of tests," *Psychometrics* 16:297.

Dahlstron, W. G., and G. S. Welsh (1960), *An MMPI Handbook*. Minneapolis: University of Minnesota Press.

Derogatis, L. R. (1977), *SCL-90.R. (Revised) Version Manual I*. Baltimore: Clinical Psychometrics Research Unit, Johns Hopkins University School of Medicine.

Dohrenwend, B. P., and B. S. Dohrenwend (1969), *Social Status and Psychological Disorder*. New York: Wiley.

Dohrenwend, B. P., B. S. Dohrenwend, M. Schwartz-Gould, B. G. Link, R. Neugebauer, and R. Wunsch-Hitzig (1980), *Mental Illness in the United States: An Epidemiological Analysis*. New York: Wiley.

Dohrenwend, B. P., L. Oksenberg, P. E. Shrout, B. S. Dohrenwend, and D. Cook (in press), "What brief psychiatric screening scales measure," in S. Sudman (Ed.), *Proceedings of the Third Biennial Conference on Health Survey Research Methods, May 1979*. National Center for Health Statistics.

Dohrenwend, B. P., P. E. Shrout, G. Egri, and F. C. Mendelsohn (in press), "Measures of non-specific psychological distress and other dimensions of psychopathology." *Archives of General Psychiatry*.

Dohrenwend, B. P., T. J. Yager, G. Egri, and F. S. Mendelsohn (1978). "The Psychiatric Statis Schedule (PSS) as a measure of dimensions of psychopathology in the general population," *Archives of General Psychiatry* 35:731.

Dohrenwend, B. S. (1977), "Anticipation and control of life events: An exploratory analysis," (p. 135) in Stauss, J. S., M. Babigian and M. Roff (Eds.), *Origins and Course of Psychopathology*. New York: Plenum Press.

Dohrenwend, B. S., L. Krasnoff, A. Askenasy, and B. P. Dohrenwend (1978), "Exemplification of a method for scaling life events: The PERI Life Events Scale," *Journal of Health and Social Behavior* 19:205.

Dohrenwend, B. S., D. Cook, and B. P. Dohrenwend (in press), "Measurement of social functioning in community populations," in J. K. Wing and P. Bebbington (Eds.), *The Concept of a "Case" in Psychiatric Epidemiology*. London: Grant, McIntyre.

Duncan-Jones, P., and S. Henderson (1978), "The use of a two-phase design in a prevalence survey," *Social Psychiatry* 13:231.

Eastwood, M. R. (1975), *The Relation Between Physical and Mental Illness*. Toronto: University of Toronto Press.

Endicott, J., and R. L. Spitzer (1978), "A diagnostic interview: The schedule for affective disorders and schizophrenia," *Archives of General Psychiatry* 35:837.

Feighner, J. P., E. Robins, S. B. Guze, R. A. Woodruff, G. Winokur, and R. Munoz (1972), "Diagnostic criteria for use in psychiatric research," *Archives of General Psychiatry*, 26: 57.

Fiske, D. W., (1971), *Measuring the Concepts of Personality*. Chicago: Aldine.

Frank, J. D. (1973), *Persuasion and Healing*. Baltimore: Johns Hopkins University Press (originally published, 1961).

Galen, R. S., and S. R. Gambino (1975), *The Predictive Value and Efficiency of Medical Diagnoses*. New York: Wiley.

Goldberg, D. P. (1972), *The Detection of Psychiatric Illness by Questionnaire*. London: Oxford.

Gurin, G., J. Veroff, and S. Feld (1960), *Americans View Their Mental Health*. New York: Basic Books.

Hagnell, O. (1966), *A Prospective Study of the Incidence of Mental Disorder*. Stockholm: Svenska Bokforlaget Norstedts-Bonniers.

Ilfeld, F. W., Jr. (1978), "Psychological status of community residents among major demographic dimensions," *Archives of General Psychiatry* 35:716.

International Classification of Diseases (I.C.D.9). Geneva: World Health Organization, 1977.

Kramer, M. (1976), "Issues in the development of statistical and epidemiological data for mental health services research," *Psychological Medicine* 6:185.

Lachenbruch, P. A. (1975), *Discriminant Analysis*. New York: Hafner Press.

Leighton, D. C., J. S. Harding, and D. B. Macklin (1963), *The Character of Danger*. New York: Basic Books.

Lin, T. (1953), "A study of the incidence of mental disorder in Chinese and other cultures," *Psychiatry* 16:313.

Mendelsohn, F. S., G. Egri, and B. P. Dohrenwend (1978), "Diagnosis of non-patients in the general population," *American Journal of Psychiatry* 135:1163.

Nunnally, J. C. (1967), *Psychometric Theory*. New York: McGraw-Hill.

Riessman, C. K. (1977), *Interviewer Effects in Psychiatric Epidemiology: A Study of Medical and Lay Interviewers and Their Impact on Reported Symptoms*. Ph.D. Dissertation, Graduate School of Arts and Science, Columbia University.

Rutter, M., J. Tizard, and K. Whitmore (1970), *Education, Health and Behavior*. London: Longman.

Shrout, P. E., and B. P. Dohrenwend (1979), "A Multivariate Analysis of Symptom Level Differences Across Groups Defined by Ethnicity, Education, Sex and Interviewer Type." Unpublished manuscript.

Spitzer, R. L. (1978), Personal communication at meeting of National Institute of Mental Health Division of Biometry and Epidemiology, on the Psychiatric Epidemiology Catchment Area Program, March 20.

Spitzer, R. L., J. Endicott, J. L. Fleiss, and J. Cohen (1970), "The Psychiatric Status Schedule: A technique for evaluating psychopathology and impairment in role functioning," *Archives of General Psychiatry* 23:41.

Spitzer, R. L., J. Endicott, and E. Robins (1978), *Research Diagnostic Criteria (RDC) for a Selected Group of Functional Disorders* (3rd Ed.). New York: Biometrics Research, New York State Psychiatric Institute.

Srole, L., T. S. Langner, S. T. Michael, M. K. Opler, and T. A. C. Rennie (1962), *Mental Health in the Metropolis*. New York: McGraw-Hill.

Star, S. A. (1950), "The screening of psychoneurotics in the army: Technical development of tests," (Vol. 4, p. 486) in S. A. Stouffer *et al.* (Eds.), *Measurement and Prediction*. Princeton: Princeton University Press.

Stokes, J. (1976). *The Psychological Symptoms of Drug Addicts*, mimeographed, Eagleville Hospital and Rehabilitation Center, P. O. Box 45, Eagleville, Pennsylvania 19408.

Tessler, R. (1977). *Reliability of Selected Measures Derived from the Psychiatric Epidemiology Research Interview: A Preliminary Report Based upon a Study of Psychaitric Patients*, mimeographed, Department of Sociology, University of Massachusetts, Amherst, Massachusetts 01002.

Weissman, M. M., J. K. Myers, and P. S. Harding (1978). "Psychiatric disorders in a U.S. urban community: 1975–1976," *American Journal of Psychiatry* 135:459.

Wing, J. K., J. E. Cooper, and N. Sartorius (1974), *The Measurement and Classification of Psychiatric Symptoms*. London: Cambridge.

Wing, J. K., A. S. Henderson, and M. Winckle (1977), "The rating of symptoms by a psychiatrist and a non-psychiatrist," *Psychological Medicine* 7:713.

Wing, J. K., S. A. Mann, J. P. Leff, and J. M. Nixon (1978), "The concept of a "case" in psychiatric population surveys," *Psychological Medicine* 8:203.

Part IV

SOCIETAL ISSUES

Compulsory Sterlization Statutes:
Public Sentiment and Public Policy

Rosalie A. Cohen and Anita M. Cohen

INTRODUCTION

Traditional notions of mental illness are simplistic, locating its cause in moral or constitutional inadequacies of individuals, either genetic or otherwise unchangeable, and requiring the constraint or removal of the individuals affected from society for its protection. Contemporary efforts are based in the conviction that the causes of mental illness are complex, that some important causal factors lie outside the individuals affected in the social and/or societal millieu, and that these conditions can be changed, thereby justifying individual or group treatment and/or social reform. (Bellack, 1963; Caplan and Caplan, 1967; Cohen, Gardner, and Zax, 1967; Marks, 1974). Since laws provide society's most formal statements of the logic which links such assumptions to public policy, this paper proposes that the persistence of compulsory sterilization statutes is an indicator that traditional assumptions about the causes and control of mental illness are still widely held in society.

Research in Community and Mental Health, Volume 2, pages 327–357
Copyright © 1981 by JAI Press, Inc.
All rights of reproduction in any form reserved.
ISBN: 0-89232-152-0

Links between assumed causes of mental illness and public policy are provided in a two-step process. Firstly, compulsory sterilization statutes are presented in historical context as indicators of one possible causal explanation for mental illness (and the other conditions covered in them). Statutes in the 50 states in the United States were subjected to content analysis in 1968, five years after the federal concern with the community mental health concept began, and again in 1973, after the states' examinations of their codes. Data from the revised codes are presented in nine appended charts with 1968 to 1973 changes discussed in the text of this paper. Post-1973 developments were also monitored and will be commented on in the text. Secondly, assumptions underlying compulsory sterilization statutes are placed in a general theoretical framework, contrasting them with other causal explanations, some of which characterize dominant contemporary efforts. From these causal explanations are derived the range of management and control options available, thereby proposing a logic of public policy.

Contemporary efforts in mental health depend increasingly upon community support. It is suggested that the continuing support for compulsory sterilization statutes demonstrates persistent public sentiment for traditional assumptions which may limit or constrain the effectiveness of these new efforts.

The Origins and Persistence of Compulsory Sterilization Statutes in the U.S.

Compulsory sterilization statutes in the U.S. arose in the late 19th and early 20th centuries out of the Eugenics movement, an effort to control scientifically the inter-generational transmission of undesirable traits in the population. It accompanied the scientific and industrial revolutions at the turn of the century; its pronouncements were couched in the language of Darwin and Mendel; and it expressed the confidence of the age that social engineering could be carried out using similar approaches to those that had brought modern societies some measure of control over their physical environments. These statutes were formal statements of the beliefs dominant at the time—i.e., that individuals are "what they are born." The Eugenics movement was world-wide among industrial nations although not all countries in which it was in vogue were successful in enacting sterilization laws.[1]

Michigan and Pennsylvania were the first states in the U.S. to make efforts to enact compulsory sterilization statutes in 1897 and 1905 respectively, but they were unsuccessful. Pennsylvania's law had passed both houses, but it was vetoed by the Governor, making Indiana the first state to succeed in 1907. Other states followed suit: Connecticut, Washington, and California in 1909; New Jersey and Iowa in 1911; Nevada and New York in 1912; North Dakota, Michigan, Kansas, and Wisconsin in 1913; Nebraska in 1915; Oregon, South Dakota, and New Hampshire in 1917; North Carolina and Alabama in 1919; Montana and Delaware in 1923; Virginia in 1924; Idaho, Utah, Minnesota, and Maine in 1925; Mississippi in 1928; West Virginia and Arizona in 1929; and Vermont and

Oklahoma in 1931. Notable in other countries were those laws enacted in Canada, in the Scandinavian countries, in Germany, and in British Columbia between 1928 and 1933.[2] In the U.S., 31 states have had compulsory sterilization statutes at one time or another since 1907; and although some were discarded when challenged on constitutional grounds, others were replaced with stronger laws, better constructed to withstand constitutional challenges.[3]

It is apparent that there is no special commonality among the states that enacted these laws. They represent all regions of the country and both rural and urban dominances. Those laws passed in several states in the same years also provide no evidence of collaboration among their developers or of common lacks or needs which might explain the emergence of the statutes at that specific point in time. The common force that appeared to be acting upon their drafters was the widespread belief of the time that the conditions named were heritable, and that these conditions could be controlled inter-generationally through sterilization and the contemporaneous marriage controls.[4] Indeed, the categories of individuals to whom the statutes applied—most commonly, the mentally retarded, the mentally ill, and the epileptic—were conservative in their scope. A Model Eugenic Sterilization Law that was proposed by prominent eugenicists of the time included also the criminalistic, the delinquent and wayward, inebriates and drug habitues, the diseased (tuberculous, syphlitic, leprous, and others with chronic, infectuous and legally segregatable diseases), the blind and partially sighted, the deaf and partially hearing, the deformed and the dependent, including orphans, ne'er-do-wells, homeless tramps, and paupers.[5] That these statutes embodied the genetic beliefs extant at the time is evidenced by the following statement of the prominent jurist, Oliver Wendell Holmes. In writing the majority opinion of the U.S. Supreme Court which upheld Virginia's compulsory sterilization statute in 1927, he wrote:

> ... for those who sap the strength of the State ... instead of waiting to execute degenerate offspring for crime, or to let them starve for their imbecility, society can prevent those who are manifestly unfit from continuing their kind ... Three generations of imbeciles are enough. . . [6]

The persistence of compulsory sterilization statutes has been remarkable. They have survived a variety of constitutional challenges ... as cruel and unusual punishment, as bills of attainder, and as violations of both procedural and substantive due process.[7] An additional ground, deprivation of the equal protection of the laws, has been a barrier to the mentally ill and handicapped in obtaining voluntary sterilization as well as in their protection from its compulsory application; that is, as legal incompetents, they are as unable to give valid consent for voluntary sterilizations as they are to resist its compulsory application. Even during the peak use of the statutes during the 1930s,[8] legislators were not influenced by reports issued by both the American Neurological Association[9] and the American Medical Association[10] concluding that scientific knowledge about the genetic transmission of the conditions covered did not justify the use of sterilization as a method of control. During the 1950s and 1960s, newer punitive forms of the statutes also emerged, resulting in a 1969 critical study of the codes of six of the states by the federal Supreme Court.[11] Major revamping of some of the codes did result from constitutional challenges in the past decade. Improved provisions for due process, additional protections for participants and provisions for hospitals and their staffs to refuse to perform sterilizations were added to the statutes in a number of states. However, few states were willing to give up these codes as mechanisms of social control.

In 1968, twenty-seven states still had compulsory sterilization statutes on the books. Unlike the criminal codes, which having developed from ancient common law had become partially obsolete without recodification, compulsory sterilization statutes had had a known origin in modern law; and they were reviewed between 1968 and 1973 by the states for purposes of repeal or recodification. Nine charts which appear in the Appendix analyze the content of these statutes as they appeared in 1973. These charts summarize: (1) the stated intents of legislatures in enacting these laws; (2) those individuals who fall under their provisions; (3) where sterilization of individuals certified for the listed conditions is conditional to marriage or discharge from custodial institutions; (4) the agencies which are to initiate action; (5) those individuals who are authorized to examine candidates for certification; (6) agencies which authorize the sterilization; (7) compensation of participants for their duties; (8) the characteristics of due process; and (9) whether immunity from prosecution is provided to participants in the legal or medical procedures of compulsory sterilization. Of special note is the continued inclusion of the mentally ill by most of the states as a category of individuals to be covered.

Between 1968 and 1973, eight states repealed or modified their original compulsory statutes, enacting Planned Parenthood or otherwise more broadly based, primarily voluntary, population control measures in their stead.[12] Arkansas was added to the charts, having passed a voluntary sterilization law which authorized parents and guardians to request sterilization for their children, making the involuntary sterilization of these dependents possible. Most other changes were responsive to due process challenges. As a result of these reviews, the number of states in which the statutes established Eugenics Boards had shrunk from six to three.[13] While in 1968, only two states had had "voluntary only" statutes (consent of the individuals affected was required), in 1973, eleven states required either the consent of the individual or of a parent or guardian.[14] While earlier, 24 states had had "compulsory only" statutes (consent not being required), in 1973 only 15 such laws remained,[15] in three cases naming the District Court or the Director of Health to provide authorization in the absence of consent.[16] Four states, one state having been added in the interim period, provided for both voluntary and compulsory cases.[17] While among those earlier states having compulsory laws, the designated agency was *required* to initiate proceedings against those appropriately certified, in 1973, there were only eight remaining.[18] Among those in which the designated agency was *authorized* to initiate proceedings against those appropriately certified, there was one less state in 1973, the number having been reduced from 12 to 11.[19] Among those states in which there were provisions for the sterilization of individuals who were not institutionalized, however, (extramural laws), the trend was reversed, their number having increased from nine to 17.[20]

The review process conducted by the states also revealed that population and economic stresses in society had created new interest in compulsory sterilization statutes. While early laws had arisen out of beliefs that the conditions covered by the statutes were genetically transmitted, more recent interest in them was punitive and economic. The 1960s marked an emergence of proposals in a number of states—some with, and others without, compulsory sterilization statutes, to establish punitive legislation for welfare mothers. Some of these proposals included sterlization, in conjunction with fines and imprisonment, the loss of welfare benefits and the loss of the custody of their children.[21] States most interested in punitive sterilization during these years were California, Delaware, Georgia, Illinois, Iowa, Louisiana, Mississippi, North Carolina, and Virginia.[22] The general foci of the proposed statutes were toward control of comparatively powerless segments of society—the poor and women in particular. Their efforts were largely concerned with controlling the rising costs of welfare; and justification for withdrawing the power to have children cited the ''immorality'' of those to be affected, or their lack of responsibility or self-control, along with their inability properly to parent their children. Louisiana and Mississippi did pass punitive criminal laws to control the costs of illegitimate births, but they did not include sterilization among their provisions. North Carolina and Virginia passed the first voluntary sterilization laws; and the former added ''grossly sexually delinquent persons'' to its compulsory coverage, becoming the state with the most comprehensive sterilization program in the country.[23]

Some states have been clearly ambivalent in the matter of compulsory sterilization. Pennsylvania, one of the earliest states to consider such a law at the turn of the century, has repeatedly considered compulsory and punitive proposals in the intervening years (including a punitive proposal in 1963 which did not include sterilization as one of its provisions) enacting none of them. There is evidence, however, that 270 sterilizations were performed without benefit of law on patients at its Elwyn State School between 1889 and 1931.[24] In Ohio, Judge Holland Gary ordered a number of sterilizations in the absence of a law until prohibited through suit;[25] and periodic law suits during the review years brought to light instances of involuntary sterilizations of dependent children whose parents have applied for the use of a state's voluntary sterilization provisions without the knowledge or consent of the children themselves. Although most of the recent punitive laws that were proposed failed to be enacted, their presentation and discussion in both political and scientific communities again made explicit the sentiments and beliefs necessary to support compulsory sterilization as a method of social control.

Since 1973, two major trends in applying the intent of the statutes are apparent. One trend is the simple continuation of those processes already described. Some states are pressed to limit their laws and other states to extend them. For example, at the time of writing, Oklahoma is considering a proposal to add convicted rapists to its compulsory coverage.[26] The second trend is for the application of compulsory sterilization statutes to be masked by the generalized acceptance of voluntary sterilization as a method of population control. Where legal consent is obtained, the use of the appropriate surgical procedures would be unremarked as compulsory sterilizations, even though those affected might be involuntary subjects. Thus, parents and guardians, guardians *ad litem* (those appointed by the Court), and institutional boards or superintendents, having received broad powers to apply procedures which they believe to be in the best interests of their charges, can give legal consent to sterilizations for those certified as incompetent by virtue of age or physical conditions. Those affected may be involuntarily sterilized under the voluntary laws, thus, legal consent having been obtained from recognized or appropriately appointed third parties.

Problems in the voluntary consent procedures have been less concerned with the substantive issue of involuntary sterilization than with shifts in "Rights" legislation in related matters. Changes in the legal "age of consent," (an earlier assumption of adult status for children than that previously defined by state laws), or the acquisition of limited areas of legal competency by the mentally ill following deinstitutionalization are examples of new ambiguities. In one case, a father claims that the court's refusal to grant his request to sterilize his retarded daughter deprives her of the equal protection of the law; that is, having been certified as legally incompetent, she cannot herself sign consent to the operation; and, if consent of a parent and legal guardian cannot be accepted, she is deprived of sterilization obtainable by others.[27]

Despite the issues raised in such cases, guardian consent provisions of the voluntary population control measures enacted in all states make difficult the assessment of the extent to which the involuntary sterilizations of third persons is employed. Of the 400 to 500 walk-in, walk-out vasectomies performed in the New York City Planned Parenthood Clinics each year,[28] or those low-cost, one-day operations for women reported to be similarly available in other cities,[29] the number of third party consents are unable to be estimated without an analysis of the clinics' records. Thus, there appears to be a shift from compulsory to "legally voluntary" but in fact involuntary sterilization for many individuals affected by sterilization statutes, reflecting little change in methods of social control or in the sentiments which underlie them. In fact, the codes appear to have been strengthened to withstand constitutional challenges rather than abandoned as mechanisms of social control.

The distribution of support for compulsory sterilization statutes, rather than its numerical weight, is of special interest. The wide range of states in which proposals continue to be considered is one measure of such distribution. In addition, when only one chamber passes such legislation, it is usually the Senate, the members of which are drawn from communities geographically distributed across the states. Shared beliefs have been found as well among the general public, although empirical research in this area is limited. In a 1962 Gallup Poll, for instance, roughly 20 percent of respondents who were asked what should be done about unwed mothers on relief answered that the solution was to sterilize them.[30] The most important evidence of the underlying beliefs about the causes of mental illness, however, are found in the codes themselves, which persist despite professional redefinition and judicial criticism. What beliefs about the causes of mental illness underlie these developments? And how are these beliefs linked to the public policy of management and control?

Public Sentiment and Public Policy

It is apparent that whatever beliefs are held about the causes of mental illness or the nature of the condition, certain specific assumptions are necessary before sterilization is considered as a method of control. One such necessary assumption is that the problem is locatable in the individuals affected. There would be no justification for using so intrusive a method of control unless based on the empirical or theoretical grounds that the problem is completely reachable in the individual and that the individual is the appropriate unit for intervention. Whether the effort of the statutes is to contain specific genetic imperfections or to serve as punishment for the constitutionally immoral or incompetent who might otherwise abuse the privilege to bear children, those characteristics must be viewed as locatable in the individuals to be sterilized. A second kind of assumption has to do with the conviction that changing the offending conditions in some alternative way is impossible or impractical. Sterlization becomes, then, a logical extension of beliefs or sentiments about the conditions covered by the statutes as being caused by unchangeable characteristics of the individuals involved.

Most management and control efforts, whether individual or social, can be incorporated into a 2x2 matrix, using the variables mentioned above—namely, (1) the cause is "in the individual" or "in his social groups" and (2) the cause is either "changeable" or "unchangeable," as expressed in the diagram below.

The Derivation of Management Strategies from Perceived Sources and Changeability in Cause of Mental Illness

	In the individual	In his social groups
Changeable	Psychotherapy Medical Treatment	Group therapy Social Reform
Unchangeable	Confinement Sterilization	Re-placement

The logical unit for intervention is that unit in which the cause is located; e.g., in the individual or in his social groups or society; and intervention strategies are logically directed toward the unit of analysis in which the cause is theoretically locatable. The second variable, the changeable-unchangeable dimension, however, determines whether intervention strategies of any sort may be viewed as potentially effective, or whether removal of the individuals affected is called for. When an assumption of unchangeability is made, hospitalization limited to long-term custodial care is no more than an expedient method to contain the impact of the mentally ill on the community rather than an effort to manage the mental illness itself; and sterilization is an extension of this containment principle inter-generationally.

Intervention strategies designed to cure mental illness find a role only where an assumption can be made that the causes of the condition can be removed or modified. Treatment decisions which follow this assumption of changeability include identifying the *locus* of the causes as the *point* of intervention and the *kinds* of causes to determine the *nature* of the intervention. Given an assumption of changeability, thus, the locus of intervention is focused on the individual only when the causes are located in the individual, and the kinds of intervention follow systematically from analysis of what kinds of problems have been located there. For example, individual psychiatry is indicated where the kinds of problems found in the individual are of psychiatric origin. Where the causes are of physiological origin, medical treatment may be called for; a reeducation or reso-cialization process may follow from an analysis that initial education or socializa-tion processes have been faulty and so forth. In each case, three assumptions have been made, namely that (1) the condition is changeable, (2) the causes lie in the individual, and (3) they are of particular kinds, specific intervention strategies for which are identifyable.

Similar levels of analysis are called for where the causes of an individual's problems are found to be changeable and in his social groups, or more generally, in society. If the loci of an individual's problems are found in improper or pathological family or peer group relationships, for instance, intervention into his family or peer groups is called for; and family or peer group therapy may be selected as a treatment modality. Similarly, where the causes are found in societal conditions, only intervention into society, using the kinds of intervention strategies logically derived from specific identifiable causes, can be justified.

It is important to note that, where pathology is found in an individual's groups, and where these groups are seen as *un*changeable, intervention for affected individuals is nevertheless possible by removing them from the offending groups and re-placing them in other more constructive ones. The foster family, divorce, or job change are intervention strategies of this type; and the current move toward deinstitutionalization may be seen as involving a similar analytic process. Indeed, the only instance in which sterilization and institutionalization of the long-term custodial type may be viewed as logically derived management modalities is when it is believed that the causes of mental illness lie solely in the individual and that it is impossible or impractical to affect them.

Compulsory sterilization statutes reflect the above assumptions; i.e., the causes of mental illness (and related conditions as covered by these statutes) lie solely in the individuals affected, and the conditions are unchangeable. Withholding public support for prevention and for curative, educative or rehabilitative efforts or new directions of group or social reform is thereby justified. It is suggested that, when the assumptions of complex causality and changeability which underlie contemporary social psychiatric research and practice are more widely shared by the public, such public resistance will tend to disappear along with the compulsory sterilization statutes in which conflicting assumptions about the causes of mental illness are made apparent.

SUMMARY

Compulsory sterilization statutes are 20th century products, and they continue to be refined and modified to meet challenges to their constitutionality. New laws embodying similar beliefs about the nature of human nature are continually being developed, whether or not they are enacted; and, on rare occasions, sterilizations have been ordered in the absence of a law. During the past several decades, despite the absence of convincing scientific evidence that most conditions covered by these statutes are transmitted genetically, sterilization continues to be seen by many as a viable method of control. Because these statutes reflect certain important assumptions made by the public about the causes of mental illness—namely, that it is caused by unchangeable characteristics of individuals—compulsory sterilization statutes are used here as indicators of the persistence of these assumptions—assumptions that contradict the thrust of contemporary public policy.

NOTES

Entitled, "Resistance to Contemporary Mental Health Developments; Compulsory Sterilization Statutes as Indicators of Public Sentiment," this paper was read at the 9th World Congress of Sociology in Upsala, Sweden, August 14-19, 1978 in the section of Theory and Praxis of Mental Health and Mental Health Care.

1. England was one such country.
2. See discussion in Haller, Mark H. (1963), *Eugenics: Hereditarian Attitudes in American Thought*. New Brunswick, N.J.; Rutgers Univ. Press. p. 139.
3. For example, North Carolina's 1919 law was never used, but its 1929 and 1933 revampings became state policy for the institutionally mentally retarded, and its newer forms are still in use for a range of disabilities.

4. In 1935, 41 states also had marriage control laws prohibiting marriages by the insane and feeble minded, 17 by epileptics, four by confirmed drunkards; and some states provided criminal penalties for having sexual intercourse with defective individuals.

5. Laughlin, J. (1922) *Eugenical Sterilization in the United States*, pp. 446–447 original. Ref. Burgdorf, R. L. and Burgdorf, M. P., "The Wicked Witch is Almost Dead: Buck v. Bell and the Sterilization of Handicapped Persons," *Temple Law Quarterly* 50:4. p. 1000.

6. Buck v. Bell, 274 U.S. 200, 201 (1927).

7. Burgdorf & Burgdorf, *op. cit.* p. 1000–1001. There is also a detailed discussion in McKinley, Patrick J. (1967–8), "Comment: Compulsory Eugenic Sterilization: For Whom Does Bell Toll?" *Duquesne Univ. Law Review* 6:2 pp. 145–156.

8. Paul, Julius, (1968), "The Return of Punitive Sterilization Proposals: Current Attacks on Illegitimacy and the AFDC Program," *Law and Society Review* III: 1 August, p. 78.

9. Comm. Am. Neurological Ass'n. (1936), *Eugenical Sterilization*.

10. Comm. to Study Contraceptive Practices & Related Problems, (1937), *American Medical Association Proceedings* 54.

11. The states reviewed by the court were California, Nebraska, Indiana, Maine, Wisconsin, and North Carolina.

12. 'Georgia, Idaho, Kansas, Montana, Nebraska, North Dakota, Oregon and Virginia.

13. Georgia, Idaho, Iowa*, Montana*, North Carolina*, and Oregon. Those with * remained in 1973.

14. Originally Minnesota and Vermont. Added were Arkansas, Colorado, Georgia, Idaho, Montana, North Dakota, Oregon, Tennessee and Connecticut.

15. Alabama*, Arizona*, Connecticut, Delaware*, Georgia, Indiana*, Kansas, Iowa*, Michigan*, Mississippi*, Nebraska, New Hampshire*, North Dakota, Oklahoma*, South Carolina*, Utah*, Virginia, West Virginia*, Wisconsin*, Idaho, Iowa, Montana, Oregon, California*, added was Washington. Those with *'s remained in 1973.

16. Iowa, Michigan, and California.

17. Maine, South Dakota, North Carolina. Virginia was added.

18. Alabama*, Connecticut, Georgia, Idaho, Iowa*, Kansas, Maine*, Michigan*, Montana, Nebraska, North Carolina*, North Dakota, Oregon, South Dakota*. Added were South Carolina and West Virginia. Those with *'s remained in 1973.

19. Arizona, California, Delaware, Indiana, Mississippi, New Hampshire, Oklahoma, South Carolina, Utah, Virginia, West Virginia, Wisconsin. South Carolina, and West Virginia were not included in 1973, but Washington was added.

20. The original states were Idaho, Iowa, Michigan, North Carolina, Oregon, South Dakota, Vermont, Delaware, and Utah. Added were Arkansas, California, Connecticut, Colorado, Georgia, Maine, Montana, and Virginia.

21. Paul *op. cit.* p. 78.

22. *Ibid.* p. 79.

23. *Ibid.* p. 92.

24. Paul *op. cit.* p. 96.

25. No 70–225, slip op. at 6 (S. D. Ohio August 7, 1970). A discussion of this case appears in Burgdorf and Burgdorf, *op. cit.* pp. 1014–1016.

26. Oklahoma Senate Bill 79.

27. Ruby v. Massey. Fed. DC 1978 452 F.Supp. 361.

28. Announcement by Alfred F. Moran, Executive Vice President of Planned Parenthood of Greater New York, reported in The Philadelphia *Bulletin* newspaper, March 20, 1979.

29. *Ibid.* The cities listed were Columbus, Ohio; Nashville, Tennessee; Augusta, Georgia and, by the time of writing, New York, New York. The technique is a new, non-surgical one—mini-laparotomies.

30. *Washington Post* news item, Jan. 27, 1965. See discussion in Paul, *op. cit.* p. 100.

REFERENCES

Bellak, Leopold (1963), "Community Psychiatry: The Third Psychiatric Revolution," pp. 1-11, *Handbook of Community Psychiatry and Community Mental Health*. New York: Grune and Stratton.

Burgdorf, Robert L., Jr., and Marcia Pearce Burgdorf (1977), The Wicked Witch Is Almost Dead. Buck v. Bell and the Sterilization of Handicapped Persons," *Temple Law Quarterly* 50(4):995-1034.

Caplan, Gerald, and Ruth Caplan (1967), "The Development of Community Psychiatric Concepts in the U.S.," pp. 1499-1516 in A. M. Freedman and H. I. Kaplan (Eds.), *Comprehensive Textbook of Psychiatry*. Baltimore: Williams and Wilkins.

Cohen, E. J., E. A. Gardner, and M. Zax (1967), *Emergent Approaches to Mental Health Problems*. New York: Appleton-Century-Crofts.

Haller, Mark H. (1963), *Eugenics: Hereditarian Attitudes in American Thought*. New Brunswick, N.J.: Rutgers University Press.

Marks, John H., Patricia Riecker, and David L. Ellison (1974), "The Sociology of Community Mental Health: Historical and Methodological Perspectives," pp. 9-40 in Paul M. Roman and Harrison Trice (Eds.), *Sociological Perspectives in Community Mental Health*. Philadelphia: F. A. Davis.

McKinley, Patrick J. (1967-68), "Comment: Compulsory Eugenic Sterilization: For Whom Does Bell Toll?", *Duquesne University Law Review* 6(2):145-156.

Paul, Julius (1968), "The Return of Punitive Sterilization Proposals: Current Attacks on Illegitimacy and the AFDC Program," *Law and Society Review* III(1):77-106.

Wood, Curtis, Jr. (1964), "A Prescription for the Alleviation of Welfare Abuses and Illegitimacy," *Henry Ford Hospital Medical Bulletin* 12(March):75-81.

STATE CODES 1968—1973

Ala. Code Tit. 45 Sec. 243 (1959)

Ariz. Rev. Stat. Ann. Sec. 36-531 (1956)

Arkansas M.H. 59-501-02 (Supp. 1978)

California Welf. & Inst'ns. Code Sec. 6624 (West. 1966) Penal 2670 (1974)

Conn. Gen'l. Stat. Rev. Sec. 17-19 (Suppl. 1965)

Del. Code Ann. Tit. 16 Sec. 6701-05 (1953)

Georgia Code Ann. Sec. 99-1301 (1955)

Idaho Code Ann. Sec. 66-801-16 Sec. 5701-5705 (1953)

Ind. Ann. Stat. Sec. 22-1601 (1964)

Iowa Code Sec. 145.9 (1966)

Maine Rev. Stat. Ann. Tit. 34 Sec. 2461 (1964)

Mich. Stat. Ann. Sec. 14-381-82 (Supp. 1965)

Minn. Stat. Ann. Sec. 256.07 (1965)

Miss. Code Ann. Sec. 6957 (1942)

Mont. Rev. Codes Ann. Sec. 38-601-08 (1947)

Neb. Rev. Stat. Sec. 83-501-09 (1943)

N. Hampshire Rev. Stat. Ann. Sec. 174:1 (1964)

N.Car. Gen. Stat. Sec. 35-36 (1966)

N. Dakota Cent. Code Sec. 25-04.1-13.1

Okla. Stat. Ann. Tit. 43a Sec. 341-46 (1961)

Oregon Rev. Stat. Sec. 436.070 (1965)

S. Car. Code Ann. Sec. 32-671-80 (1962)

S. Dak. Code Sec. 30.1501-14 (1939)

Utah Code Ann. Sec. 64-10-1-14 (1953)

Ver. Stat. Ann. Tit. 18, Sec. 3201-04 (1959)

Va. Code Ann. Sec. 37-231 (Supp. 1966)

Wash. Rev. Code 9.92.100

W. Va. Code Ann. Sec. 16-10-1 (1966)

Wisc. Stat. Sec. 46.12 (1965)

(Arkansas added in interim)

APPENDIX I.   Stated Intents of the Laws

	Alabama	Arizona	Arkansas	California	Connecticut	Delaware	Georgia	Idaho	Indiana	Iowa	Maine	Michigan
Punitive				X								
Therapeutic*		X						X	X	X	X	X
Preventive of wards of the state		X					X	X		X		X
Prevention of mental illness		X	X			X	X	X	X	X	X	X
Prevention of feeble minded		X				X	X	X	X		X	X
Prevention of epilepsy		X								X	X	
Prevention of delinquency, crime							X				X	
Prevention of sex perverts												X
Prevention of moral degenerates										X		X
Prevention of other forms of maladjustment							X	X				
Prevention of physical harm							X	X				
Prevention of syphilis										X		
To protect society from menaces, or for the public good		X								X		X
Person incapable of comprehending consequences of his actions					X							

*If the statement of intent included "... in the welfare..." or "best interests of the individual..." as well as of the state, a "therapeutic" intent was recorded. No state looked upon statutes as directed toward sexual causality of the conditions covered by them.

Minnesota	Mississippi	Montana	Nebraska	N. Hampshire	N. Carolina	N. Dakota	Oklahoma	Oregon	S. Carolina	S. Dakota	Utah	Vermont	Virginia	Washington	W. Virginia	Wisconsin	TOTALS
														X			2
X	X			X	X	X	X		X		X	X	X		X		17
				X			X	X									8
X	X			X	X		X	X	X	X		X	X		X		20
X	X			X	X		X		X			X	X		X		16
X				X			X		X						X		8
							X										3
																	1
																	2
											X						3
																	2
										X							2
		X			X	X	X		X		X	X	X		X		12
																	1

APPENDIX II. Individuals Affected

	Alabama	Arizona	Arkansas	California	Connecticut	Delaware	Georgia	Idaho	Indiana	Iowa	Maine	Michigan
Mentally ill		X	X	X	X	X	X	X	X	X	X	X
Mentally defective or deficient	X	X	X	X	X	X	X	X	X	X	X	X
Criminally insane												X
Epileptic		X			X	X			X	X		
Perverted or abnormal mentality												
Sexual deviants or perverts				X						X		X
Moral degenerates				X						X		X
Syphilitic										X		
Habitual criminals				X		X				X		
Nonphabitual criminals												
Menaces to society										X		
Those unlikely to perform functions of a parent							X	X				
Those whose children are likely to be social menaces										X		X
Those whose children are likely to be wards of state										X		X
Those whose children are likely to have physical, mental, or nervous disorders or deficiencies		X		X			X	X	X	X	X	X
Those whose children are likely to be socially inadequate		X							X			
Those subject to discharge								X			X	
Marriage license application by those certified for listed conditions												

Minnesota	Mississippi	Montana	Nebraska	N. Hampshire	N. Carolina	N. Dakota	Oklahoma	Oregon	S. Carolina	S. Dakota	Utah	Vermont	Virginia	Washington	W. Virginia	Wisconsin	TOTALS
X	X	X		X	X	X	X	X	X	X	X	X	X		X	X	26
X	X	X		X	X	X	X	X	X	X	X	X	X		X	X	27
																	1
	X			X			X		X		X				X		11
										X							1
											X		X				5
																	3
								X									2
							X				X		X			X	7
													X			X	2
																	1
		X						X		X	X						6
																	2
								X									3
	X	X		X	X		X	X	X	X		X	X		X		19
	X			X			X		X								6
X					X		X				X						6
					X			X									2

APPENDIX III. Sterilization of Individuals Certified for Listed Conditions is Conditional to Marriage or Discharge from Custodial Institution

	Alabama	Arizona	Arkansas	California	Connecticut	Delaware	Georgia	Idaho	Indiana	Iowa	Maine	Michigan	Minnesota
Marriage													
Parole or discharge								X			X		X

APPENDIX IV. Agency which Initiates Action

	Alabama	Arizona	Arkansas	California	Connecticut	Delaware	Georgia	Idaho	Indiana	Iowa	Maine	Michigan
Individual or parent or guardian, spouse, next-of-kin			X				X	X			X	
Super or board of institution for the mentally ill		X		X	X	X			X	X	X	X
Super or board of institution for the feeble-minded and/or epileptic	X	X		X	X	X			X	X	X	X
Director of state dept. of family & children services							X					
Any charitable institution or Super of any institution supported wholly or in part by public funds												X
Medical staff or institutional physician					X						X	
A physician									X		X	
Warden of penal institution										X		X
Super or warden of any training camp, corrective or reform school, detention home or camp										X		X

APPENDIX III—(Continued)

Mississippi	Montana	Nebraska	N. Hampshire	N. Carolina	N. Dakota	Oklahoma	Oregon	S. Carolina	S. Dakota	Utah	Vermont	Virginia	Washington	W. Virginia	Wisconsin	TOTALS
				X					X							2
				X	X				X							6

APPENDIX IV—(Continued)

Minnesota	Mississippi	Montana	Nebraska	N. Hampshire	N. Carolina	N. Dakota	Oklahoma	Oregon	S. Carolina	S. Dakota	Utah	Vermont	Virginia	Washington	W. Virginia	Wisconsin	TOTALS
		X			X	X				X		X	X				10
X		X					X		X	X			X		X	X	16
X		X				X	X		X	X			X		X	X	18
																	1
						X	X		X								4
																	2
								X					X			X	5
						X	X		X							X	7
							X						X		X		5

(continued)

APPENDIX IV. Agency which Initiates Action (Continued)

	Alabama	Arizona	Arkansas	California	Connecticut	Delaware	Georgia	Idaho	Indiana	Iowa	Maine	Michigan
Board (or div.) of public health							X	X				
Dept. (or Committee) of public welfare												X
State Brd. of eugenics (or of public protection)												
Court				X								
Any two persons												
Any family member												X
Sheriff												X
Super. of the poor												X
Super. of any township												X
Any state resident												
Commissioner or board of mental health or clinic						X						
Friend												

Minnesota	Mississippi	Montana	Nebraska	N. Hampshire	N. Carolina	N. Dakota	Oklahoma	Oregon	S. Carolina	S. Dakota	Utah	Vermont	Virginia	Washington	W. Virginia	Wisconsin	TOTALS
																	2
X					X											X	4
																	0
														X			2
								X									1
																	1
																	1
																	1
																	1
										X							1
												X					2
													X				1

APPENDIX V. Those Authorized to Examine Candidates for Certification

	Alabama	Arizona	Arkansas	California	Connecticut	Delaware	Georgia	Idaho	Indiana	Iowa	Maine	Michigan
A. *Who Examines*												
Psychiatrists			X									
General physician(s)			X				X	X	X			X
Institutional physician(s)			X		X		X				X	
Board of the institution and/or super.						X		X	X			
Board of physicians					X	X					X	
Subcommission for mentally retarded												
Mental hygiene clinic						X						
Surgeons					X							
Alienist						X						
Social worker												
Psychologist												
Dept. of state brd. of health or eugenics, or protection						X				X		
B. *Approval, if a board*												
Two members												
Majority or quorum					X		X			X		
Unanimous						X						

Minnesota	Mississippi	Montana	Nebraska	N. Hampshire	N. Carolina	N. Dakota	Oklahoma	Oregon	S. Carolina	S. Dakota	Utah	Vermont	Virginia	Washington	W. Virginia	Wisconsin	TOTALS
					X											X	3
X			X								X	X					9
										X							5
X										X						X	6
						X											4
										X							1
																	1
						X						X				X	4
																	1
						X						X					2
X						X						X					3
		X							X	X							5
																	0
								X		X							5
						X										X	3

APPENDIX VI.　Agency which Authorizes the Sterilization

	Alabama	Arizona	Arkansas	California	Connecticut	Delaware	Georgia	Idaho	Indiana	Iowa	Maine	Michigan
State board of eugenics or control or public or social protection										X		
State board of health or mental hygiene or medical examiners		X		X					X		X	
Super. or board of Initiating Institution	X											
State hospital board												
Brd. of directors of institution(s)											X	
A board of physicians											X	
A psychologist or social worker												
Public Welfare Dept.						X						
Courts			X	X	X		X	X	X	X		X
Physicians & surgeons												
Hospital sterilization committee		X										
Board of county commissioners												
Subcommission for mentally retarded												

Minnesota	Mississippi	Montana	Nebraska	N. Hampshire	N. Carolina	N. Dakota	Oklahoma	Oregon	S. Carolina	S. Dakota	Utah	Vermont	Virginia	Washington	W. Virginia	Wisconsin	TOTALS
		X			X												3
							X	X	X						X		8
				X						X	X						4
													X				1
	X																2
						X											2
						X											1
X																X	3
					X								X	X			11
												X					1
																	1
				X													1
										X							1

APPENDIX VII.   Compensation for Duties

	Alabama	Arizona	Arkansas	California	Connecticut	Delaware	Georgia	Idaho	Indiana	Iowa	Maine	Michigan
A. To:												
Examining board or examiner					X	X		X		X		
Surgeon or physician					X			X		X		X
Counsel								X		X		X
Hospital						X						X
Guardian ad litem		X							X	X		
B. For:												
Miscellaneous fees & expenses												
Publication												
C. Amount of compensation:												
Set fee												X
Reasonable fee								X		X		
Reasonable warden's or superintendent's discretion					X							
Reasonable according to authorizing agency			X							X		X
Actual & necessary										X		
Not exceeding a certain sum		X							X	X		X
C. Cost to be borne by:												
Individual or his family			X					X				X
Institution		X				X			X			
State					X			X		X		X
County												
Petitioner			X									

Minnesota	Mississippi	Montana	Nebraska	N. Hampshire	N. Carolina	N. Dakota	Oklahoma	Oregon	S. Carolina	S. Dakota	Utah	Vermont	Virginia	Washington	W. Virginia	Wisconsin	TOTALS
		X				X		X								X	8
				X		X			X	X		X					9
																	3
					X							X					4
	X			X			X		X	X	X		X		X		11
										X							1
															X		1
		X				X									X	X	5
					X					X	X	X					6
																	1
									X	X					X		6
		X							X	X							4
	X			X			X										7
									X	X							5
	X			X	X	X	X		X		X				X		11
								X				X	X				7
					X					X					X		3
																	1

APPENDIX VIII.   Characteristics of Due Process

	Alabama	Arizona	Arkansas	California	Connecticut	Delaware	Georgia	Idaho	Indiana	Iowa	Maine	Michigan
A. Notice sent to:												
Dept., bureau, agency, inst. or charitable org. which has custody or control		X										X
Individual		X	X	X					X	X	X	X
Person individual last resided with						X						
Parent, spouse or legal guardian		X	X	X	X	X	X	X	X	X	X	X
Adult children				X								
Nearest kin			X		X				X	X	X	X
Public defender												
Individual's attorney												X
Guardian ad litem		X				X	X	X	X	X		X
Custodial guardian or Comm. of Public Welfare			X									X
Personal friend										X		
Publication in newspaper												
Petitioner for commitment				X								

Minnesota	Mississippi	Montana	Nebraska	N. Hampshire	N. Carolina	N. Dakota	Oklahoma	Oregon	S. Carolina	S. Dakota	Utah	Vermont	Virginia	Washington	W. Virginia	Wisconsin	TOTALS
																	2
X	X	X		X	X		X	X	X	X	X	X	X		X		20
																X	2
X	X	X		X	X	X	X	X	X	X	X	X	X		X	X	26
																	1
X	X				X			X	X						X		12
								X									1
								X		X							3
	X			X	X		X			X	X		X				14
		X						X									4
								X									2
															X		1
																	1

(*continued*)

APPENDIX VIII. Characteristics of Due Process (*Continued*)

	Alabama	Arizona	Arkansas	California	Connecticut	Delaware	Georgia	Idaho	Indiana	Iowa	Maine	Michigan
B. Rights of individuals affected:												
Right to legal hearing		X	X	X	X		X	X	X	X		X
Right to counsel		X	X				X	X	X	X	X	X
Right to jury trial							X			X		X
Right to subpoena witnesses										X		
Right to appeal		X	X				X	X	X	X	X	X
Individual must be present at hearing		X		X						X		
Indivual may be present at hearing			X						X			X
Examining physician(s) must be present								X				X
Legal guardian must be present, or parent, spouse or next of kin												
Legal guardian may be present, or parent, spouse or next of kin				X					X	X		
Guardian ad litem must be present												
Guardian ad litem may be present												
Friend may be present										X		

Minnesota	Mississippi	Montana	Nebraska	N. Hampshire	N. Carolina	N. Dakota	Oklahoma	Oregon	S. Carolina	S. Dakota	Utah	Vermont	Virginia	Washington	W. Virginia	Wisconsin	TOTALS
				X													10
	X			X	X		X	X	X	X	X		X		X		18
																	3
									X								2
	X			X	X		X	X	X	X	X		X		X		18
		X							X		X						6
	X			X	X		X		X		X		X		X		11
																	2
																	0
	X			X	X	X	X		X	X	X		X		X		13
										X	X				X		3
				X								X	X				3
																	1

APPENDIX IX. Immunity from Prosecution of
Participants in the Legal or Medical
Procedures of Compulsory Sterilization

	Alabama	Arizona	Arkansas	California	Connecticut	Delaware	Georgia	Idaho	Indiana	Iowa	Maine	Michigan
Exemption from liability or immunity from prosecution of participants in the legal or medical procedures		X	X	X			X	X	X		X	X

Minnesota	Mississippi	Montana	Nebraska	N. Hampshire	N. Carolina	N. Dakota	Oklahoma	Oregon	S. Carolina	S. Dakota	Utah	Vermont	Virginia	Washington	W. Virginia	Wisconsin	Tennessee	TOTALS
X	X	X		X	X	X	X	X	X	X			X		X		X	21

CURRENT PUBLICATIONS FROM JAI PRESS

Annual Series

Consulting Editor: **RITA J. SIMON,** Director, Program in Law and Society, University of Illinois.

ADVANCES IN EARLY EDUCATION AND DAY CARE
Series Editor: Sally Kilmer, Bowling Green
State University

ADVANCES IN SPECIAL EDUCATION
Series Editor: Barbara K. Keogh, University of California,
Los Angeles

ADVANCES IN SUBSTANCE ABUSE
Series Editor: Nancy K. Mello,
Harvard Medical School

COMPARATIVE SOCIAL RESEARCH
Series Editor: Richard F. Tomasson, The University
of New Mexico

CURRENT PERSPECTIVES IN SOCIAL THEORY
Series Editors: Scott G. McNall and Gary N. Howe,
University of Kansas

PERSPECTIVES IN ORGANIZATIONAL SOCIOLOGY
Series Editor: Samuel B. Bacharach,
Cornell University

POLITICAL POWER AND SOCIAL THEORY
Series Editor: Maurice Zeitlin, University of California,
Los Angeles

RESEARCH IN COMMUNITY AND MENTAL HEALTH
Series Editor: Roberta G. Simmons, University
of Minnesota

RESEARCH IN ECONOMIC ANTHROPOLOGY
Series Editor: George Dalton,
Northwestern University

RESEARCH IN LAW AND SOCIOLOGY
Series Editors: Rita J. Simon, University of Illinois,
and Steven Spitzer, Harvard Law School

RESEARCH IN POLITICAL ECONOMY
Series Editor: Paul Zarembka, State University of
New York, Buffalo

RESEARCH IN RACE AND ETHNIC RELATIONS
Series Editors: Cora B. Marrett, University of Wisconsin,
and Cheryl Leggon, University of Illinois, Chicago Circle

**RESEARCH IN SOCIAL MOVEMENTS, CONFLICTS
AND CHANGE**
Series Editor: Louis Kriesberg, Syracuse University

RESEARCH IN SOCIAL PROBLEMS AND PUBLIC POLICY
Series Editor: Michael Lewis, University of
Massachusetts

RESEARCH IN SOCIAL STRATIFICATION AND MOBILITY
Series Editors: Donald J. Treiman, National Academy of
Sciences, and Robert V. Robinson, Indiana University

**RESEARCH IN SOCIOLOGY OF EDUCATION AND
SOCIALIZATION**
Series Editor: Alan C. Kerckhoff, Duke University

**RESEARCH IN SOCIOLOGY OF KNOWLEDGE, SCIENCES
AND ART**
Series Editors: Robert Alun Jones, University of Illinois,
and Henrika Kuklick, University of Pennsylvania

RESEARCH IN THE INTERWEAVE OF SOCIAL ROLES
Series Editor: Helena Z. Lopata, Loyola University
of Chicago

RESEARCH IN THE SOCIOLOGY OF HEALTH CARE
Series Editor: Julius A. Roth, University of
California, Davis

RESEARCH IN THE SOCIOLOGY OF WORK
Series Editors: Ida Harper Simpson, Duke University,
and Richard L. Simpson, University of North Carolina,
Chapel Hill

STUDIES IN COMMUNICATIONS
Series Editor: Thelma McCormack, York University

STUDIES IN SYMBOLIC INTERACTION
Series Editor: Norman K. Denzin, University of Illinois

Journal

SYMBOLIC INTERACTION
Official journal of the Society for the Study of Symbolic Interaction
Editor: HARVEY FARBERMAN, School of Social Welfare, Health Sciences Center,
State University of New York-Stony Brook.

Beginning with volume 4 (1981), JAI Press Inc. will become the publisher of **Symbolic Interaction**. All subscriptions
should be sent to the publisher. All matters relating to submission of manuscripts should be sent to the editor. Please
ask for full details.

Volume 4 (2 issues) 1981

Institutions:	$27.50
Non-Members:	$15.00
Members:	$12.50

Please add $2.00 for postage in the United States, and $4.00 for foreign.

Monograph Series

CONTEMPORARY STUDIES IN SOCIOLOGY
Editorial Board: Rita J. Simon, Robert Althauser, Clark McPhail, John Clark, and John D. Kasarda

Index

SOCIAL CASEWORK CUMULATIVE INDEX 1920-1979
Compiler: Katherine A. Kendall, former Executive Director of the Council on Social Work Education and Secretary-
General of the International Association of Schools of Social Work

July 1981	Cloth	ca. 704 pages	Institutions: $65.00
ISBN: 0-89232-194-6			Individuals: $40.00

The cumulative index will cover all issues from 1920, when the journal was known as *The Family*, through 1979, at which
time the title became *Social Casework: The Journal of Contemporary Social Work*. It will contain an historical overview of
the journal and its significance to the field and four separate indexes —by subject, author, title, and book review.

Please ask for detailed brochure on each publication

 JAI PRESS INC.
P.O. Box 1678, 165 West Putnam Avenue
Greenwich, Connecticut 06830
Telephone: 203-661-7602   *Cable Address:* JAIPUBL

Advances in Behavioral Pediatrics

A Research Annual

Series Editor: **Bonnie W. Camp, M.D.**,
University of Colorado Medical School

This series will cover topics relating behavioral outcome to care and management of neonates and infants, psychological issues surrounding diagnosis and management of children with chronic disease or disability and hospitalized children, developments in the field of learning disabilities and school problems, psychosocial aspects of child and adolescent medicine, disorders of parenting, behavioral aspects of anticipatory guidance, and primary prevention of behavioral disorders. This series will be of interest to pediatricians, psychiatrists, behavioral scientists and others who are concerned with behavioral aspects of pediatric medicine and the clinical application of child and adolescent psychology.

Volume 1.   **Published 1980**   **Cloth**   **Institutions: $ 31.00**
ISBN 0-89232-076-1   **266 pages**   **Individuals: $ 15.50**

CONTENTS: Foreword, Bonnie W. Camp. **Studies on Long-Term Outcome in Newborns with Birth Weights Under 1500 Grams,** Beverly L. Koops and Robert J. Harmon, University of Colorado Health Science Center. **Nonorganic Failure to Thrive: The Status of Interactional and Environmental Etiologic Theories,** Milton Kotelchuck, Children's Hospital Medical Center, Boston. **Predicting Cognitive Development from Assessments in Infancy,** Michael Lewis and Nathan Fox, Institute for the Study of Exceptional Children. **Language Lateralization and Developmental Disabilities,** Marcel Kinsbourne, Hospital for Sick Children, Toronto. **Long Term Follow-up Studies of Hyperactive Children,** Roscoe A. Dykman and Peggy Ackerman, University of Arkansas College of Medicine. **Dietary Treatment of Behavioral Disorders,** J. Preston Harley, University of Wisconsin Clinical Science Center. **Development in Black Children,** Ura J. Oyemade and Pearl L. Rosser, Howard University College of Medicine. **Stages and Phases in the Response of Children and Adolescents to Illness or Injury,** Dane G. Prugh and Lloyd O. Eckhardt, University of Colorado Health Sciences Center. **Adolescent Suicide,** Barbara Herjanic and Zila Welner, Washington University School of Medicine. **Effects of Television on the Developing Child,** Ronald G. Slaby, Harvard University and Gary R. Quarfoth, City of Seattle Law and Justice Planning Office.

JAI PRESS INC., P.O. Box 1678, 165 West Putnam Avenue, Greenwich, Connecticut 06830.

Telephone: 203-661-7602   **Cable Address: JAIPUBL**

Advances in Early Education and Day Care

An Annual Compilation Of Theory And Research

Series Editor: **Sally Kilmer**
Department of Home Economics
Bowling Green State University

This annual series is designed to provide an academic forum for the publication of original research, critical reviews and conceptual analyses of theoretical and substantive issues related to the education, care and development of young children. The series is intended to stimulate research and to enhance communication among scholars in early childhood education, child development, social work, public administration and related fields. Volume 1 focuses on critical issues in attaining and maintaining quality in programs for young children. Leaders in early childhood education, child development, social work and government discuss the rationale and relative effectiveness of various quality control mechanisms and agents as well as recommendations for research and policy. The roles of consumers and government, licensing and other regulation, redentialling and professionalization of personnel, and evaluation are reviewed in relation to both group programs and family day care. This series is the only academic reference work for faculty and graduate students engaged in research and theoretical analyses of issues related to early education and day care for young children.

Volume 1.   **Published 1980**   Cloth   **Institutions: $ 31.00**
ISBN 0-89232-127-X   **225 pages**   **Individuals: $ 15.50**

Volume 2.   May 1981   Cloth   Institutions: $31.00
ISBN 0-89232-149-0   Ca. 300 pages   Individuals: $15.50

CONTENTS: Interdisciplinary Preparation for Leaders in Early Education and Child Development, Millie Almy, University of California — Berkeley. Causal Models in Early Education Research, Sueann Ambron, Stanford University. Observation and Experiment: Complementary Strategies for Studying Day Care and Social Development, Allison Clarke-Stewart, University of Chicago. Building Prerequisite Learning Skills for Reading and Mathematics, Eileen Earhart, Michigan State University. Different Roles for Mothers and Teachers: Contrasting Styles of Child Care, Robert Hess, and Mary Conroy, Stanford University, W. Patrick Dickson, Wisconsin Center for Research & Development, and Gary G. Price, University of Wisconsin — Madison. The Roles of Home, Nursery School and Kindergarten in Preschool Development, J. McVicker Hunt, University of Illinois — Champaign. Teacher Education in Action: Student and Instructor Behavior in Adult Learning Environments, Elizabeth Jones, Pacific Oaks College. Current Research in Day Care Personnel Preparation, Donald Peters, Pennsylvania State University, Marjorie Kostelnik, Michigan State University, Relations Between Physical Setting and Adult/Child Behavior in Day Care, Elizabeth Prescott, Pacific Oaks College.

Volume 3.   In Preparation   Cloth   Institutions: $ 31.00
ISBN 0-89232-206-3   Ca. 300 pages   Individuals: $ 15.50

TENTATIVE CONTENTS: Children at Play between Cultures/Home and School Environments, Eva Balke and Bjorn Berg, Oslo, Norway. Intergrating Handicapping Children into Preschool Programs, Gayle M. Clapp, Miami University and Nancy Carlson, Michigan State University. A Comparative Study of Group and Family Infant Day Care, Henry J. Policare, Mark Golden and Lucille Rosenbluth, Medical and Health Research Association of New York City. Urban Parents' Strategies for Finding Child Care Services, Douglas Powell, Merrill-Palmer Institute. Day Care and the Disadvantaged Family: Effects on the Child, the Family and the Community, Craig T. Ramey and FPG Colleagues, Frank Porter Graham Child Development Center. The Professional Development of the Teacher of Young Children, Jane Schwartfeger, University of Michigan. Mainstreaming Handicapped Children in the Early Years: An Analyses of Research from Various Theoretical Perspectives, Bernard Spodek, University of Illinois. Evaluation Strategies for Early Childhood Title I Programs, Mary Jane Yurchak, The Huron Institute.

INSTITUTIONAL STANDING ORDERS will be granted a 10% discount and be filled automatically upon publication. Please indicate initial volume of standing order
INDIVIDUAL ORDERS must be prepaid by personal check or credit card. Please include $1.50 per volume for postage and handling.
Please encourage your library to subscribe to this series.

JAI PRESS INC., P.O. Box 1678, 165 West Putnam Avenue, Greenwich, Connecticut 06830.

Telephone: 203-661-7602   Cable Address: JAIPUBL